Your PGCME, an Amateur Guide to Medical Education.

An experiment in AI-human collaboration.

Dr Mark Burgin

Disability Analyst and General Practitioner

Published by New Generation Publishing in 2023

Copyright © Dr Mark Burgin 2023

First Edition

ISBN   978-1-83563-020-4

www.newgeneration-publishing.com

New Generation Publishing

This book was created using BARD and ChatGPT as teachers for a human who was learning the content of the Post Graduate Certificate in Medical Education (PGCME). The methodology used is largely described in this book's chapter of AI learning. The human has a professional interest in medicine and an amateur interest in education and AI. The theory that is being tested is that human AI collaboration is an emergent property.

No special prompts were used apart from 'step by step' and the generated text was checked and edited by the human. The final text was not proofread by an expert in medical education and references were limited to those necessary to make the main points. The result is evidence of both the limitations of and the strengths of AI as a teacher and the power of collaboration.

For full disclosure

I have been involved in education most of my life studying medicine, law and ethics. I have studied part time, distance learning including managing health service through the OU. I have lived abroad learning to speak another language and have self-taught for the diploma of child health. I applied for and studied a distance learning PGCME but for personal reasons was not able to proceed.

I have written a number of articles for lawyers which have been published in non peer reviewed journals. I have previously written a book called the Art of Personal Injury report writing. Those who are interested in the extent to which LLMs can improve the quality of writing can read this other book as evidence of my best efforts without assistance and compare the two books.

The decision to write this book.

The decision to write this book rather than one I planned on disability is that I wanted to choose a subject that I do not have expertise in. Although I have been involved in education as a student most of my life and as a teacher occasionally, I readily accept that my skills are very limited. I felt that this was a fairer test of the AI as I would not always know the correct answer although I could ask educated questions.

Another reason was that it was something that I had genuine interest in and would not otherwise have had a chance to study. Having the motivation necessary to complete the task and self-publish the book was an important factor. Although I do not currently have many opportunities to do formal teaching I feel that the skills I would learn could be useful in future projects so the effort would be worthwhile.

I have always found system analysis to be easier than other people appear to and I did well at A level Maths. I have always enjoyed the feeling of cognitive dissonance and this again may alter the experiment. Any analysis should recognise that the human in this experiment may have unusual aspects that mean the findings do not apply to all human AI collaborations.

Contents

INTRODUCTION TO THE CHAPTERS.

This section is an innovation suggested by BARD to improve the interest and usability of the book. The four elements are an alternative title for those that do not like formal titles, a hook to grab the reader's interest, a short description to focus attention and an objective written as a short task.

BARD gave these suggestions in response to a prompt 'how can I improve the book'. This introduction to the chapters may be useful before reading the book to orientate the reader. Others be useful after reading the book to help them revise or as a list of bonus activities to consolidate learning.

1: Introduction to Medical Education.

Alternative title: What does it take to become a doctor?

The hook: The average doctor spends over 10,000 hours in medical school. That's a lot of time and money invested in an education that should prepare them to provide safe and effective care to patients. But is the current medical school curriculum meeting this goal?

Description: Medical education has evolved over time in response to the changing needs of healthcare. This chapter provides an overview of the history of medical education, the goals and principles that underpin effective medical education and considers the possible futures of medical education.

SMART objectives: Discuss the strengths and weaknesses of different curricula.

2: The Role of the Teacher in Medical Education

Alternative title: The Teacher's Role in Shaping the Future of Medicine.

Hook: Teachers are responsible for not only imparting knowledge, but also for shaping the future of medicine.

Description: Teachers who are skilled communicators, caring and passionate about teaching create a supportive and stimulating learning environment. They use the simple approaches of feedback, knowledge of teaching techniques and assessment of the student's progress.

SMART objectives: Identify strengths and weaknesses in your teaching skills.

3: Developing Educational Objectives

Alternative title: How to Write SMART Educational Objectives

Hook: Do you want to ensure that your students are learning what they need to learn? If so, you need to write SMART educational objectives.

Description: Educational objectives are statements describing what students should be able to do after a learning experience. Understanding the curriculum is crucial for effective teaching. Educators can read the syllabus, review reading lists and talk to students to gain insights into their needs. Scoping surveys can help identify important topics and align them with teaching episodes.

SMART objectives: Practice creating educational objectives using a scoping survey.

4: Interprofessional education

Alternative title: Interprofessional Education: A Collaborative Approach to Improving Patient Care

Hook: Doctors cannot achieve the best possible care for their patients alone. They must understand the roles of nurses, social workers and pharmacists. Interprofessional education (IPE) is a unique opportunity for doctors to gain insights that can improve their performance.

Description: IPE can be delivered through various methods such as joint lectures, case-based discussions, simulations, community-based projects and more. To ensure the success of IPE, educators should focus on promoting positive social interactions among different professional groups. This involves encouraging open communication, addressing conflicts and emphasising common goals for high-quality patient care. It is crucial to avoid tribalism and to respect the needs and preferences of each group.

SMART objectives: List 3 insights (positive or negative) about other professional groups.

5: Instructional Design in Medical Education

Alternative title: Instructional Design Models for Effective Learning in Medical Education

Hook: Can we find a simpler and clearer instructional design model?

Description: Instructional design models provide a systematic approach to creating effective learning experiences. These models can help educators to identify the learning objectives, design the learning activities and assess the learning outcomes. There are many different instructional design models available, each with its own strengths and weaknesses. The choice of model depends on the specific needs and goals of the learning experience.

SMART objectives: Write a summary of the key steps in instructional design.

6: Assessment and Evaluation in Medical Education

Alternative title: Assessment and Evaluation: The Key to Effective Medical Education

Hook: Assessment motivates students and helps them identify areas for improvement.

Description: Assessment and evaluation in medical education can be divided into two main categories: formative and summative. Formative assessment is used to provide feedback to students on their learning, while summative assessment is used to measure student achievement at the end of a course or program. Choosing the best methods will depend upon the specific learning objectives of the topic.

SMART objectives: Consider the strengths and weaknesses of using three assessment techniques to assess knowledge of assessment.

7: Designing MCQ questions.

Alternative title: An introduction to MCQ Question Design.

Hook: How to design effective and fair MCQ questions.

Description: This chapter provides an overview of the key principles of MCQ question design. It covers topics such as the structure of MCQ questions, the use of clinical vignettes and the different types of MCQ questions. It provides practical advice on how to write MCQ questions that are clear, challenging and fair.

SMART objectives: Design a MCQ question that is effective and aligned with learning objectives.

8: Portfolio based evidence.

Alternative title: Portfolio-Based Assessment: A Holistic Approach to Measuring Student Learning.

Hook: How Portfolio-Based Assessment can identify the exceptional student.

Description: Portfolio-based evidence is an assessment method that allows students to demonstrate their learning through a variety of formats, including essays, projects, presentations and artifacts. This approach to assessment is holistic, meaning that it takes into account all aspects of student learning, including knowledge, skills and abilities. Portfolio-based evidence can also help students develop self-assessment and self-directed learning skills.

SMART objectives: Create a list of performance criteria for a rubric.

9: OSCE type clinical assessment.

Alternative title: The OSCE: Developing a Tool for Assessing Clinical Skills

Hook: OSCE - as good as real life or plastic and artificial? How to make better OSCEs.

Description: The OSCE is a series of stations, each of which tests a different clinical skill. OSCEs are typically used to assess students' skills in history taking, physical examination, diagnosis and communication. OSCEs offer objectivity, validity, reliability, efficiency and comprehensiveness. However challenges include cost, time and artificiality.

SMART objectives: Create a detailed medical template of a patient.

10: Preclinical education: Becoming a scientist.

Alternative title: The Foundation of Clinical Medicine.

Hook: The answers to clinical problems often lie in the science that underlies medicine rather than improvements in clinical skills.

Description: Preclinical studies provide students with the foundation they need to understand the causes of disease, the mechanisms of action of drugs and the effects of disease on the body. They also help students develop critical thinking skills and the ability to apply their knowledge to real-world problems.

SMART objectives: Provide a compelling answer to the question 'why study preclinical sciences?'

11: Clinical Teaching.

Alternative title: Clinical Teaching: A Student-Centered Approach.

Hook: How to create more efficient clinical teaching.

Description: Clinical teaching provides students with real-world patient care settings. Bedside teaching uniquely allows students to interact with patients. A clinical teaching policy document can provide guidance on expectations of students behaviour and educators performance. It should also contain remediation strategies for slower learners.

SMART objectives: Critically appraise a Clinical teaching policy document.

12: Clinical rotations.

Alternative title: Clinical Rotations: Apprenticeship for independent practice.

Hook: Do CPD and appraisal support doctors in clinical rotations?

Description: Clinical rotations are an apprenticeship for independent practice. They offer doctors the opportunity to develop skills and knowledge. They also involve long hours, a stressful environment and emotional strain. CPD can help fill gaps in training on important topics such as management, teaching, ethics or regulations. CPD can also help the doctors pass knowledge examinations.

SMART objectives: Create a Personal development plan for an example case.

13: Teamwork skills.

Alternative title: The Importance of Teamwork Skills in Healthcare

Hook: Understanding your role in a group and improves team performance.

Description: The chapter explains the importance of teamwork skills in healthcare and provides tips for educators on how to teach these skills to medical students. The transition from merely working together to collaboration increases performance significantly. The key to unlocking the unique skills and expertise is avoiding dysfunctional interactions. This includes both being aware of the emotional and intellectual needs which in turn reduces staff stress and burnout.

SMART objectives: Identify the team roles in a scenario using the Belbin Team Roles Model.

14: Situational judgement and ethics.

Alternative title: Making Ethical Decisions in a Complex World.

Hook: In today's healthcare environment, healthcare professionals are often faced with complex ethical dilemmas. How can they develop the skills they need to make sound ethical decisions?

Description: Learning to make ethical decisions involves learning the theory such as the Four Principles of Biomedical Ethics or GMC guidance and practice on real life problems. One surprisingly complex example is how to write good medical records. There are many areas in medicine where a balance must be made between available resources, including doctors time and patient rights.

SMART objectives: Develop an ethical challenge teaching plan for a PBL session.

15: Postgraduate Life.

Alternative title: The Transformative Journey of Postgraduate Life for Doctors

Hook: Would you choose a job that has some of the highest rates of drug and alcohol abuse, depression and suicide?

Description: Medicine is an extraordinary career which gives opportunities and experiences that are incredible. Post graduate doctors need to align their values, skills and interests with their aspirations. Setting SMART goals, finding a mentor and maintaining a healthy work-life balance are important. Maintaining a sense of self is essential if the doctor wishes to avoid medicine's unique occupational risks.

SMART objectives: Consider the symptoms and signs that indicate that a doctor should leave their current role and find another role.

16: Communication skills

Alternative title: Effective Communication Skills for Doctors

Hook: Communication is the power to persuade!

Description: Teaching communication skills involves learning about communication models which in turn focus on performing tasks. Achieving these tasks leads to good communication but they have limits. To develop further the doctor needs professionalism which includes personal skills such as clarity of thought, respect and emotional insight. Identifying what the doctor wants to achieve or the content of the communication gives different ways of looking at the task.

SMART objectives: Write a paragraph about an idea to improve communication skills training.

17: Preparing Lectures

Alternative title: Creating a compelling and inspiring lecture.

Hook: Why are so many lectures boring?

Description: This chapter provides educators with ideas on how to prepare effective lectures. The basic topics are setting learning objectives, conducting research and creating a well-structured outline. The key is to reduce the number of points and make them clearer by omitting irrelevant information. Adding a hook, using visuals using humour and active learning e.g. answering questions can add polish to good lecture and make it great.

SMART objectives: Take a lecture that failed and make it engaging and inspiring.

18: Small Group Teaching and Facilitation

Alternative title: The Power of Small Group Teaching.

Hook: How to use facilitation to control the power of small groups.

Description: Small group teaching offer numerous benefits for both students and educators. It can foster active learning, individualised instruction and increased opportunities for practice. Good facilitation leads to a positive and supportive learning environment that promotes collaboration, critical thinking, problem-solving skills, social skills and self-esteem. Facilitating uses techniques such as discussion, problem solving, role playing and brainstorming.

SMART objectives: Identify a problem you have had when trying to facilitate a small group and consider what technique was being used.

19: Problem-based learning (PBL)

Alternative title: Problem-Based Learning: A Student-Centered Approach to Learning

Hook: Is Problem-based learning (PBL) the answer to all medical learning problems?

Description: PBL is a student-centered instructional method that presents students with real-world problems and challenges them to find solutions. Used correctly it can engage students, promote critical thinking, communication and collaboration. If there is insufficient time, lack of teacher support, poorly designed problems and poor group dynamics it can fail.

SMART objectives: In the educator's current role are there any factors that could alter the effectiveness of PBL?

20: Distance learning in medical education:

Alternative title: Distance Learning: A New Era in Medical Education

Hook: Can Distance Learning ever be accepted as mainstream Medical Education?

Description: Distance learning in medical education offers a number of benefits, including flexibility, tailored learning, convenience, affordability and improved resources. However, there are also challenges to overcome, such as the lack of interaction with peers and faculty, technical difficulties and the need for self-discipline. Distance learners increasingly have access to appropriate learning materials but formal assessment remains a barrier.

SMART objectives: Could large language models (LLM) replace the need for peer support and improve engagement for distance learning?

21: Educational technology in medical education

Alternative title: The Promise and Challenges of EdTech in Medical Education

Hook: What can EdTech do that LLMs cannot?

Description: The advantages of EdTech include enhanced accessibility, personalised learning experiences and the ability to overcome traditional educational constraints. There are challenges that need to be addressed for EdTech to reach its full potential, such as cost, specificity and automation. EdTech's success will be limited until it addresses the practical problems, provide appropriate solutions and is able to adapt to meet the specific needs education has.

SMART objectives: Look for an EdTech tool that is available or promised that will not be replaced by LLMs.

22: Using LLMs in Medical Education.

Alternative title: How LLMs will Revolutionise Medical Education.

Hook: Large language models (LLMs) are a powerful new technology that students are already using to revolutionise medical education.

Description: LLMs can be used to provide personalised learning experiences, adaptive assessments, clinical decision support and research capabilities. By learning to use LLMs appropriately medical educators can harness the power of LLMs. This means enhancing teaching, learning and even patient care in the field of medicine.

SMART objectives: Ask a student how they are using LLMs and use an LLM to list pros and cons of the way they use the technology.

23: Global health in medical education

Alternative title: Global Health: A Holistic Approach to Medicine

Hook: Healthcare in the UK is part of global health, no more 'us and them'.

Description: Global health is a complex and multifaceted field that encompasses a wide range of topics, from epidemiology and public health to ethics and international development. By integrating global health principles into medical education, students can develop the knowledge and skills they need to address the global health challenges at home and abroad.

SMART objectives: Identify a global health problem that affects the UK and consider whether the UK could learn from countries facing more severe versions of the same problem.

24: The Causes of Health disparities

Alternative title: Solving Health Disparities: A Multifaceted Approach

Hook: Solving society's most intractable problems.

Description: This topic provides an overview of the complex issue of health disparities. These differences can be caused by a variety of factors, including social determinants of health, such as poverty, discrimination and lack of access to healthcare. It also discusses the importance of a multifaceted approach to address health disparities, as well as some specific strategies that can be implemented to improve health equity.

SMART objectives: Consider the effects of universal access to primary care - which disparities would be resolved and which would remain.

25: Learning Professional standards.

Alternative title: Professionalism in Medical Education: Challenges and Opportunities

Hook: A personal journey to professionalism.

Description: This chapter discusses the different models of professional standards, the benefits and problems of professional standards and the role of educators in teaching professional standards. Professionalism is a flawed concept as it tries to dictate the personal qualities required. Learning to align behaviours whilst staying true to core values is possible and can be taught.

SMART objectives: Consider how you have overcome a personal quality that conflicts with ethical codes or current practice.

26: Patient safety

Alternative title: Patient Safety: A Complex but Crucial Issue

Hook: There are 800,000 clinical errors in the UK every year, this is 4 per every doctor on the GMC register. We all make mistakes, learning from those mistakes makes doctors better.

Description: Patient safety is a complex issue, but it is one that is essential to address. Healthcare providers, administrators and policymakers all have a role to play in preventing system failure. This chapter will explore the challenges of teaching patient safety, as well as some practical tips for educators in addressing the risk factors.

SMART objectives: Consider a department that you are familiar with and identify the possible risk factors for poor safety.

27: Quality improvement

Alternative title: QI: A Crucial Process with Significant Challenges

Hook: Despite the potential benefits of QI, such as improving patient outcomes, reducing costs and enhancing the quality of care, these benefits often do not materialise in practice.

Description: This chapter discusses the challenges of quality improvement in healthcare and how to overcome them. It explores the reasons why QI is often not successful and discusses strategies for improving stakeholder engagement and resource allocation. An existential challenge is a failure to achieve alignment of perspectives between managers and clinicians.

SMART objectives: Choose one QI method and try to phrase it as a clinical rather than managerial goal.

28: Evidence-based medicine

Alternative title: Evidence-Based Medicine: A Practical Approach to Improving Patient Care

Hook: Do patients want Evidence-based medicine (EBM) or individualised care?

Description: Evidence-based medicine (EBM) is a valuable approach to clinical decision-making that can help ensure that patients receive high-quality care based on the best evidence. EBM which integrates the best available research evidence with clinical expertise and patient values. However, there are also challenges to using EBM, doctors do not have the time to do their own research and guidelines can lack generalisability.

SMART objectives: Consider if a patient wants a new promising cancer treatment but it is not yet in the guidelines, can a doctor refuse to consider this option until it is in the guidelines? What if your research of the evidence suggests that it is a significant advance in similar patients but there is no evidence for that specific patient?

29: Professional Development for Medical Educators

Alternative title: The Importance of Professional Development for Medical Educators

Hook: Medical Educators lack time to keep up with all the areas they cover.

Description: The chapter outlines a systematic approach to professional development, including steps such as reviewing current practice, identifying gaps, planning steps to address those gaps, implementing training, networking with colleagues and assessing the effectiveness of the training. It identifies a synergy with production of teaching materials which can reduce the gap between available time and study needs.

SMART objectives: Calculate how much time you need to keep up to date in all the areas assuming that you require 50 hours a year for each discipline.

30: Scholarship and Research in Medical Education

Alternative title: Scholarship and Research: The Foundations of Excellence in Medical Education.

Hook: Are you feeling stuck in your teaching despite reading up on the topic and cannot seem to achieve your goals?

Description: Scholarship and research in medical education can take many forms, including self-funded role-based research, pursuing a Master's degree, or seeking scholarships. Some educators will want to find an answer to a difficult problem, others will want to advance their career and others will want to broaden their experience to help their students.

SMART objectives: Reflect on your experience as an educator and think of problem that you found challenging. How could it be researched?

31: Reflecting in Medical Education

Alternative title: Reflection: A Key to Patient-Centered Care

Hook: What types of resistance are there to reflection?

Description: Reflection is a process of thinking about and analysing an experience to learn from it. In medical education, reflection is an important tool for developing clinical skills, judgment and self-awareness. The method chosen should be easy to use and meaningful and relevant to the individual student.

SMART objectives: Write questions as you are reading this chapter, what do you want to know more about? Is there anything that stops you from writing the questions?

32: Teaching leadership skills.

Alternative title: Leadership Development in Medicine.

Hook: Whether you're a junior doctor or a senior consultant, all doctors are leaders.

Description: Leadership development is the process of learning and developing the skills and knowledge necessary to be an effective leader. Leadership development can be formal or informal. Formal leadership development programs provide learners with the opportunity to learn about leadership theories, skills and techniques. Informal leadership development can occur through on-the-job experience, mentoring and self-study.

SMART objectives: Rate your leadership qualities (Communication, decision making, problem solving, motivation, vision, teamwork) on a scale from one to 10. Do you have any qualities of special leaders?

33: Medical humanities:

Alternative title: The Human Experience of Medicine.

Hook: The experience of illness changes understanding more fundamentally than learning alone can achieve.

Description: There are many resources available for students to explore the experience of illness with compelling and emotional accounts. The choice of whether to read descriptions, look at art, film, read philosophy and history of medicine is personal. Experiential learning can help the learner develop empathy.

SMART objectives: Choose one example of experiential learning to engage with and try to identify your own insights from the piece.

34: Using models from Sociology, Psychology and Anthropology.

Alternative title: The Social, Psychological and Cultural Dimensions of Medicine.

Hook: How different perspectives offer valuable insights into intractable problems.

Description: This chapter provides an overview of the models from sociology, psychology and anthropology that have been used to understand health and illness. It discusses the strengths and limitations of these models and it explores how they can be used to improve medical education and practice.

SMART objectives: Consider how an anthropologist would address homelessness. What are the barriers to people having a home in the UK?

35: Disabled doctors and reasonable adjustments.

Alternative title: Disability and Inclusion in the Healthcare System.

Hook: Anyone can be disabled by a dysfunctional system; reasonable adjustments help all workers.

Description: The challenges faced by disabled doctors in the healthcare system are similar to their non-disabled peers. Creating an inclusive environment for disabled doctors through reasonable adjustments has a broader effect. Systems become less dysfunctional and benefit healthcare with improved care, job satisfaction and less mistakes.

SMART objectives: Consider an example of a problem that you have with your work and whether there is something that would make that easier. Would disabled doctors be able to perform better if it was solved?

36: Challenges and Future Directions in Medical Education

Alternative title: The Future of Medical Education

Hook: Will the predicted changes to Medical Education improve or worsen the student experience?

Description: There is a gap between the priorities of students and those of educational institutions. Progress is often slowed by failures of universities to adapt to the modern world. Educators should engage with students to understand their visions and priorities for the future.

SMART objectives: Prepare a briefing document for the education department on one innovation that has not been incorporated. E.g. YouTube videos of lectures.

37: Medical law

Alternative title: Medical Law for Healthcare Professionals.

Hook: Without an understanding of the law it is difficult to make sure that documents the doctor signs are not false or misleading

Description: There is no single source of all the laws that apply to clinical practice. A doctor may have to refer to statute law and government advice to find all the relevant details. The language in these documents can be unfamiliar and will need breaking down into parts to fully understand. Doctors need help to find and understand the laws that apply to clinical practice.

SMART objectives: Prepare a summary of the law on an area you commonly are involved, e.g. death certificates, sick notes or consent.

38: Political issues in Medical Education

Alternative title: The Politics of Medical Education

Hook: The way we train doctors is changing, but is it changing for the better?

Description: Political issues in medical education are about standards, ideology, funding and curriculum. There is pressure to reduce standards so that more students pass and less drop out. Ideology is moving from doctors as independent professionals to parts of multidisciplinary teams. Funding is not increasing as fast as student numbers leading to less money per student. Curricula are being changed from knowledge and skills towards attitudes and diversity.

SMART objectives: Choose one issue and give arguments for and against the proposition that change is needed.

39: How to plan CME

Alternative title: How to Organise Effective CME.

Hook: Understanding your collaboration style can unlock your potential for continuing learning.

Description: The doctor needs to decide whether their goal in CME is to maintain or expand their knowledge. Identifying their learning style will allow them to assess what activities they will enjoy most. Small adaptions to activities can improve engagement and reduce drop out rates. Feedback, whether from self-reflection, assessment or comments from others can help plan future CME.

SMART objectives: Identify your collaboration style and how a lecture could be adapted to include this style.

40: The Dissertation, Thesis or Essay.

Alternative title: The Supervisor's Role in Dissertation or Thesis Writing

Hook: Ask the right questions: How supervisors can help researchers gain deeper insight.

Description: The writing of a thesis is a complex process that can be broken down into a series of stages. The skills required for each stage can be taught, but students also need ongoing support in the form of questions. Learning to ask the right questions takes time and practice. Supervisor's roles also include helping students to identify and solve problems and by providing clear boundaries for the project.

SMART objectives: Read an article and write a question that would help the author improve their work.

Chapter 1: INTRODUCTION TO MEDICAL EDUCATION:

Medical education is the process of training doctors to provide safe and effective care to patients. It is a complex and challenging process that requires a combination of knowledge, skills and attitudes. The costs are high due to the length of the course, production of learning materials, creation of learning experiences, direct teaching and assessment.

Changes occur slowly in medical education because of the risks of changing a successful system. The costs of providing remediation to a cohort of students who fail to make progress would be high. Understanding the goals of medical education can ensure that educators are not afraid to incorporate new advances.

The goal of medical education is to produce doctors who are able to:

- Understand the basic sciences of medicine: Medical students must have a deep understanding in the basic sciences of medicine, such as anatomy, physiology, biochemistry, microbiology and pharmacology. This knowledge is essential for understanding how the body works and for diagnosing and treating diseases.

- Apply this knowledge to the diagnosis and treatment of patients: Medical students must be able to apply their knowledge of the basic sciences to recognise patterns for the diagnosis and treatment of patients. This requires the ability to think critically, to solve problems and to make decisions under pressure.

- Communicate effectively with patients and their families: Medical students must be able to communicate effectively with patients and their families. This includes the ability to explain medical concepts in a clear and understandable way and to answer their questions. Doctors also need to be able to work with patients and their families to develop a treatment plan that is both effective and acceptable.

- Work effectively as part of a team: Medical students must be able to work effectively as part of a team. This includes the ability to collaborate with other healthcare professionals, such as nurses, pharmacists and social workers, to provide the best possible care for patients.

- Demonstrate professionalism and ethical behaviour: Medical students must demonstrate professionalism and ethical behaviour in all aspects of their work. This includes the ability to maintain patient confidentiality, to treat patients with respect and to make decisions that are in the best interests of patients.

These 5 goals should underpin the educator's systems of assessment. They should be aware of weaknesses in the cohort and make changes to address them. This overall view of the progress can be lost when assessing specific topics. The goals also provide an excellent overview of performance.

They could and perhaps should be on every dean of medicine's wall to help them track progress. As an individual educator it may not be possible to arrange formal assessment in each area but an estimate is also useful. The insight that this information gives can help direct the educator's efforts in their specific areas.

Principles of Effective Medical Education

There is a debate at the heart of medical education as to the balance between patient and doctor centred care. The educator cannot take sides on this debate but can ensure that the students have the right tools to deal with the consequences. A technique called casuistry can help protect students from burnout.

Doctor centred care was the dominant model for almost the entire history of medicine. This model protected doctors from becoming emotionally damaged by the treatment of their patients. Before good quality nursing and healthcare departments the experience of illness and death was truly horrific.

Patient centred care is possible in the controlled clinical environments of western healthcare systems. The doctors do not face the horror of uncontrolled pain or the smells and sounds and sights of a dying person. They can listen to patient and understand their suffering, they can consider the options and involve the patient, they have time to learn and maintain their professional standards.

There are a number of principles that underpin effective modern medical education. These include:

- A focus on the patient: Medical education should be patient-centered. It should focus on the needs of patients and on how doctors can provide the best possible care.

- A focus on evidence-based medicine: Medical education should be based on evidence. Doctors should be taught how to evaluate the evidence and how to use it to make decisions about patient care.

- A focus on lifelong learning: Medical education should prepare doctors for a lifetime of learning. Doctors should be taught how to learn new information and how to adapt to change.

- A focus on professionalism: Medical education should instil in doctors a commitment to professionalism. Doctors should be taught the importance of ethical behaviour and of upholding the highest standards of care.

Few would deny that doctors should focus more on the patient's needs, evidence-based medicine (EBM), lifelong learning and professional behaviour than has historically been the case. Social changes in the West have led to improvements in the way that patients are treated by doctors. However, these changes, rather than improving the quality of life of healthcare professionals, appear to be causing burnout and driving them out of the profession.

These four principles have also led to an increasing pressure on the medical curriculum. Medical students complain that they do not feel prepared for the actual work. Some doctors question whether the focus on these principles is leading to adverse effects on the quality of education and whether we are expecting too much from the humans that study medicine.

At the same time, there are further pressures on the curriculum. Some argue for the importance of cultural competence and teaching doctors how to deal with difficult patients. Others argue that medical education could do more to teach doctors how to deal with uncertainty and the patient's experience of care. These additional demands may push out some traditional skills.

Medical schools should also address the needs of healthcare professionals. This includes providing support for stress management, burnout prevention and work-life balance. Doctors who are patient centred need substantial training to deal with the greater emotional burdens of patient centred care. They must learn how to deal with moral injury e.g. where they see suffering they cannot relieve or have to refuse a patient a necessary treatment.

Casuistry

A model to managing the conflict between ethical principles and the real world is casuistry. Casuistry is a method of ethical decision-making that involves examining similar cases to the one at hand to find a solution. By looking at how other people have dealt with similar ethical dilemmas, healthcare professionals can gain insights into how to resolve their own dilemma.

The students need appropriate examples, learn how to analyse the situation, facilitate a list of options and how to choose the best option. Finding the right examples can be difficult and is an area ripe for further research. Working through examples is straight forward with techniques such as problem-based learning PBL and situational judgement SJ.

The key skill is getting the student to generate enough options. Often the moral injury occurs because the student feels that they have no choice. By moving their thinking from general principles to specific examples they can find different choices. This deals with the criticism of casuistry as being patient centred means that the doctor is focused on the specific rather than the general.

One example of how casuistry applies to clinical practice is the use of the guideline. Guidelines are doctor-centred evidence-based generalisations. This means that many or even most patients will not receive patient-centred care if doctors follow guidelines. Casuistry gives an ethical explanation of why they should not follow the guideline for that patient.

A key learning task is the difference between casuistry and sophistry (which is the use of clever but false arguments, especially with the intention of deceiving). The educator should explain that the doctor considers all the options and listens to the patient. It is through this process that they find a different management.

The process protects the doctor from moral injury because they are not blindly following instructions but finding a solution. The logic underpinning the decisions are sound and defensible and the patient is involved in the decisions. Unlike sophistry the doctor using casuistry will often refer to self-evident and simple principles.

History of Medical Education

The history of medical education is long and complex. The first medical schools were established in Europe in the 12th century. These schools were based on the apprenticeship model, where students learned by observing and assisting more experienced doctors. They would also learn by reading medical texts and by practicing on cadavers.

The apprenticeship model was the dominant form of medical education for centuries. It had several advantages. First, it allowed students to learn from experienced doctors. Second, it allowed students to learn in a practical setting. Third, it was relatively inexpensive as a system. Fourthly supervision and doctor centred approaches protected students from the psychological trauma of illness.

However, the apprenticeship model also had several disadvantages. First, it was not a very systematic approach to learning. Second, it was not very rigorous. Third, it was not very accessible to people from poor backgrounds as it was based upon personal relationships. Fourthly it was a slow and inefficient way to learn.

In the 18th century, medical schools began to adopt a more formal curriculum. This curriculum included lectures, laboratory work and clinical rotations.

The introduction of a formal curriculum was a major step forward in medical education. It made medical education more systematic and rigorous. It also made medical education more accessible to people without connections.

Lectures were used to teach students the basic sciences of medicine. Clinical rotations were used to teach students how to diagnose and treat patients through history and examination. Laboratory work was used to broaden the monitoring of patients beyond clinical symptoms and signs.

However, the formal curriculum also had some disadvantages. First, it was more expensive than the apprenticeship model as it required an academic staff. Second, it was not as practical as the apprenticeship model. Third, it was not as individualised as the apprenticeship model.

In the 19th century, medical education began to change. New medical schools were established and the curriculum began to include more scientific subjects. There was an increasing recognition of the need to get the best students and Edinburgh led the way in offering places to women. The clinical laboratory allowed students to learn about the diagnosis and treatment of diseases through the scientific method.

In the 20th century, medical education underwent a major transformation. This transformation was driven by advances in medical science and technology. As a result of these advances, medical schools began to focus on training doctors who could specialise in the new treatments that became available.

One of the most important developments in 20th century medical education was the introduction of the clinical clerkship. The clinical clerkship or rotation is a period of time when medical students rotate through different clinical departments, such as internal (general) medicine, surgery and paediatrics.

The clinical rotation allows medical students to gain experience in the clinical setting. It also allows them to learn from specialist doctor by working with them. This postgraduate training in several areas replaces the doctor immediately entering their specialism. The rotation gives them relevant experiences that they can apply to their own specialty.

Today, medical education is a global enterprise. There are over 15,000 medical schools in the world and they educate over 1 million students each year. Many changes are driven by the new technologies so there is increasing subspecialisation which in turn increases the demand for specialist doctors.

More specialists mean a reduction in the number of generalists who can look holistically at the patient. As medicine becomes more expensive so does training to be a doctor. Those who have the skills in patient-centered care but come from poor backgrounds are struggling to find the funding.

There are constant pressures on medical schools to reduce the time taken to train a doctor, to reduce the costs associated with training.

Medical education is typically divided into three phases:

- Preclinical education: This phase of education focuses on the basic sciences of medicine, such as anatomy, physiology and pharmacology.

- Clinical education: This phase of education focuses on the application of the basic sciences to the diagnosis and treatment of patients.

- Postgraduate education: This phase of education focuses on the further development of the doctor's knowledge, skills and attitudes.

There is a risk that the curriculum will attempt to exclude topics that are more relevant for another phase in the teaching. This is understandable because the curriculum is packed and diversions may take time away from the current phase. However, it is important to remember that learning is not a linear process. Students need to be able to see how the different parts of medicine fit together and they need to be able to apply what they are learning to real-world situations.

Those students who do not master the basic science may struggle later to provide safe and effective care to patients. They may find it harder to understand how the human body responds to disease or recognise variations of clinical patterns. They may lack the critical thinking skills that allow students to analyse patient data and to make sound decisions about treatment.

Techniques such as the spiral curriculum where the student repeatedly encounters the same material has been tried. Students dislike this approach as they get bored and it takes away from their other learning. Including revision elements when teaching new aspects of a medical problem can be useful in complex topics such as diabetes.

The problem-based learning (PBL) approach can help students integrate knowledge across phases. PBL is a student-centered approach to learning that involves students working in small groups to solve problems. PBL can help students to develop critical thinking skills and to learn how to apply the basic sciences to the diagnosis and treatment of patients.

Another way to address this challenge is to use clinical rotations from the start of the course. Clinical rotations can help students to see how knowledge from different phases combines to produce good care. However, it is important to make sure that students have a strong foundation in the basic sciences before they start clinical rotations.

In a subject as complex as medicine it is easy for a student to prefer areas that they are good at whether the sciences, clinical or management. Helping students to achieve a balance may be more difficult in some curricula and teaching systems than others. The educator should identify individuals who are becoming too clinical or science oriented and offer individualised teaching.

The Future of Medical Education

Learning to be a medical educator involves being prepared for the future and the following are a few suggestions as to the likely changes and challenges. The healthcare students of today will be the leaders and educators and clinicians of the future. They need to be prepared for what they will face over their careers.

> Increased use of technology: Generative AI is likely to be transformative as it has the potential to improve speed and complexity of learning, make learning individualised and allow students who have previously been excluded to learn. For example, generative AI can be used to create personalised learning with a collaborative approach at much lower cost.

> Interprofessional education (IPE) is the process of educating students from different healthcare professions together. IPE is expected to become increasingly important in the future as healthcare is increasingly delivered by multidisciplinary teams. For example, IPE can help students to understand the roles and responsibilities of other healthcare professionals and to develop the skills they need to work effectively as part of a team.

Increased focus on lifelong learning: In the future, doctors will need to be lifelong learners. They will need to be able to keep up with the latest advances in medicine and to adapt to the changing needs of patients. Medical educators will need to focus on teaching students how to learn, rather than just teaching them specific facts and information.

The growing demand for healthcare services. The global population is aging and as a result, the demand for healthcare is increasing. There is a shortage of healthcare workers in many parts of the world. This will put a strain on the healthcare system and it will require medical educators to find new ways to train more doctors.

The need for more personalised and preventive care: In the future, doctors will need to be able to provide more personalised and preventive care. This will require them to have a deep understanding of the individual patient's needs and to be able to involve patients with their own healthcare choices to find the best treatment plans.

Preparing for each of these changes involves understanding the impact upon medical education. Changing the rules for the new technology, expanding the role of the educator to work with other professionals, provide lifelong learning and establish new medical schools will all change how educators work. The educator can start writing the new learning materials needed for training in patient centred and inclusive methods.

No-one can predict the future least of all doctors but we can all be better prepared for those changes that are coming. Educators are often guilty of being lost in the past they should remember teaching is about listening to their students. Students have an excitement of the future and can help the educator address the gaps in their own knowledge.

Conclusion

In conclusion, medical education is a complex and challenging process that aims to train doctors who can provide safe and effective care to patients. The goals of medical education include developing a deep understanding of the basic sciences, applying knowledge to diagnose and treat patients, effective communication with patients, working as part of a team and demonstrating professionalism and ethical behaviour.

Principles of effective medical education include a patient-centered approach, evidence-based medicine, lifelong learning and professionalism. However, there are ongoing debates about the potential adverse effects of these principles on the quality of education and the well-being of healthcare professionals. Medical schools must give students tools such as casuistry to survive these changes.

The history of medical education has evolved from the apprenticeship model to a more formal curriculum, incorporating lectures, laboratory work and clinical rotations. Advances in medical science and technology have further transformed medical education, leading to a global enterprise with increasing specialisation and demands on the curriculum.

The future of medical education will likely involve increased use of technology, interprofessional education, a focus on lifelong learning, addressing the growing demand for healthcare services and the need for more personalised and preventive care. Being prepared for these changes and actively involving students in shaping the future of medical education is crucial for producing well-equipped healthcare professionals.

Overall, medical education continues to evolve to meet the demands of a changing healthcare landscape, with the ultimate goal of providing the best possible care to patients while supporting the professional growth and well-being of doctors.

Top tips.

- Track the 5 goals of understand, apply, communication, teamwork and professionalism as informal targets for individual and cohort skills.
- Casuistry. Explain how to use casuistry to resolve real world problems which general principles cannot solve and the importance of listing choices.
- Prepare for the future. Identify steps that can be taken to adapt to LLMs and expand the educator's role. Create the learning materials to future proof medical education.

Chapter 2: THE ROLE OF THE TEACHER IN MEDICAL EDUCATION

Teachers in medical education (educators) are a key part of the shape of future doctors and the health service in general. The cost of a doctor's training is many hundreds of thousands of pounds and that investment may take decades to repay. Doctors can treat 10s of thousands of patients each year and they are responsible for substantial resource allocation.

The goal of the teacher in medical education is to provide students with the knowledge, skills and attitudes that they need to become safe and effective doctors. Small differences in doctor's skills can have significant impact in patient's outcomes and costs.

Effective teachers in medical education have a deep understanding of the basic sciences and the clinical practice of medicine. They are also passionate about teaching and about helping students to learn. Effective teachers are skilled communicators who are able to communicate complex information in a clear and concise way.

The teacher's role in medical education is to create a learning environment that is conducive to student learning. This environment should be supportive, challenging and stimulating. The teacher should create opportunities for students to learn in a variety of ways, including through lectures, small group discussions, problem-based learning and clinical rotations.

Becoming a doctor is a long and challenging process even for the most talented of students. The educator can significantly influence the difficulty that a student faces during their training. Recognising when a student requires more support can allow the student to bridge a difficult area. Being able to signpost help when appropriate can avoid the risk of crisis.

Giving Feedback.

The teacher should provide students with feedback on their learning. This feedback should be constructive and helpful. The teacher should also be available to answer students' questions and provide them with support. It can also help students to develop a sense of self-efficacy and to feel confident in their abilities.

Feedback should be constructive and helpful and it should be given in a timely manner. This feedback should be specific and actionable and can help students to identify their strengths and weaknesses. It should help students develop a plan for improvement.

Asking questions about the student's work is often better than pointing out errors or giving a mark. Asking the student to reconsider an element that was not well covered is more engaging than a negative comment. The student is given a clear idea of how to improve their work and can make progress more quickly.

This is particularly important in longer or more complex pieces of work such as a dissertation where the student may be getting lost in the text. Encouraging a story like answer can help the student see the bigger picture. The question guides the student back to the issues without giving them the answer.

An educator may wish to provide formal feedback in the form of an assessment however often informal feedback is more effective. A student who is struggling may benefit more from an immediate 'have you covered …?' than waiting for the marked work. This approach also encourages self-critical understanding.

Having a virtual classroom is an advance as the educator can record informal advice individually to the students. Being able to read what the students are doing in real time can give a better understanding of the student's progress than a finished piece of work.

Feedback is time-consuming and cognitively complex for the educator but is essential for many students to make progress. The skill of giving good feedback takes time to learn and perfect. Feedback can even slow learning if it is very poor but the best feedback can increase learning speeds dramatically.

Teaching Techniques

Many teaching techniques have been upgraded to use the latest technology. This is due in part to the increasing availability of high-quality educational resources online, as well as the growing popularity of mobile devices. These technologies can make it easier for students to access and participate in learning and they can also help to make learning more interactive and engaging.

Lectures can be a valuable way to introduce students to new concepts and ideas. However, they are not as effective for developing critical thinking skills. This is because lectures are typically one-way communication, where the teacher is the only one doing the talking. This can make it difficult for students to actively participate in the learning process and to develop their own critical thinking skills.

There are a few ways to improve lectures to make them more effective for developing critical thinking skills. These include asking questions throughout the lecture, using case studies and visual materials. These changes can be distracting, making it harder to follow the concepts. It may be better to uploading the lectures for video streaming. The university should ensure that they are well-produced and that they are easy to watch, engaging and interactive.

Uploading the lectures can improve accessibility by adding subtitles for those who are hard of hearing or who are learning English as a second language to understand the video. Students who are sick or who live far away from campus can continue to be able to access their lectures. Providing transcripts allows students with e.g. ASD who find listening difficult to read the material instead. Some students need to watch the lecture more than once and video provides more flexibility.

Small group discussions are still a valuable way for students to develop critical thinking skills. They can help learn how to apply the basic sciences to the diagnosis and treatment of patients. However as these problems become more complex the students have to shoulder more responsibility for solving them without a facilitator. The educator can assist by providing appropriate learning materials to support this type of study.

Collaborative work with AI is a new teaching technique that is still in its early stages. However, it has the potential to revolutionise medical education by providing students with access to personalised learning experiences and by helping them to develop new skills. Students often require training to use AI correctly.

Clinical rotations are a valuable way for students to gain experience and responsibility in the clinical setting. These rotations are becoming more integrated, with students working with other healthcare professionals to provide care to patients. Interprofessional education (IPE) increases the efficiency and breadth of the learning that can be achieved.

Assessment of student's progress.

Teachers in medical education can use a variety of assessment methods to evaluate student learning. Some common formal assessment methods include:

- Multiple choice exams
- Case-based exams

- Clinical skills assessments
- Portfolios

Effective teachers in medical education also assess their student's progress in following qualities using informal measures:

- Critical thinking is the ability to think clearly and rationally about a problem or issue. Effective teachers in medical education help students to develop critical thinking skills by exploring how they see the issues from different perspectives and how they apply evidence. Students may excel when providing their answers verbally, written or even visually so opportunities for different methodologies should be available.

- Problem-solving is the ability to identify a problem, to generate solutions and to evaluate the effectiveness of those solutions. Students need to learn to solve problems collaboratively as a team. They should all contribute but may have different roles.

- Communication is essential for effective patient care. Opportunities for developing communication skills include speaking with patients, practical sessions with communication skills theories and

- Teamwork is essential in the healthcare setting. Effective teachers in medical education help students to develop their teamwork skills by providing them with opportunities to understand the work and values of colleagues. This can be through inviting different professionals to provide teaching.

The use of multiple assessment techniques allows a more comprehensive understanding of the student's performance. This allows the educator to modify their teaching methods, improve the learning materials and arrange remedial teaching.

The formal assessments provide evidence mainly about knowledge. The informal assessments provide evidence mainly about skills. The educator should be prepared to investigate problems with additional assessment as required. The more evidence available the easier it is to work out how to make things better.

Conclusions.

In conclusion, the role of the teacher in medical education is of utmost importance in shaping competent and compassionate healthcare professionals. Effective teachers not only impart knowledge and skills but also play a pivotal role in developing the attitudes and values necessary for delivering safe and effective patient care.

This chapter has explored various aspects of the teacher's role in medical education. Teachers need to have a deep understanding of the basic sciences and clinical practice, as well as their passion for teaching and helping students learn. It is important to create a supportive and stimulating learning environment that encourages active participation and critical thinking.

Of key significance is providing constructive feedback that addresses the emotional consequences of decisions and actions. By understanding the stresses felt by students and encouraging them to actively seek feedback, teachers can better support their students and facilitate their professional growth.

Having a comprehensive toolbox of both teaching techniques and assessment methods is essential. These allow the educator to adapt their teaching as required and diagnose the student's difficulties promptly.

The impact of teachers in medical education extends far beyond the classroom. By instilling a sense of professionalism, promoting lifelong learning and serving as role models, teachers can shape the future of healthcare by nurturing competent and compassionate doctors.

In conclusion, the role of the teacher in medical education is challenging but immensely rewarding. Through their dedication and expertise, teachers can make a profound difference in the lives of patients and contribute to the advancement of healthcare. Let us recognise and celebrate the pivotal role that teachers play in moulding the next generation of healthcare professionals.

Top Tips

Ask questions about students' work using insights to engage them and encourage critical thinking.

Create a learning environment that is supportive, challenging and stimulating by using an array of teaching methods and materials.

Encourage collaborative work particularly with AI to ensure access to personalised learning experiences and help develop new skills.

Chapter 3: DEVELOPING EDUCATIONAL OBJECTIVES

Educational objectives are statements that describe what students should be able to do at the end of a learning experience. They are important because they help to ensure that students are learning what they need to learn. They have the additional function of providing a framework for assessment. Some educators even try to include the way that they will be taught in their objectives.

The risk is that the educator will develop an educational plan and lose sight of the objectives. Equally they may focus on the objectives without reference to the nature of the material that they need to teach. For many subjects it is straightforward to create SMART educational objectives. The educator can see what is important and how to arrange it logically.

Often the educator will need to understand the curriculum and undertake a scoping survey to be able to identify good objectives. These processes will inform the creation of objectives by identifying the key concepts. The correct objectives to choose may not be obvious and the educator should be prepared to reconsider it they are not effective.

In this chapter, for instance, the key concepts are how to create a list of concepts, how to organise them into a coherent whole and how to develop the objectives. These are listed as the three top tips section and the scoping survey is the SMART objective in the chapter section above.

The reason I chose these rather than other elements of creation of educational objectives is because they are SMART. They are specific tasks that can be achieved in a reasonable timescale and the outcome is measurable and relevant. A list of the key concepts which are organised and developed are the outcome that the educator requires.

SMART educational objectives

There are a number of different approaches to developing educational objectives. They do not have significant advantages and the approach most commonly used is designated the SMART acronym, which stands for:

Specific: The objective should be specific and clearly defined. They should not be vague or general and should be written in the active voice. They should describe what students will be able to do, not what the teacher will do.

Measurable: The objective should be measurable. How will you know if students have achieved the objective?

Achievable: The objective should be achievable for the students. It should be challenging and not be too difficult or too easy for students to achieve.

Relevant: The objective should be relevant to the students' learning goals and the learning experience. They should be aligned with the learning goals of the course or program.

Time-bound: The objective should have a deadline. This will help students to stay focused and motivated.

Here are some examples of educational objectives:

- After reading this chapter, students will be able to define the term "educational objective" and give three examples of objectives.

- After completing the practice, students will be able to create a feedback form based upon their objectives.

- After working with their group the student will be able to list the reasons why some educational objectives failed.

Developing educational objectives is an important part of the preparation for any learning experience. By taking the time to write clear and specific objectives, teachers can help to ensure that students are learning what they need to learn.

Educators can use these objectives to guide their planning and instruction. Selecting instructional materials, activities and assessments that are aligned with the objectives.

Understanding the curriculum.

Understanding the curriculum is an essential part of being an effective educator. The curriculum is the blueprint for the course and it outlines the learning goals, objectives and content that students will be expected to learn. By understanding the curriculum, educators can ensure that they are teaching the material that is most important and that they are meeting the needs of their students.

There are a few things that educators can do to understand the curriculum. First, they should read the course syllabus carefully. The syllabus should outline the learning goals, objectives and content for the course. Second, they should review the reading lists for the course. The reading lists will provide additional information about the material that will be covered in the course. Third, they should talk to their students. Students can provide valuable insights into their own learning needs and expectations.

Once educators have a good understanding of the curriculum, they can begin to plan their teaching. They should consider the learning goals and objectives, the content that will be covered and the needs of their students. They should also consider the best way to deliver the material. There are a variety of teaching methods that can be used and the best method will vary depending on the material and the students.

My experience of the PGCME is that the university's websites were very vague about the nature of their study curriculum. The course descriptions give little information as to their content. Even as a student I was given little guidance beyond what was on the website and my tutors also struggled to give clarification.

As an educator there may be more information available however, I will assume for the purpose of this chapter that the educator is in no better position than I was. Identifying the learning goals can be challenging because it may not be clear what the curriculum designers intended. There may be substantial overlap between different topic in any course including the PGCME.

The course syllabus documents are not always kept up to date and may have omissions. The reading lists are variable with some topics having recommended reading including tens and others none or one. The past papers may give some details as to what is expected from the students but occasionally the structure of the course will change.

Scoping Survey

If the objectives remain elusive then a scoping survey will be required, LLMs will often provide a good range of topics relevant to the subject. Start from the subject as a whole, rather than the course because it is a helpful to recognise overlaps. Iterating until there are 30-40 different topics will give sufficient differentiation between concepts as well as a manageable list. Ordering the areas logically so that they tell a story is also a good way to make the course more understandable.

Once the topics to be covered have been scoped and assigned as part of the course, they need to be assigned to teaching episodes. It is likely that the educator has access to the subject of each of the planned teaching episodes or at least the number. A further scoping survey will provide another list of topics this time aiming for a similar number to the number of teaching episodes. Hopefully they can be more or less assigned to the teaching planned during the course.

At this point it may be clear which group of topics need to be covered in each part of the course however there will usually be areas of overlap. These are often at the boundaries of subjects and it may not be possible to separate them. An example of this problem is headaches which has generalist, psychological, neurological, ENT and cardiovascular causes. Each specialty should provide its own version of the headache story.

At this stage the best approach is to take the provisional list to a relevant subject matter expert to resolve any inconsistencies remaining. This should allow some tweaking of the topic areas so that the boundaries are clear and the content requirements are understood. This preparation takes less time than it sounds and improves the educator's performance.

Further steps that can be taken as to identify the most important concepts for prioritisation and repetition. Asking students to rate each subject can determine any resistance to learning and where increased work will be needed. The educator should now have a comprehensive list of teaching episodes, a short description of what the teaching episode is about and the concepts that they are intended to teach.

Practical steps towards identifying objectives.

The educator will start with the topic list and may be able to write a list of objectives for each teaching episode using the SMART approach. There may be objectives that cannot be allocated to any specific teaching session. These are 'emergent objectives' that arise as a consequence of undertaking the course. These are not achievable in any one session but emerge out of participation in the whole course.

If the educator is struggling with the creation of educational objectives then they should work backwards. Studying the curriculum should allow the educator to work out what the author of the curriculum intended. This should in turn clarify the necessary objectives to achieve these aims.

The educator may still find it difficult to identify educational objectives and bring them into a coherent whole. Conducting a scoping survey allows the educator to work out how the curriculum fits together. They will then be able to map the educational objectives and the teaching episodes and write the educational objectives.

The educational objectives should then be tested to check that they are both necessary and sufficient for the student to gain an understanding of the topic. This is a thought experiment where the educator imagines the student only achieving the educational objectives. If the student would fail the assessment then the reason for that issue should be considered.

The reason may be that the student needs a grounding in another area, they may also need to learn a list of facts or the educational objectives are incorrect. Other issues are that there are problems with the assessment process or that there are student factors that need addressing.

The purpose of objectives is to provide a structure to the teaching, an achievement that the student may reasonably reach and a measure for success. Objectives can be used to guide instruction, to select appropriate teaching methods and to assess student learning.

Evidence that students are aware of the teaching objectives is limited even when they are written down. Although classically there have always been three objectives this is not immutable and there will times when it is better to have fewer. The students should be both aware of the objectives and find them useful.

This means that the educator needs to develop the educational objectives and share them with their students. They should get feedback on the educational objectives and be prepared to explain why they were chosen. They can be shared with other educators to ensure that the objectives are accurate and aligned with the content standards.

Conclusions.

Developing educational objectives is a crucial aspect of effective teaching and learning. Educational objectives serve as a roadmap for both educators and students, guiding the teaching process and ensuring that students are learning what they need to know. The SMART approach, emphasising specificity, measurability, achievability, relevance and time-bound nature, provides a valuable framework for creating clear and focused objectives.

Understanding the curriculum plays a vital role in crafting meaningful educational objectives. Educators must familiarise themselves with the course syllabus, reading lists and student perspectives to ensure they meet the learning needs and expectations of their students. Conducting a scoping survey may be required to identify key concepts and organise them logically, enhancing the coherence and effectiveness of the course.

Throughout the process of developing objectives, educators should continuously evaluate and refine them. Identifying emergent objectives that emerge as a consequence of the course and ensuring they align with the curriculum's intentions further enhances the educational experience. Additionally, seeking feedback from students and collaborating with other educators can help validate and improve the objectives, ensuring they are both necessary and sufficient for student learning.

Ultimately, educational objectives provide a structure for teaching and learning, guiding educators in selecting appropriate teaching methods and assessments. The active involvement of students in understanding and being aware of the objectives is crucial, fostering a more engaging and effective learning environment. By investing the time and effort into developing clear, meaningful and student-oriented educational objectives, educators can foster successful learning experiences that empower students to achieve their goals.

Top tips.

Conduct a scoping survey to create list of all the concepts you will need to cover in your teaching and organise the list based upon students learning needs and importance of topics.

Develop educational objectives that are logical and cohesive, aligned with content and engage the students emotionally and mentally.

Test the educational objectives in a thought experiment, would a student who has achieved the educational objectives pass the assessment process?

Chapter 4: INTERPROFESSIONAL EDUCATION (IPE)

Interprofessional education (IPE) is a collaborative educational approach that brings together students from different healthcare professions to learn about and from each other. IPE is designed to help students develop the knowledge, skills and attitudes necessary to work effectively as members of interprofessional teams.

interprofessional education (IPE) can be delivered in a variety of ways. Here are common methods ranked from low to high risk:

- Joint lectures: Joint lectures allow students from different healthcare professions to learn sane topics together. This can help students to develop an understanding each group of healthcare professionals have different roles and responsibilities.

- Case-based discussions: Case-based discussions allow students from different healthcare professions to discuss real-world cases. This can help students to learn how each will contribute to collaborate with other healthcare professionals to provide patient care.

- Simulation exercises: Simulation exercises allow students from different healthcare professions to practice their skills in a safe and controlled environment. This can help students to develop their confidence and competence in working with other healthcare professionals and conflict resolution.

- Community-based projects: Community-based projects allow students from different healthcare professions to work together to address a community health issue. This can help students to develop their understanding of the role of healthcare professionals in the community.

The common thread in these methods is team building built by understanding, communication and mutual respect. Whilst professions are often tribal there is often infighting and this can spill over in IPE sessions. The success of an IPE session depends upon managing the social interactions.

This starts before the groups meet with exercises designed to improve the way that the individuals behave in groups. This involves teamwork skills and identifying the roles that individuals are most comfortable with.

Forming groups within the profession and getting them to meet and interact can be helpful.

The more skilled each of the groups is at incorporating new members and recognising their skills the more successful the IPE session will be. Educators should meet with their opposite numbers to ensure that the other professional group is properly prepared. Where possible the educator should attend as session with the other professional group.

Managing intergroup social interactions.

The key method that IPE improves outcomes is social rather than educational as it promotes interprofessional teambuilding. The educator should be aware that simply learning together will not be as effective as if the professionals communicate with each other. This is particularly important if there is a history of conflict between different professions.

Where the groups show challenging behaviour, the educator can use the rivalry to improve understanding about each other's cultures and values. The most vocal members of each group can be asked to come to the front and debate their issues. Experience of facilitating this type of interaction will increase the chance of success. Even if there is no agreement the next IPE will be less fraught because they will feel listened to.

This means that the educator should be careful avoid tribalism or making jokes that show lack of respect. They should try to avoid any professional group feeling that they are getting a worse deal, for instance if the groups are larger than they would be. Offering benefits, for instance with two lecture times rather than one or starting later can improve cohesion between the groups.

Emphasising the similarities between groups and focusing on the common goal of high-quality patient care can improve cohesion. Providing a safe space where students share their thoughts and feelings can uncover misunderstandings or lack of sensitivity. If the IPE is not working being flexible by making changes can help the students develop the confidence to adapt to IPE.

Where the topic appears irrelevant to one of the professional groups it may be better to avoid use IPE and teach it separately, at least at first. When teaching a subject that appears to have little relevance it is always important to explain the rationale but more so when using IPE. Each professional group can feel that they are only learning that subject because of the other professional group.

Educators can be role models by getting to know students from different healthcare professions and introducing them to each other. Using active learning methods can provide opportunities to interact and reflect on the learning. Collecting feedback both formally and informally can help the educator work out what is effective.

It is worth reflecting on the educator's own feelings about IPE as often it is out of their comfort zone and experience. Sitting in on the other professional groups teaching can be a first step towards the educator breaking down their own barriers. When IPE is being introduced it is important for all educators to share their previous experiences.

IPE should be optional to avoid those who do not have the right skills feeling pushed into joint teaching. Apart from the distress that enforced participation causes to the educator it often damages the process and increases tribalism. With sensitivity and respect IPE can be introduced and achieve the many benefits that are possible.

It takes time to build relationships and create a positive and supportive learning environment. Each conversation between the groups or about IPE is one step closer to acceptance of the approach. Sell IPE as a chance to learn about areas that are usually out of bounds and explain what the students have to gain from the interaction. The use of stories can be compelling and influential in reducing reluctance.

The benefits of IPE.

Students are more interested in how IPE improves their chances of passing their examinations than saving the NHS money. Managers often list the following advantages apparently unaware that they are not persuasive to the students. Consider which of these are relevant to the student's needs in a high stakes course such as medicine.

- Enhanced patient-centered care: IPE can help to improve patient care by increasing communication and collaboration between healthcare professionals. This can lead to better decision-making and more effective care.

- Enhanced patient safety: IPE can help to reduce medical errors by promoting communication and collaboration among healthcare professionals. This can benefit patients if for instance an incorrect dose is prescribed the pharmacist will feel less inhibited to raise the issue with their medical colleagues.

- Reduced costs of healthcare delivery: IPE can help to reduce costs by reducing the need for duplication of services. For example, if students from different healthcare professions are learning together, they can share resources such as textbooks and clinical facilities.

- Increased knowledge of the roles of other healthcare professions: IPE can help to reduce professional isolation by increasing social interaction between professions. This can lead to improved communication and collaboration when working together as a team.

- Increased job satisfaction: IPE can help to increase job satisfaction by providing students with a more well-rounded education. This can lead to students feeling more confident and competent in their chosen profession.

Educators need to present these advantages of IPE to the students in a way that motivates them to participate in the process. It is important not to mistake compliance with engagement because the former will not achieve the benefits that the latter will. A particular trigger point is the suggestion that different groups should share resources to save money.

Before IPE is started the students should recognise that they have needs that another professional group can help with. Assessment of their knowledge of the roles and responsibilities of other health care professionals, ability to communicate in a team environment, ability to collaborate, understanding of the patient experience and professionalism can demonstrate gaps.

Whilst many students will have excellent skills in many of these areas there will be some who lack in one or more of these areas. This will provide a reason for these students to engage with IPE as they will see the need to improve their scores. The initial learning can be focused on addressing the issues in the assessment. The progress that the students make in their score will then be a source of reward.

Those who are initially reluctant will see their colleagues improving and wish to engage. It may be possible to offer selected students the chance to have an attachment in another professional's speciality such as dentistry, pharmacy or physio. This will allow students to experience these different lifestyles and may even lead to a desire to swap courses.

It is also important to remove sources of resistance to IPE such as additional time commitments, making the learning fun and fear of failure. Students often feel overloaded with their workload and resist any attempt to add more. Equally removing other tasks does not remove the need for the students to learn. Persuading students that they can learn more effectively in a shorter time period will improve engagement.

There are a number of challenges to implementing IPE, including:

- Lack of time

- Lack of resources
- Lack of faculty expertise
- Lack of commitment from faculty
- Lack of understanding of the benefits of IPE

However, these challenges can be overcome with careful planning and coordination. IPE is a valuable investment in the future of healthcare. By educating students to work together as members of interprofessional teams, IPE can help to improve the quality of care for patients.

Introducing IPE.

Where IPE is not formally arranged by the university an educator may wish to organise some IPE activities. They can ask for volunteers which reduces the costs and workload associated with the IPE. This can act as a test run for formal IPE to be introduced into the curriculum.

The following examples are a shopping list for students who are keen to be involved in IPE. Each example has advantages and disadvantages but the student's preference is the key determinant. Tailoring an activity to fit the student's preferences appears to involve more work. The students who have chosen to volunteer will be more engaged and prepared to make the activity work.

- Simulations: Simulations allow students to practice working together in a safe environment. For example, students from medicine, nursing and social work might participate in a simulation of an emergency room. This would allow them to practice working together to assess and care for a patient.
- Case studies: Case studies allow students to learn about the challenges of caring for patients with complex needs. For example, students from medicine, nursing and social work might participate in a case study about a patient with a disability. This would allow them to learn about the different challenges that this patient faces and how different healthcare professionals can work together to provide care.
- Joint learning in community settings: Joint learning in community settings allows students to learn about the challenges of providing care in the community. For example, students from medicine, nursing and social work might participate in a joint learning experience at a homeless shelter. This would allow them to learn about the challenges that homeless people face and how different healthcare professionals can work together to provide care.

- Interprofessional clinical rotations: Students from different healthcare professions rotate through the same clinical setting, working together to provide care to patients. This type of IPE allows students to learn how to collaborate with each other and to understand the different roles that each profession plays in the delivery of care.
- Interprofessional case conferences: Students from different healthcare professions meet to discuss a particular patient case. This type of IPE allows students to share their perspectives on the case and to learn from each other's experiences.
- Interprofessional team-based learning: Students from different healthcare professions work together in small groups to learn about a particular topic. This type of IPE allows students to learn how to work together as a team and to develop their communication and problem-solving skills.
- Shadowing: In shadowing, students observe healthcare professionals at work. This type of learning helps students to gain a better understanding of the different roles of healthcare professionals and to see how they work together to provide care to patients.

Students have an important role in IPE because they can help the educator develop the process. Their insights are often generalisable and lead to important improvements being part of the process. The educator can work collaboratively with students to develop the correct learning materials and adapt to problems.

This type of organic growth in an educational program is very different from the complete transformation that usually occurs when making a change. Whilst this can be a welcome change of pace it is also an opportunity to learn new skills such collaborative development. Rapidly iterating on teaching materials can lead to a steep learning curve.

Conclusion

Interprofessional education (IPE) is a collaborative educational approach that brings together students from different healthcare professions to learn about and from each other. IPE is designed to help students develop the knowledge, skills and attitudes necessary to work effectively as members of interprofessional teams.

IPE can be delivered in a variety of ways, including joint lectures, case-based discussions, simulation exercises and community-based projects. Each of these methods has its own advantages and disadvantages and the best approach will vary depending on the specific needs of the students and the healthcare setting.

There is a growing body of evidence that supports the benefits of IPE. Studies have shown that IPE can lead to improved patient care, reduced medical errors and increased job satisfaction for healthcare professionals.

However, there are also some challenges to implementing IPE, including lack of time, lack of resources, lack of faculty expertise and lack of commitment from faculty. These challenges can be overcome with careful planning and coordination.

IPE is a valuable investment in the future of healthcare. By educating students to work together as members of interprofessional teams, IPE can help to improve the quality of care for patients.

Top tips.

- Pilot IPE. Introducing IPE to a few students first can help to identify any challenges or areas for improvement before rolling it out to a larger group. The students who participate in the pilot can also provide valuable feedback that can be used to shape the future of IPE at the institution.
- Foster Social Interaction: Encourage informal communication and social engagement to breakdown barriers. This can reduce stress and improve morale and may even lead to study groups.
- Encourage Collaboration: Promote collaborative learning experiences to help students understand their different roles and build effective team dynamics. Offer the chance to work on a problem together or have peer learning.

Chapter 5: INSTRUCTIONAL DESIGN IN MEDICAL EDUCATION

In medical education, Instructional design (ID) is used to design courses, programs and simulations that help students learn the knowledge and skills they need to be safe and effective healthcare professionals. ID models can be helpful for medical educators because they can help them to create instruction that is aligned with the learning objectives and that is effective in helping students to learn.

There are a number of instructional design (ID) models that are used to create effective learning experiences. These models share some similarities, but they also have different strengths and weaknesses. To understand these models better, it is helpful to summarise and compare them.

ID models also differ in their focus. Some models focus on the cognitive domain, which is concerned with the learner's knowledge and understanding. Other models focus on the affective domain, which is concerned with the learner's attitudes and emotions. Still other models focus on the psychomotor domain, which is concerned with the learner's skills and abilities.

Instructional design (ID) can be seen as a series of choices between different technologies that are then fitted together to create a learning episode. Good teaching materials can be expensive, so most educators will be limited to technologies that are cheap. It is also rare that individualised teaching materials can be provided for different groups of students, which further limits the choices.

In practice, educators will get the greatest value from understanding their topic and the different approaches that can be taken. Creating a story to explain the approach chosen will provide hooks for students to learn. Materials essential to the teaching may not be expensive or complex.

The most common mistake is to overcomplicate the learning episode. Students will only take away a small part of the information presented, so there is no point in providing additional information that is not essential. Keeping the messages simple and the evidence provided clear reduces the stress on the student and maximises their understanding.

The ADDIE model.

The ADDIE model is a systematic approach to instructional design that can be used to create effective learning experiences. The model is divided into five phases: analysis, design, development, implementation and evaluation.

The analysis phase is the first step in the ADDIE model. In this phase, the instructional designer identifies the needs of the learners and the goals of the learning experience. The designer also gathers information about the learners' prior knowledge and skills, learning styles and preferences.

The design phase is the second step in the ADDIE model. In this phase, the instructional designer creates a plan for the learning experience. This plan includes the learning objectives, the instructional methods and the learning materials.

The development phase is the third step in the ADDIE model. In this phase, the instructional designer creates the learning materials. This can be done by the designer themselves, or by a team of instructional designers, writers, graphic designers and other experts.

The implementation phase is the fourth step in the ADDIE model. In this phase, the learning experience is delivered to the learners. This can be done in a variety of ways, including face-to-face instruction, online courses, or blended learning.

The evaluation phase is the fifth and final step in the ADDIE model. In this phase, the instructional designer evaluates the effectiveness of the learning experience. This includes collecting data on the learners' progress and making changes to the learning experience as needed.

The ADDIE model is a versatile and effective approach to instructional design. It can be used to create learning experiences for a variety of audiences and in a variety of settings. The model is also flexible enough to be adapted to the specific needs of each learning experience.

The advantages of using the ADDIE model are that it is easy to understand and use. The system creates a well-designed and effective learning episode. It is also flexible and can be adapted to the specific needs of each learning experience.

The disadvantages of using the ADDIE model are that it can be time-consuming and expensive. It can be difficult to get agreement on the needs of the learners and the goals of the learning experience. The educator may need several iterations before an optimal design emerges.

The Dick and Carey Model

The Dick and Carey Model is a widely used instructional design model that is known for its step-by-step approach to creating effective learning experiences. The model consists of eight steps:

Identify instructional goals. The first step in the model is to identify the instructional goals. This involves determining what learners should be able to do after completing the instruction.

Analyse learners. The next step is to analyse the learners. This involves identifying the learners' prior knowledge, skills and abilities, as well as their learning styles and preferences.

Write performance objectives. The third step is to write performance objectives. Performance objectives specify what learners should be able to do after completing the instruction. They should be specific, measurable, achievable, relevant and time bound.

Develop instructional strategies. The fourth step is to develop instructional strategies. Instructional strategies are the methods and activities that will be used to help learners achieve the performance objectives.

Develop and select instructional materials. The fifth step is to develop and select instructional materials. Instructional materials can include textbooks, computer-based training programs, online courses and other resources.

Develop and conduct formative evaluation. The sixth step is to develop and conduct formative evaluation. Formative evaluation is used to assess the effectiveness of the instruction during development. This feedback can be used to improve the instruction before it is delivered to learners.

Revise instructional materials. The seventh step is to revise instructional materials based on the results of the formative evaluation.

Conduct summative evaluation. The eighth step is to conduct summative evaluation. Summative evaluation is used to assess the overall effectiveness of the instruction after it has been delivered to learners. This information can be used to improve the instruction for future learners.

The Dick and Carey Model's advantages are that it a comprehensive and systematic approach and provides a clear framework for planning and developing instruction. The model is flexible and can be adapted to a variety of learners and learning situations. It obtains feedback from both summative and formative evaluation.

The disadvantages are that it can be time-consuming and expensive requiring several iterations. The model can be difficult to use for complex or challenging learning objectives. The model is not always flexible enough to adapt to changing learning needs.

Mager's ISD Model

Mager's ISD Model is a well-known and widely used instructional design model. It is based on the idea that instructional design should be focused on the learner and their needs. It is popular as it is known for its simplicity and focus on performance. It is a goal-oriented approach that starts with identifying the desired outcomes of instruction and then works backwards to develop the necessary learning activities.

The model consists of six steps:

- Identify the terminal objective. What do you want the learner to be able to do at the end of the instruction? The terminal objective should be specific, measurable, achievable, relevant and time bound.
- Identify the enabling objectives. What skills and knowledge does the learner need to achieve the terminal objective? The enabling objectives are the steps that the learner must take to reach the terminal objective. The enabling objectives should be specific and measurable and they should be arranged in a logical sequence.
- Write performance statements for each objective. A performance statement is a clear and concise description of what the learner will be able to do. Performance statements should be written in the learner's perspective and should be specific, measurable, achievable, relevant and time bound.
- Develop test items for each objective. The test items should assess the learner's ability to meet the performance statements. Test items can be written in a variety of formats, such as multiple choice, true/false, fill-in-the-blank and essay.
- Develop instructional materials. The instructional materials should be designed to help the learner achieve the performance statements. The instructional materials can include a variety of resources, such as textbooks, articles, videos and simulations. The materials should be engaging, relevant and easy to understand. They should also be consistent with the learning objectives.
- Conduct evaluation. Evaluate the effectiveness of the instruction to ensure that the learner is meeting the objectives. This can be done by giving the learner a pre-test and a post-test, surveys or by observing the learner's performance. The evaluation results can be used to improve the instruction.

Mager's ISD Model has several advantages. It is well-structured and systematic and it is easy to understand and use. The model is focused on the learner's ability to perform a specific task or skill. This focus on performance can help to ensure that instruction is relevant and effective.

However, Mager's ISD Model also has some disadvantages. It is not appropriate for all types of learning. Its simplicity means that it may not be comprehensive and struggles with complex learning objectives. It can also be unclear whether all the objectives have been met, particularly if the learner has a variety of needs.

Gagne's Nine Events of Instruction

Gagne's Nine Events of Instruction is a model of instructional design that can be used to create effective learning experiences. The model is based on the idea that learning is a complex process that involves a number of cognitive and affective factors. The nine events are:

1. Gain attention. The first step in any learning experience is to gain the learner's attention. This can be done by using a variety of techniques, such as asking a question, telling a story, or showing a video.

2. State objectives. Once the learner's attention has been gained, the next step is to state the objectives of the learning experience. This will help the learner to understand what they are expected to learn and how they will be assessed.

3. Recall prior learning. Before new information can be learned, it is important to activate the learner's prior knowledge. This can be done by asking questions about the learner's previous experiences or by reviewing relevant concepts.

4. Present the stimulus. The next step is to present the new information to the learner. This can be done in a variety of ways, such as through lectures, demonstrations, or hands-on activities.

5. Provide guidance. As the learner is presented with new information, it is important to provide them with guidance and support. This can be done by answering questions, providing feedback, or offering hints and suggestions.

6. Elicit performance. Once the learner has been presented with new information, it is important to elicit their performance. This can be done by asking them questions, having them complete exercises, or giving them opportunities to practice what they have learned.

7. Provide feedback. This event is about providing the learner with specific and constructive feedback on their performance. This feedback helps the learner identify their strengths and weaknesses and adjust their learning strategy.

8. Enhance retention and transfer. The final step in Gagne's model is to enhance retention and transfer. This can be done by providing practice opportunities, reviewing the material regularly and providing opportunities to apply the information in real-world settings.

The advantages of Gagne's model are that it comprehensive and covers all the important steps in the learning process. It can provide a stimulating learning experience and enhanced learner engagement. It can be more effective than other ID models for teaching difficult topics.

The disadvantages are that it is highly user dependant requiring good timing and planning. Can be difficult to implement all nine events in a learning experience. The additional effort required to implement the technique may not be necessary if the students already have prior knowledge. It does not work well with some learners and is less effective in groups already exposed to the technique.

The SAM Model

The SAM Model is a learner-centered approach to instructional design. It focuses on the individual needs of the learner and the learning environment. It can be used to design a wide variety of learning experiences, from traditional classroom instruction to online courses. The SAM Model is also well-suited for use with learners with diverse needs.

The SAM Model consists of four steps:

- Select: The first step is to select the appropriate instructional materials and activities. This involves considering the learner's needs, the learning objectives and the learning environment.
- Adapt: The second step in the SAM Model is to adapt the instructional materials and activities to meet the individual needs of the learner. This may involve providing additional support for struggling learners or challenging more advanced learners. The instructional materials and activities can also be adapted to meet the needs of different learning styles.
- Mediate: The third step in the SAM Model is to mediate the learning process. This involves providing feedback to the learner, answering questions and resolving any problems that the learner may

encounter. The instructional designer can also mediate the learning process by providing additional support materials, such as tutorials or practice exercises.

- Measure: The fourth step in the SAM Model is to measure the learner's progress. This can be done through a variety of methods, such as quizzes, tests, or performance assessments. The results of the assessment can be used to identify areas where the learner needs additional support and to adjust the instructional materials and activities.

The advantages of using the SAM Model are that it is learner-centered and delivers education tailored to that individual's learning style and needs rather than on the content to be learned. It is particularly useful when designing materials for learners with diverse needs. It can improve an individual's performance dramatically as the SAM Model is iterative and can make changes as needed based on the learner's feedback.

The disadvantages include the model is less good at providing group than individual learning. The approaches are not always generalisable and it can be more time-consuming than other instructional design models. The SAM Model requires a high level of expertise from the instructional designer. It requires a high level of collaboration between the instructional designer and the learner which is often impracticable.

The Backward Design Model

The Backward Design Model is a process for creating curriculum that starts with the end in mind. It is a three-step process that helps educators identify what students should know and be able to do by the end of the learning cycle, create an assessment to measure that learning and plan a sequence of lessons that will prepare students to successfully complete the assessment.

- Identify desired results: The first step in the Backward Design Model is to identify the desired results of the learning. This includes identifying the knowledge, skills and understandings that students should have by the end of the learning cycle. Educators can use a variety of resources to identify desired results, such as educational standards, curriculum guides and professional learning communities.
- Determine acceptable evidence: Once the desired results have been identified, the next step is to determine how students will be assessed. This involves creating an assessment that will measure students' knowledge, skills and understandings. The assessment

should be aligned with the desired results and should be fair and equitable.

- Plan learning experiences: The final step in the Backward Design Model is to plan the learning experiences that will help students achieve the desired results. This includes selecting the instructional strategies, resources and activities that will be used to teach the content. The learning experiences should be engaging and relevant to students' lives.

The Backward Design Model has advantages as it allows the educator to focus on the desired results of learning and align materials with those desired results. It can help improve student achievement because materials are aligned with the desired results. The materials can be simplified as educators can be more intentional about their teaching and to make sure that they are teaching what is important.

Disadvantages include the risk that the educator will leave out important content because the model uses a variant of teaching to the test. This can limit learning to the desired results rather than all the content that students need to know. Focus on results can lead to less emphasis on critical thinking skills and other skills not easy to measure on tests. It can be difficult to identify the desired results and acceptable evidence once the curriculum has been developed.

Reigeluth's Elaboration Theory.

Reigeluth's Elaboration Theory is an instructional design theory that argues that content to be learned should be organised from simple to complex order, while providing a meaningful context in which subsequent ideas can be integrated. The theory is based on the following principles:

- Sequencing: Content should be sequenced in a way that builds on prior knowledge and gradually increases in complexity. This means starting with the most basic concepts and gradually adding more complex information.

- Elaboration: Content should be elaborated upon by providing examples, analogies and other supporting information. This helps learners to understand and remember the information better.

- Meaningful context: Content should be presented in a meaningful context that helps learners to understand and remember it. This can be done by using real-world examples, stories, or case studies.

- Learner control: Learners should be given some control over the pace and sequence of instruction. This allows them to learn at their own pace and focus on the areas that they need the most help with.

Reigeluth's Elaboration Theory has been used to design a variety of instructional materials, including textbooks, computer-based training programs and web-based courses. The theory has been shown to be effective in improving student learning outcomes.

Here are some examples of how Reigeluth's Elaboration Theory can be applied to instruction:

Pre-instruction: In the pre-instruction phase, the learner is prepared for the instruction by activating prior knowledge and providing motivation. This can be done by asking questions, reviewing previous lessons, or providing a brief overview of the topic to be covered.

Instruction: In the instruction phase, the learner is presented with the new information in a gradually elaborated way. This means starting with the most basic concepts and gradually adding more complex information. The information should also be presented in a meaningful context that helps learners to understand and remember it. Use analogies and metaphors to help the learner understand new concepts. Provide opportunities for the learner to ask questions and get feedback.

Post-instruction: In the post-instruction phase, the learner is given opportunities to practice and apply the new information. This can be done through activities, exercises, or projects. Summary and synthesis is the process of summarising and integrating new information with prior knowledge.

Elaboration Theory has the advantage of being based on an established learning theory and can help learners to develop a deep understanding of the material. It is learner centred and develops upon learners' prior knowledge by providing opportunities to actively participate in the learning process. Elaboration Theory is efficient because it helps learners to learn more in less time. This is because it focuses on what the learner needs to know next and it provides opportunities for learners to practice and apply what they have learned.

Disadvantages of the theory include that it requires a high level of expertise from instructional designers This is because it requires a thorough understanding of the subject matter and the learner's needs. Elaboration Theory can be difficult to apply to some learning topics particularly in a mixed ability learning episode. It can be difficult to assess as progress may align with the learner's needs rather than the curriculum and it is more difficult to measure the depth of understanding.

Branching theory

Branching theory is a learning theory that uses a branching tree structure to present information to learners. The tree structure is created by dividing the material to be learned into a series of nodes, or units of instruction. Each node contains a brief overview of the material, followed by a set of questions. Learners are asked to answer the questions and their responses are used to determine which node they should proceed to next.

As computer-based learning improves, game developers may be able to create more effective learning experiences by using a branch-like structure. This type of structure allows learners to choose their own path like in a game, which can help them to learn at their own pace and in a way that is most engaging for them.

Learners could choose to follow the branch that interests them most and they could also go back and explore other branches later. This type of structure can help them learn more effectively because it allows them to be more engaged in the learning process.

Branching theory is divided into two phases: selection and presentation.

- Selection: In this phase, the learner is given a pre-test to assess their knowledge. The pre-test results are used to determine the learner's starting point and the appropriate level of instruction. Each node requires its own pre-test to identify the correct instruction.
- Presentation: In this phase, the learner is presented with the instruction that is appropriate for their level of knowledge. The instruction is presented in a series of branching paths, with each path leading to a different level of difficulty. The learner can choose the path that is most appropriate for their needs.

Branching theory is based on the idea that learners learn at different rates and in different ways. By individualising instruction, branching theory can help learners to learn more effectively.

The advantages of using branching theory include individualising the learning to the learner. The learner can progress at their own pace and take on the level of challenge that they feel happy with and avoid feeling frustrated or boredom and can lead to deeper learning. They stay in the learning zone for more the time and get feedback to support their continued engagement with the material.

The disadvantages of using branching theory are it can be complex to develop a large enough tree to cover all possible choices. This can become expensive and inflexible as the number of choices increases exponentially. Difficulties with modulating the challenge for each path can risk a learner becoming trapped in an area that is too difficult or easy and being asked the same questions repeatedly.

The 4C/ID model

The 4C/ID model is a newer instructional design model that is based on the idea of complex learning. Complex learning is the ability to apply knowledge and skills in new and unfamiliar situations. It is mainly used to teach skills as other methods may be better for teaching knowledge.

The 4C/ID model is designed to help learners develop complex learning skills by providing them with the opportunity to practice and apply their knowledge and skills in a safe and supportive environment. The model is also designed to help learners develop the ability to transfer their learning to new and unfamiliar situations.

The 4C/ID model consists of four components:

1. Learning tasks: Learning tasks are the heart of the 4C/ID model. They are authentic, complex tasks that require learners to use their knowledge and skills to complete them. Learning tasks should be designed to be challenging but achievable and they should be progressive in difficulty.

2. Supportive information: Supportive information is provided to help learners bridge the gap between their prior knowledge and the learning tasks. Supportive information can include definitions, examples, explanations and demonstrations.

3. Procedural information: Procedural information is provided to help learners learn how to perform specific tasks. Procedural information can include step-by-step instructions, checklists and troubleshooting guides.

4. Part-task practice: Part-task practice is provided to help learners master specific skills before they attempt to complete the entire learning task. This type of practice can help learners to master the skills that they need in order to complete the learning task. Part-task practice should be followed by whole-task practice, in which learners practice the entire learning task.

The 4C/ID model has several advantages. First, it is effective for developing complex learning skills. Second, it allows learners to practice skills in a safe environment. Third, it can help learners transfer their learning to new and unfamiliar situations.

However, the 4C/ID model also has some disadvantages. First, it can be complex and time-consuming to create the necessary materials, particularly supportive and procedural information. Second, it requires expert instructional design support. Third, it can be difficult to create authentic learning environments.

Discussion of the models.

These models contain the same 5 steps although put different levels of priority upon those steps. Each of the steps are important to a successful learning episode and the educator should know how to perform all the steps. In any individual learning episode there may only be time and resources to achieve one of these steps.

- Understand the learners. The first step in the teaching and assessment process is to reflect on the learners. This involves understanding the learners' needs, skills and prior knowledge, as well as their motivations and interests.
- Understand the content. Once you understand your learners, you need to understand the content that you need to teach. What are the objectives of the learning? What are the key concepts that need to be covered?
- Write a summary of the key steps. This includes the learning objectives using SMART criteria and a testing approach that will provide evidence of learning. Writing down what needs to be achieved keeps the aims clear during the learning episode.
- Prepare the learning environment. This involves providing context, feedback and strategies to engage the learners in the process. The context should be relevant to the learners' lives and interests. The feedback should be timely and specific. The strategies should be designed to keep the learners engaged and motivated.
- Assess the effectiveness of learning. This involves assessing the learners' progress during and after the learning episode against a variety of methods, including tests, surveys and learner responses. The assessments should be used to identify areas where the learners need additional support and to adjust the teaching and assessment process as needed.

The models identify the need to prepare by reflecting on and understanding the fit between, the learners and the content. There are times when the learners have little chance of learning the material or equally that they are already in advance of what is being taught. The advantage of this reflection is to prepare the educator properly for the challenge.

Writing down a summary of the important steps in the teaching and assessment process provides a simple guide for the educator to follow in the learning episode. This ensures that the process goes smoothly and each of the tasks is completed. Many educators leave the assessment of learning to the end however this misses opportunities to improve the learning episode.

Conclusions.

Overall, instructional design models in medical education provide a systematic approach to creating effective learning experiences. Each model has its own strengths and weaknesses and the choice of model depends on the specific needs and goals of the learning experience. The models do not add anything new but they provide a system for constructing the learning experience. This ensures that the educator does not miss any steps whatever their preferred design style.

The ADDIE model is versatile and easy to understand, but it can be time-consuming and expensive. The Dick and Carey Model is comprehensive and systematic, but it may not be flexible enough for complex learning objectives. Mager's ISD Model is simple and focused on performance, but it may not be suitable for all types of learning.

Gagne's Nine Events of Instruction covers all important steps in the learning process, but it requires good timing and planning. The SAM Model is learner-centered and adaptable, but it may be more time-consuming and require a high level of expertise. The Backward Design Model focuses on desired results but may lead to a narrow focus on testable outcomes.

Ideally educators should choose the instructional design model that best fits their specific context and learning goals. In practice educators will prefer a specific design model based on their own style of teaching. Educators should be aware of the weaknesses with their preferred style of teaching so they can make adjustments.

Top tips.

Choose an instructional design model that aligns with the specific needs and goals of the learning experience and use it to plan the learning.

Use the educator's preferred instructional design model to plan the same learning experience and compare the two approaches.

Identify what is different between the two approaches and create a plan to incorporate the missing element when using preferred ID.

Chapter 6: ASSESSMENT AND EVALUATION IN MEDICAL EDUCATION

Assessment and evaluation are essential components of medical education. They are used to measure student learning, identify areas of weakness and provide feedback to students on their progress. Assessment and evaluation can also be used to improve the quality of medical education programs. As well as these formative functions they have the summative function of ensuring that graduates are competent to practice medicine.

Assessment works best when it is planned in conjunction with the learning materials. The assessment will adapt to the learning materials and vice versa. This ensures that there is good alignment and the key elements are emphasised. The educator will then decide whether the assessment should be formative or summative.

The purpose of most assessment is to provide formative feedback so is performed during the teaching experience. The students are assessed as they are learning using rough and ready approaches. These low-cost methods are not as accurate but are not pass fail. The students can then see how their performance is progressing and where they still need to learn.

Where the assessment is complex and requires formal delivery to be effective then it should be used for summative assessment. The additional costs in time and money mean that it can only be used sparingly and must be reserved for special purposes. This risks that type of assessment being unfamiliar to the student and less reliable.

There is increasing use of blended approaches such as continuing assessment where the students have hundreds of summative assessments during their course. This has substantial negative effects on the students who report high levels of anxiety. Having each piece of work count to the overall mark also inhibits the student from using a variety of learning methods.

Educators should be mindful of these negative consequences and alert to students with disabilities. There are a few students who will become unwell if they are subjected to continuing assessment. Continuing assessment is an artificial construct and against many educational principles. Reasonable adjustments would include using alternative assessment methods for disabled students.

Types of Assessment and Evaluation

There are many different types of assessment and evaluation methods that can be used in medical education. Some common methods include:

- Written examinations: Written examinations are a common way to assess student knowledge. They can be used to measure student understanding of basic concepts, as well as their ability to apply knowledge to real-world situations. They can be used to assess knowledge, skills and attitudes.

- Multiple-choice tests are a common type of assessment that can be used to measure students' knowledge of a particular topic.

- Clinical examinations: Clinical examinations are used to assess student skills in patient assessment and management by direct observation. They can be conducted in a simulated clinical setting, or in a real-world clinical setting. These tests are used to assess student skills in history taking, physical examination and diagnosis.

- Simulations: Simulations are used to create realistic learning experiences for students and to assess skills when performing clinical procedures. They can be used to assess students' knowledge, skills and attitudes in a safe environment.

- Portfolios: Portfolios are collections of student work that demonstrate their learning over time. Portfolios can include written assignments, clinical reports and other evidence of student learning.

- 360-degree feedback: This feedback is gathered from a variety of sources, such as faculty, peers and patients, to assess student performance.

The choice of assessment and evaluation methods will vary depending on the specific learning objectives of the medical education program. Although a wide range of methods will be required during the course the educator will have to choose one for any learning experience. Generally the cheapest and simplest is the likely to be the best.

Assessment and evaluation should be used to improve the quality of medical education. They can be used to identify areas where students need additional support and to make changes to the curriculum or teaching methods. Assessment and evaluation can also be used to track student progress over time and to ensure that students are meeting the learning objectives of the program.

The purpose of assessment in medicine is to help students to develop their skills and understanding. The feedback should be formative that is to support students rather than summative which is to check progress. Students should feel that they have control over the assessment process and have access to additional assessments as required.

Summative assessment is to check that students have reached the required level of performance. In an ideal system the results would already be known before the students sat the tests. The students who were going to fail would have received remedial teaching and had their problems diagnosed. It would be a carrot rather than a stick as it would offer a chance to gain a merit rather than the risk of failing.

Benefits of Assessment

All of the benefits of assessment can be achieved through formative assessment. The costs of assessment can be reduced by using formative assessment. The greater the delay between learning and assessment the less effective that assessment is. Educators should advocate for systems of assessment that increase the benefits and decrease the burden of assessment.

Here are some of the benefits of using assessment and evaluation in medical education:

- Improved student learning: Assessment and evaluation can help students to learn more effectively. When students know that they will be assessed, they are more likely to study and prepare for the assessment. This can lead to deeper understanding of the material.

- Identification of areas of weakness: Assessment and evaluation can help to identify areas where students need additional support. This information can be used to provide students with the help they need to succeed.

- Improved teaching: Assessment and evaluation can help to improve the quality of teaching. When teachers know how their students are performing, they can make changes to their teaching methods to better meet the needs of their students.

- Improved patient care: Assessment and evaluation can help to ensure that medical graduates are competent to practice medicine. By identifying areas where students need additional support and by providing them with the help they need, we can help to ensure that they are able to provide safe and effective care to their patients.

Where an assessment system is failing to deliver for students the educator must advocate for a better system. This means that they should highlight the problems with the system for instance poor student mental health and restricted learning. They should also provide solutions such as increased formative assessment.

Burdens of assessment.

The main burdens of assessment are as a direct result of using summative rather than formative assessments. Summative assessment is by its nature unwieldly, inflexible and wasteful of resources. The need to be rigorous means that previously used assessments cannot be reused. Students can be distracted from their learning by the need to learn for the test.

- Cost: Assessments can be expensive to develop, administer and score. The cost of assessments can be a burden on schools and districts, especially those with limited resources.

- Time: Assessments can take a significant amount of time to develop, administer and score. This can be a burden on teachers, who are already under pressure to cover a lot of material in a short amount of time.

- Impact on student learning: Assessments can have a negative impact on student learning if they are not well-designed or if they are used in a way that is not aligned with the curriculum. When students are constantly being assessed, they may feel stressed and anxious, which can make it difficult for them to learn.

- Teaching to the test. There is a risk that educators and students will focus on passing the assessment rather than learning the material. If the assessments are too narrow in scope or designed to reward memorisation.

- Adjustments for student learning styles and preferences: Not all students learn in the same way. Some students learn best by reading, while others learn best by doing. Assessments should be designed to be fair to all students, regardless of their learning style or preference.

- Time taken to return results: Students and parents need to know how they are doing in order to make informed decisions about their education. Assessment results should be returned in a timely manner so that students and parents can use them to make the best decisions for their future.

The balance between summative and formative assessments should be 10% to 90%. Summative assessments should be used solely as a confirmation of what the educator already knows. This means that for many students the number of formative assessments will increase. Used correctly formative assessments improve student confidence and engagement.

Principles.

Assessment and evaluation in medical education is a complex and challenging process. However, by carefully considering the principles of validity, reliability, fairness and feasibility, educators can develop assessment methods that will help to ensure that students are prepared to practice medicine.

Even when using informal formative assessments it is important to ensure that the assessments are measuring something real. Students need to have confidence in the results of the assessment even if they are not being used to measure performance. Students have a right to good quality feedback and educators must ensure that they explain if the assessment has limitations.

- Validity is the extent to which an assessment measures what it is intended to measure. For example, a multiple-choice test that asks students to identify the symptoms of a particular disease should be valid if it is designed to measure students' knowledge of the disease.

- Reliability is the extent to which an assessment produces consistent results over time. For example, if a student takes a multiple-choice test on the same topic twice, they should score similarly on both tests if the test is reliable.

- Fairness is the extent to which an assessment does not disadvantage any particular group of students. For example, an assessment that is written in a language that is not the native language of some students is not fair to those students.

- Feasibility is the extent to which an assessment can be implemented in a practical and efficient manner. For example, an assessment that requires students to complete a long research project may not be feasible if students do not have the time or resources to complete the project.

Educators will often have to use assessment methods that have weaknesses. A test that provides rapid results may not be as fair or reliable as a longer test. Using the best test means compromising on one of the principles. Transparency is key to this approach as the students can use what they understand.

Building assessments into learning experiences can ensure that students have prompt authentic feedback. The educator can monitor the student's progress and provide additional help to those who are struggling. The students can direct their learning to deal with weaknesses identified by the assessments.

Developing effective assessment methods:

When creating a learning experience the educator will have ideas about how to assess that experience. They can choose the type of assessment that they will use but then need to develop an effective method. Any pre-prepared assessments will be too general and making up new assessments is time consuming.

By adapting pre-prepared assessments or developing assessments from the learning materials the educator can create an effective assessment. The first step is consider what is wrong with the materials, whether they test the material and whether the principles are achieved. This diagnosis indicates what needs to be done to develop the method.

The steps below outline the different approaches that the educator can take to improve existing materials. The correct steps can be determined by the diagnosis so an educator will not need to use all the steps in every case. For instance, an assessment that has poor student approval could benefit from student involvement.

- Alignment: The assessment should be aligned with the learning objectives and provide useful information on the student's progress in the skills and knowledge that were taught.
- Varied methods: Different assessment methods can measure different things. Choose assessment methods that give a comprehensive view of the materials for instance including skills and knowledge.
- Feedback: Consider how the performance on the assessment can be used to provide feedback. Provide the results of the assessment in a way that is relevant to the student's goals.
- Improve teaching: Consider whether the assessment can provide feedback about the quality of the teaching. For instance, if all students have poor performance in an area then it may be better to change the learning experience.
- Professional development: Where assessment methods fail to provide good feedback or identify weaknesses the educator may consider learning more about assessment methods. New ideas may help the educator to develop better assessments.
- Student involvement. Students can give an alternative insight into the strengths and weaknesses of the assessments. For instance, students can help the educator create processes which are fair to those with disability.
- Multiple assessments: It is better to develop several different assessment approaches to a difficult learning experience. The

68

educator can then experiment with these methods and find the best approach.

- Resources and time: The development of assessment methods takes time and money. Focus available resources on key areas of where students need the most feedback.
- LLM collaboration: Use LLMs to collaborate when developing assessments. Use prompts to check for weakness and give feedback. For instance, using LLMs to answer MCQ questions.

These steps can help develop better formative assessments and allow them to be integrated into the learning experience. The creation of teaching materials and the associated formative assessments are an ongoing process. The educator should be continuously developing parts of their teaching materials.

They can react to the experiences in the teaching session or work on developing neglected areas of their teaching materials. The educator must prioritise those aspects of their teaching that do not go well but can also work out why things go well.

Ideally all educators would share their teaching materials but in reality it can be difficult to find these. The university should collate all the materials that their educators produce but again this does not always happen. Some educators choose to share their learning materials online but many are prevented from doing so. There is a gap in the market for an entrepreneur to disrupt.

Think like an AI.

The theory of tokens is a way of thinking about how AI works. AI models are designed to have a large number of tokens, which are essentially small pieces of information. Each token represents a concept but is also the relationship between other concepts. This is why AI can get confused if two concepts have more than one relationship.

Using the theory of tokens can help educators to create more effective assessments. Assessments test the meaning of tokens, the usual relationships and the exceptions to rules. Educators can assess students' understanding of the material by creating tests that focus on tokens. The tokens can be drawn as a mind map and used to monitor progress.

The educator can work with AI to generate the list of tokens in their topic or provide the AI with the list. AI can then be used to generate assessments based on a list of tokens that it is given. By providing questions that have previously been used AI can recognise the structure of the questions required and generate new questions using the same structure.

The complexity of the relationships between tokens increases and then reduces as the number of tokens increases. For instance it is difficult to diagnose a disease from two or three symptoms but it is usually easy with 5. This means that questions designed for inexperienced can be made more difficult and suitable for experienced students simply by removing tokens.

1. Identify the tokens. The first step is to identify the tokens that are relevant to the topic being tested. This can be done by brainstorming a list of concepts and facts that are related to the topic.

2. Create test questions. Once the tokens have been identified, the educator can create test questions that require the student to demonstrate their understanding of the tokens. The questions can be of various types, such as multiple choice, fill-in-the-blank, or short answer.

3. Use the model to generate test questions. If the educator has access to a large language model, they can use the model to generate test questions automatically. The model can be trained on a dataset of medical texts and it can then be used to generate questions that are relevant to the topic being tested.

4. Ask the model to answer the questions. If the question is good the model will be able to provide an answer that is unique.

5. Add or remove tokens from the question. This will vary the difficultly of the question and help improve weak questions.

Learning to use AI in this way takes time and practice. At present the assessment methods that LLMs can generate are limited to test questions based upon the tokens. It is likely that emergent properties in the future will include other assessment methods and broaden LLM's usefulness. Using the model to answer questions is a simple step that all educators can use now.

By leveraging the theory of tokens, educators can create assessments that focus on fundamental concepts, their meanings, interactions and exceptions. This approach encourages students to engage with the material at a deeper level, promotes critical thinking and facilitates a comprehensive understanding of the subject matter.

Conclusions.

Assessment and evaluation play crucial roles in medical education. They not only measure student learning and identify areas of improvement but also ensure that graduates are competent to practice medicine. Various methods can be employed for assessment and evaluation, including written examinations, clinical examinations, simulations, portfolios and 360-degree feedback. It is important to use a variety of methods to obtain a comprehensive understanding of student learning.

The benefits of using assessment and evaluation in medical education are numerous. They contribute to improved student learning, help identify areas of weakness, enhance teaching quality and ultimately improve patient care. However, there are also burdens associated with assessment, such as cost, time constraints, potential negative impact on student learning and the risk of focusing on "teaching to the test." These burdens need to be addressed and mitigated for effective assessment and evaluation.

Principles such as validity, reliability, fairness and feasibility should guide the development of assessment methods. Assessments should align with learning objectives, employ a variety of methods, provide feedback to students and inform teaching and learning strategies. Involving students in the assessment process and ensuring access to practice materials and clear syllabi are also important. Leveraging technology can assist in creating high-quality assessments, such as checking the clarity of multiple-choice questions.

Thinking like an AI, the theory of tokens can be applied to develop more effective assessments. By identifying relevant tokens (concepts) and designing test questions around them, educators can assess students' understanding comprehensively. AI models can be utilised to generate test questions based on token lists and the models answers can be used for quality control.

In conclusion, assessment and evaluation are vital for medical education. By employing diverse methods, adhering to principles and leveraging the theory of tokens, educators can create assessments that promote deep understanding, critical thinking and improved learning outcomes in medical students.

Top tips.

Integrate assessment. Formative assessment should be included into the learning experience to provide feedback and adapting the teaching.

Improve assessment. Use a range of steps to develop better assessments that are able to deliver the advantages without the burdens.

Tokens. Apply the theory of tokens to create more effective assessments by focusing on fundamental concepts, their meanings, interactions and exceptions.

Chapter 7:DESIGNING MULTIPLE-CHOICE QUESTIONS (MCQS)

Designing Multiple-Choice Questions (MCQs) requires careful consideration of various factors to ensure their effectiveness and fairness. It is technically demanding and costly to create good quality MCQs. Many educators rely upon others to create them or reuse previous MCQ papers.

Learning how to create and adapt MCQs is important for all educators as it improves the educator's ability to choose appropriate MCQs. Understanding how the technology works means that when an MCQ is inappropriate it can be adapted. This is particularly important when creating MCQs for formative assessment. Irrelevant or inappropriate difficulty questions can be distracting.

In formative assessment there should be no more than 3 MCQs. This is to prevent overload, decrease the time spent upon the questions and the cost of creating them. The educator can ensure that they are relevant to the material, act as a reminder to the learning and can be achieved by most students.

The importance of making the questions easy cannot be overstated. The students need to be able to answer the questions based upon the learning experience they have had. If they fail then either the learning experience has failed or the questions were badly created. Avoid the temptation to show off by asking a 'clever' or 'trick' question.

General advice for creating MCQs.

There are some basic rules for creating MCQs that are sufficient to create formative assessment MCQs. The rules are somewhat rigid but are reliable and easy to use. The pilot testing can be with LLMs rather than students. Perfecting MCQs takes several times longer than writing the initial draft and is rarely necessary.

> 1. Start with a clear and concise question stem: The stem should state the problem or issue without any extraneous information.
>
> 2. Write plausible distractors: Create incorrect answer options that could be chosen by students who do not know the correct answer. Ensure the distractors are grammatically correct and consistent with the topic.

3. Maintain a single correct answer: Each question should have only one correct answer that best solves the problem or answers the question.

4. Avoid giving away the answer in the question stem: The question stem should not contain clues or hints that give away the answer.

5. Vary the length of distractors: Distractors should have varying lengths to make it challenging for students to guess the correct answer by eliminating the obviously incorrect options.

6. Avoid using "all of the above" and "none of the above" as distractors: These options can be too easy to eliminate and may lead to guessing.

7. Pilot test your questions: Test your MCQs with a small group of students to identify any issues and ensure the questions are appropriately challenging.

8. Use a variety of question types: Incorporate different question types, such as factual, conceptual, application, problem-solving, or critical thinking questions. This variety will assess different learning outcomes and engage students.

9. Consider different levels of difficulty: Include questions of varying difficulty levels to accommodate students with different levels of understanding.

10. Utilise a variety of formats: MCQs can be presented in different formats like traditional multiple-choice, fill-in-the-blank, or extended matching formats. Using diverse formats helps maintain student engagement.

11. Align questions with learning objectives: Ensure that the questions align with the learning objectives of the course or assessment.

12. Revise based on feedback: Incorporate feedback from the pre-test and make necessary revisions to improve the clarity and effectiveness of the questions.

Educators should avoid trying to write multiple MCQs, one MCQ that is aligned and relevant is better than a number that are not. The aim of formative MCQs is to check understanding of the material and reinforce the learning. The summative MCQs are designed to separate the better students from the weaker student.

One straightforward MCQ can provide comprehensive information about the student's understanding and feedback to the students about their learning. The process of creating an MCQ is a useful way of learning about the structure of MCQs.

Analysing the structure of MCQs.

MCQs are highly structured so being able to analyse their structure can identify strong and weak questions. The question gives some pieces of information in the question stub and these provide a pattern. The student should be able to recognise the pattern based on the information and exclude other patterns.

Pattern recognition is easier with more information so the educator can make a question more challenging by removing some of the information or easier by adding information. This way of calibrating a question for different student abilities allows the same question to be used in different situations.

There should be enough information in the stub for the student to be able to propose an answer without reading the answers. This allows the student who understands the material to have the feeling of recognition when they see the answers. This feeling ensures that the MCQ does not interfere with the student's memory.

Many educators prefer questions were the student selects the single incorrect answer rather than the single correct answer. This is because the good student can identify each of the right answers using the feeling of recognition. It encourages students to read all the answers rather than pick an answer that looks right.

Medical MCQs are often phrased as clinical questions to make them more engaging. The question itself is surrounded by extraneous information to create a clinical vignette. Some consider that additional clinical information should create a separate pattern to get to the same answer.

Having two separate patterns pointing to the same answer has some disadvantages, some students will use one and others the alternative. This means that different students are tested on different knowledge. Also some students who know the correct answer will chose the wrong answer because they are distracted by the second pattern.

The relevance of the question to the topic may be unclear if it does not include relevant keywords. Often it is possible to improve the relevance of a borderline question by including distractors that are relevant. This indicates that the condition discussed is a differential of the conditions in the topic.

Questions that are worded in a way that changes their usual meaning are considered to be trick questions. Some examiners argue that they are fair as the students should be aware of the tricks and that they have to make the questions harder to identify the best candidates.

It is better to provide clues that need to be interpreted, such as test results or specific phrases than using tricks. This can get around the problem that the more information that is given makes the questions easier. Clues are in effect mini questions within the questions that need solving before the answer becomes clear.

Educators should avoid the use of trick questions although may decide to run a session on how to answer them. MCQs are simple to mark so they will be used in situations where other methods would be better. Educators have a duty to ensure that the assessment is fair for all students.

There are three types of MCQ in common use in medical assessment, meaning questions, pattern questions and exceptional questions.

Key tips for analysing MCQs.

It is possible to answer many multiple choice questions without any knowledge of the subject. The educator should analyse any MCQ for structures that give away the answer. The clues in an ideal MCQ would be solely in the information given and not the structure.

Each question should be considered to determine its suitability for the specific situation that it is being used. It is not a good idea to select a group of questions in one topic and use these. The reason is that the value of MCQs is that they look carefully at a narrow area.

It is better to create a new MCQ that addresses the precise learning issue but has flaws than use a perfect MCQ that misses the issue. It is possible to use LLMs to analyse an MCQ using these questions as a prompt. Although the answers have variable quality they can give the educator some ideas about whether to use the MCQ.

- Identify the key words in the stem. The key words are the words that provide the most important information about the question.

- Identify the clues. What information is provided about the units of measurement, the number of significant figures and the type of answer that is expected?

- Identify the pattern in the answer choices. The pattern is the way in which the answer choices are related to each other.

- Determine the level of difficulty of the question. The level of difficulty can be determined by the amount of information provided in the stem and the complexity of the pattern.

- Determine the relevance of the question. The question should be relevant to the material that is being assessed.

- Determine the fairness of the question. The question should be fair to all students. All students should have an equal opportunity to answer the question correctly.

MCQs are seen as the easiest way to provide assessment, they can be given to students with minimal work. Educators should resist this approach and consider each MCQ to determine if is relevant. They should create their own MCQ if none are suitable. They should analyse the MCQ to determine whether adaptions should be made.

Formative assessment can include reused MCQs and this reduces the amount of work required in subsequent years. Using MCQs to support learning rather than as a formal test means that students will not bother learning the answers and giving them to the year below. Some educators will present the MCQs at the beginning and end of the session as feedback on learning.

Meaning questions.

Meaning questions are typically used to assess a student's knowledge of the definitions of terms or concepts. They can be written in a variety of ways, but they typically involve asking the student to identify the correct definition for a given term or concept. They can be recognised because they explicitly state the subject of the question.

Many MCQ questions rely upon the student's knowledge of the meaning of a word or phrase. This is reasonable for core knowledge but is not a good way of assessing more esoteric aspects of the topic. It is rarely necessary for a student to remember specific details about facts that they are not likely to use.

In medicine students are expected to remember a large number of facts about a particular disease. These facts are organised into areas such as symptoms, signs, diagnosis, investigations, treatment, prognosis etc. Meaning questions are simple tests of whether the student remembers all the facts about that disease in that area.

Meaning questions have the advantage of being simple to create as they start from the disease and then ask the student to consider a list of features set out in the answer. The format can be made more interesting by adding extraneous clinical details or starting from a unique feature.

Few diseases have unique features that are not present or rarely present in other diseases. When these features are present they be used can reverse the question by asking the student to recognise that the meaning of that feature is the disease in question. One variant is of this is 'which is the most common cause of ...' type of question.

These types of questions can be effective in assessing a student's knowledge of a particular disease, but they are not the only way to assess a student's knowledge. Other types of questions, such as those that require the student to apply their knowledge to a new situation, can be more effective in assessing a student's understanding of the material.

Meaning type questions can be generated by AI using the prompt 'list 6 features of the following...' The educator then can remove two of the features and replace one of them with an incorrect answer. Then change the question to 'which of these is not a feature of...' where the incorrect answer is the right choice.

To create the alternative type where the correct answer is the right choice, change the subject of the question. For example the MCQ could be generated on symptoms of a heart attack and then the subject changed to pulmonary embolism.

Recognising the pattern.

Pattern questions test the student's ability to recognise patterns in data (not the structure of the question). The question stem will provide a set of data and the student will be asked to identify the pattern that is present.

Medical knowledge contains many patterns that the student should recognise in order to make a diagnosis, recognise a risk or understand a clinical process. These patterns are more difficult to turn into a MCQ because it may be easy to guess the answer. The student may be using patterns that the educator had not intended.

The key problem with using an MCQ for diagnosis type questions is that the answer is provided. This means that even if the student does not have all the knowledge they can work back from the answers to find the correct answer. Short notes type of questions can be better tests of this type of knowledge.

Where this type of MCQ excels in asking the student to differentiate between several different diagnoses which have similar presentations. Extended matching questions are one example of this approach. The student needs to identify the clue that makes one diagnosis more likely than the other. This means hiding the clue in a description that could apply to any on the list.

There are ways of making this type of question more complex for instance by making it a two-step problem. Giving a list of findings and asking what treatment should be given or what other feature might be present. The risk is that the student will simply guess the answer rather than work out the diagnosis.

This type of MCQ is more popular and engaging than asking about the meaning of a word of phrase because it is closer to real world problem solving. The educator can use their own experiences of clinical difficulties to provide subject matter. The best questions ask about real clinical dilemmas.

Exceptions to rules.

Exceptional questions test the student's knowledge of exceptions to general rules. The student is tested on their understanding of the limits of rules in medicine. The question stem may provide a general rule but often the rule will be implicit.

There are many implicit rules in medicine and students need to know when they do not apply. This can be due to safety issues, for instance a drug may be generally safe but not in pregnancy. There may be disease that can be missed easily because it has non-specific symptoms so it not considered in the differential.

This type of MCQ is often neglected because exceptions are by their nature exceptional. The educator wishes the student to learn the general rules and this may be more important than learning exceptions. It is however possible to create questions on exceptions that reinforce the rules.

One area that exceptional MCQs are used is when dealing with normal variants. The general rule is that this type of symptom is serious however this variant is normal and the patient can be reassured. Normal variants can be overlooked in conventional teaching if they are easily differentiated from more serious problems.

Exceptional MCQs are the most difficult to generate using AI as the educator needs to know about the exception to create the prompt. For this reason, it is better to use experience from outpatient clinics looking for common errors. These real-life examples of the difficulties can provide more compelling learning than invented questions.

Conclusions.

As an educator it is best to see the MCQ as a quick method of creating a formative assessment. This means that the educator can create simple MCQ questions testing knowledge of meaning and pattern recognition. As the students' knowledge progresses exceptional questions can be included to stretch their understanding and ability to analyse the data.

Designing effective and fair multiple-choice questions (MCQs) requires a thoughtful approach that considers various factors. By following the general advice for creating MCQs, educators can ensure that the questions are clear, challenging and aligned with learning objectives. Varying the question types and difficulty levels accommodates different student abilities and engages learners effectively.

Follow general advice for MCQ creation: Start with a clear and concise stem, create plausible distractors, maintain a single correct answer, avoid giving away the answer in the stem, vary distractor lengths, avoid using "all of the above" and "none of the above," pilot test and pre-test questions, use a variety of question types and formats, align questions with learning objectives and revise based on feedback.

When analysing the structure of MCQs, educators can calibrate questions for different levels of difficulty by adjusting the amount of information provided. It is essential to avoid using trick questions and instead focus on providing clues that require interpretation, fostering critical thinking skills in students.

In the medical context, using clinical vignettes can make MCQs more engaging. However, educators should be cautious about providing multiple patterns leading to the same answer to avoid confusion among students.

In assessing knowledge, meaning questions can be used to test core knowledge, while pattern recognition questions can challenge students to identify patterns in data and differentiate between similar diagnoses. Exceptional questions can be valuable for testing students' understanding of exceptions to general rules.

Throughout the process, educators should ensure the relevance and fairness of the questions, allowing all students to have an equal opportunity to answer correctly. By incorporating these key principles into MCQ design, educators can create valuable assessment tools that enhance students' learning experiences. Remember, the MCQ is best utilised as a tool for quick knowledge checks during early learning phases and as students progress, more complex and engaging question types can be incorporated to stretch their understanding and analytical abilities.

Top tips.

Use MCQs to check whether the student understands the meaning of words and recognises patterns but do not use it when the student is making judgements.

When creating MCQs start with a list of concepts that you wish to test and consider whether each concept is suitable for an MCQ.

AI testing of MCQs can lead to more comprehensive and insightful feedback than testing on students because the AI will give reasons for the choice.

Chapter 8: PORTFOLIO-BASED EVIDENCE

Portfolio-based evidence is a type of assessment that allows learners to demonstrate their learning in a variety of ways. It is a more holistic approach to assessment than traditional tests and exams, as it allows learners to show what they know and can do in a variety of contexts. Needing a range of skills makes creating a portfolio is more challenging.

The decision to include a portfolio in a medical education course is likely to encounter resistance. The faculty will be concerned about the workload and that it will take the students attention from other more pressing topics. The university will be concerned about the costs associated with running the portfolio and marking the work. The students will be concerned that it demands skills that they have not learned.

The portfolio approach is most effective when it is used to show that a student has had the correct experience on an attachment. In practice students are asked to get specific tasks signed off rather than provide evidence. Similarly the dissertation is often adapted to include evidence collected by the student during their studies.

Leaving portfolios out of the medical training has three main negative consequences. First the students lack the management skills that they will require when they are involved in service development tasks. Second those students that have practical experiences have no way of sharing them and the advantages of their diversity is not recognised. Third the students lack the confidence to tackle tasks that involve the same skills such as teaching, leadership and politics.

There are ways of including portfolio type activities within other learning episodes. Even if an educator decides never to formally use this teaching technique they can create tasks that build the relevant skills. For instance, ask a group of students to make a list of evidence that they could use to show a skill or to bring in artifacts in a show and tell. Discussing a practice rubric can help students understand what would be required of them if they were to create a portfolio.

What is a portfolio?

Portfolio-based evidence is a type of assessment that requires students to collect and present evidence of their learning. The portfolio also needs to be organised and reflections need to be included. For many students the amount of work needed to collect evidence can take most of their effort.

The types of evidence are complex and may require repeated attempts to gather a good example. A piece of written work is not likely to be sufficient unless further re-writes are undertaken. This disadvantages those who are weak in writing because they struggle to produce one piece of work. Asking them to produce several pieces of work is overwhelming.

The organisation of a portfolio can be outside of some student's skill sets. They may struggle to work out the connections between different pieces of evidence. This can make the portfolio untidy and disordered reducing the value of the work that they have done.

This evidence can take many forms, such as:

- Written work: This can include essays, reports, research papers, lab reports, or other types of written assignments. Written work can be a good way to assess students' knowledge, understanding and ability to communicate their ideas.

- Presentations: Presentations can be a good way to assess students' ability to communicate their ideas to an audience. Presentations can be given in a variety of formats, such as oral presentations, poster presentations, or video presentations. They can help students share learning experiences.

- Artifacts: Artifacts can include a variety of items, such as videos, photographs, drawings, models, or other creative work. Artifacts can be a good way to assess students' creativity, problem-solving skills and ability to apply their knowledge in a real-world context.

- Performances: Performances can include observed clinical skills, procedures and tests. Performances can be a good way to assess students' ability to apply their knowledge and skills in a real-world setting.

- Self-reflections: Self-reflections can be a good way for students to assess their own learning and progress. Self-reflections can be written essays, journals, or other types of reflective writing.

There are several social elements of a portfolio such as presentations and performances. The evidence required may depend on the student approaching an individual for feedback. The student may find these elements more challenging and struggle to complete the portfolio despite initially good progress.

Rubrics can be an effective tool to improve student performance in creating a portfolio. They can refer to the marking schedule and FAQ sections for ideas. The lists of what will and wont be included can help students who struggle with understanding the instructions.

Advantages of portfolios

Portfolio-based evidence is a valuable tool for assessing student learning. It can help students to demonstrate their learning in a variety of ways, reflect on their progress and develop important skills. This list can be used as a discussion point with students who want to try portfolio learning.

The students may recognise that they have knowledge or skills gaps and need to prepare for portfolio learning. They may feel uncertain about the learning methods, their ability to be holistic, self-assessment, self-directed learning and gathering evidence in a workplace.

- Varied learning methods: Portfolios allow students to demonstrate their learning in a variety of ways. This can help to ensure that students are not only learning the content, but also developing the skills and abilities that they need to be successful.
- Holistic evidence of student learning: Portfolios can provide a more comprehensive view of student learning by including a variety of evidence assessing a range of learning outcomes including those difficult to obtain in other ways such as student engagement and motivation. Portfolios give opportunities to show creativity and innovation.
- Self-assessment skills: As students collect and reflect on their work, they learn to identify their strengths and weaknesses. This can help them to engage with the learning objectives, set their goals for learning, track their own progress and encourage a growth mindset.
- Self-directed learning: Portfolio-based evidence provides students with an opportunity to develop their critical thinking, metacognitive and problem-solving skills. As they work on projects and presentations, students learn to recognise their progress, self-regulate and identify problems, gather information and learn to develop their own learning approaches.
- Workplace evidence: For those who are applying their learning to their workplace the portfolio will provide more relevant information for their assessments than the results of tests. For these students the collection of materials for the portfolio can be incorporated into their work patterns saving time and effort.
- Public relations: Portfolios can help students to develop their communication skills to the greater public. As students prepare their portfolios, they must learn to communicate their ideas clearly and effectively. Their portfolios can be used to showcase their work in a form that others can access.

The complexity of a portfolio means that many students will struggle with the organisation needed. The performance of the best and the worst students can be much broader than other tasks. This can be useful for selection processes which need to differentiate between student's abilities.

Discussing likely problems can ensure that all students have all the necessary skills to create a portfolio prior to starting. Where the students have several gaps the preparation phase may be as long as a year. The educator should avoid starting a portfolio with the hope that the students will have time to learn the skills afterwards.

Challenges with portfolios.

There are a few challenges associated with using portfolio-based evidence which need addressing before the technique is selected for a topic. The workload for preparing and running portfolios can be reduced by selecting certain students for this as an additional challenge.

- Many students have never created a portfolio before. This can be a challenge, as they may not know where to start or how to organise their work. It is a skill that takes time and practice to develop. Students may not see the value in learning this skill unless they are explicitly told that it will be useful in the future.
- Not all students will be able to create a portfolio independently. Some students may need one-on-one assistance from an educator to learn the skills of portfolio building. This can add to the cost of portfolio-based assessment and the time needed for students to achieve their targets.
- The types of knowledge and skills that are best shown in a portfolio may not match those that the curriculum requires. Portfolios can be used to assess a wide range of learning outcomes. However, it is important to make sure that the types of evidence that students collect are aligned with the learning objectives. If students collect evidence that does not align with the learning objectives, their portfolio will not be an accurate reflection of their learning.
- Collecting and presenting evidence can be a time-consuming process. Students may spend longer processing the evidence than they do performing the learning activity. This can be a distraction for some students as many have limited time to allocate and can lead to them losing interest in this learning exercise. This is particularly problematic for portfolios which require maintenance over time.
- It can be difficult for educators to assess many portfolios fairly and accurately. Students may fill their portfolios with low-quality

evidence or use tick-box approaches. This can lead to educators taking short cuts and failing to notice those who made extra efforts.

- Portfolio-based evidence can be subjective, particularly if the portfolio has an unclear purpose. It is important for educators to develop clear criteria for assessing portfolios and to provide students with feedback on their work. It is important to develop clear criteria for assessing portfolios and to provide students with feedback on their work.

- The materials that best show the evidence may be confidential or sensitive. This can make it difficult to share portfolios with others, such as parents or employers. It is important to consider the confidentiality of the materials when designing a portfolio. Students may struggle to get feedback on their portfolio from their usual sources.

The educator will therefore have to prepare the students by asking them to collect evidence as a series of specific tasks. This store of evidence then can be collated into a portfolio without need for further collection. In this way the different skills required to collect different pieces of evidence can be addressed separately.

The educator will need to interact with much of the evidence provided by the students. Although the rubric can be used for self-evaluation or peer evaluation the educator will need to check a substantial proportion personally. This involves substantial time allocation to ensure a fair evaluation.

One approach that can be helpful is to get the student to write a short summary piece on each piece of evidence. This list of evidence with a short summary can allow the educator to focus their attention on the most important parts of the portfolio.

Teaching the skills of a portfolio.

Start by explaining the purpose of the portfolio and why a collection of work samples is the best way of demonstrating the learning objectives. Students should be asked to obtain specific pieces of evidence so that they can start with a simple task. When they produce this the process of selecting, organising and presenting should be modelled.

When selecting work samples for a portfolio, it is important to choose samples that are relevant to the learning outcomes and show the best examples of work. This means that the student will have to repeat the task several times to get an ideal example. The student should ensure that they represent a variety of their skills and knowledge with different evidence for the same topics.

Feedback can include asking the students what other evidence would be helpful. Encourage the students to collaborate and work together to organise their portfolios. Once they have selected the samples they need to organise them in a way that makes sense.

Although a physical binder may be useful for collecting objects, printing out materials can lead to a large volume of material to wade through. A digital portfolio has the advantage of being able to attach the evidence as files which the educator can look at as required. Whatever the format there should be a cover page, an introduction and a table of contents.

The addition of a short summary sentence on each piece of evidence is an innovation that can help both student and educator. The student should also write a reflective essay to explain the portfolio as a whole and discuss what they demonstrate about their skills and knowledge. They should also reflect on the learning process and progression as a learner.

Rubric.

A rubric is a scoring guide used to evaluate the quality of student work. It is a set of criteria that are used to assess the work and it provides a way to communicate expectations to students. Rubrics can be used to assess a variety of student work, including essays, projects and presentations.

1. Performance criteria: These are the specific things that the student is expected to do or know. They should be clear, concise and measurable.

2. Rating scale: This is a scale that is used to measure the student's performance against the performance criteria. The scale can be numerical, descriptive, or a combination of both.

3. Indicators: These are qualitive descriptions of what work that meets each level of the rating scale would look like.

Rubrics can be used to assess a variety of different things, including:

- Knowledge: How well does the student understand the material?

- Skills: How well can the student apply the material?

- Attitudes: What is the student's attitude towards the material?

- Performance: How well does the student's overall performance meet the requirements?

Rubrics can be used by teachers, students and parents to:

- Set expectations: Rubrics can help to ensure that everyone knows what is expected of them.

- Provide feedback: Rubrics can be used to provide feedback to students on their work.

- Guide learning: Rubrics can be used to guide students in their learning.

- Assess learning: Rubrics can be used to assess student learning.

A rubric for portfolios is a tool that helps educators assess the quality of student work. It is important to create a comprehensive rubric that includes both criteria that will be included and criteria that will not be included. The rating scale and indicators should be clear and concise and they should include examples of the types of evidence that would be appropriate. The rubric should also include a discussion of the advantages and challenges of that specific portfolio.

It is best practice to include a frequently asked questions (FAQ) section in the rubric so that educators do not have to repeat their advice unnecessarily. The rubric is the most appropriate place to give general feedback on the group's performance. The educator should update the rubric to model the student's portfolio making.

Conclusions.

Portfolio-based evidence is a versatile and effective assessment approach that offers several advantages for both students and educators. It allows students to demonstrate their learning through various formats, promotes holistic assessment, develops self-assessment and self-directed learning skills and provides workplace-relevant evidence. Additionally, portfolios can serve as a means of communication and public relations, showcasing students' work to a wider audience.

However, there are also challenges associated with portfolio-based evidence that need to be addressed. Students may lack experience in creating portfolios and may require guidance and support. Aligning the portfolio content with the learning objectives is crucial to ensure accurate assessment.

The process of collecting and organising evidence can be time-consuming and educators may face difficulties in assessing a large number of portfolios fairly. Subjectivity and the confidentiality of materials are other potential challenges. The rubric can take a long time to write and perfect but can address some of these problems.

Teaching students the skills of portfolio creation involves explaining the purpose and guiding them in selecting, organising and reflecting on their work samples. Rubrics also play a vital role in assessing portfolio quality, providing clear criteria, a rating scale and indicators for evaluation. Rubrics help set expectations, provide feedback, guide learning and assess student progress.

Overall, portfolio-based evidence offers a comprehensive and meaningful approach to assessing student learning. By addressing the challenges and utilising effective teaching strategies and rubrics, educators can harness the full potential of portfolios to support student growth, reflection and skill development beyond simply learning medicine.

Top tips.

Preparation for a portfolio includes practicing evidence collection, matching the evidence with performance and writing reflections.

For educators, selecting specific students for portfolio assessment or incorporating portfolio-type activities in other learning episodes can help manage the workload.

Rubrics play a vital role in guiding students and educators, ensuring alignment with the learning objectives and including examples of appropriate evidence.

Chapter 9: OSCE TYPE CLINICAL ASSESSMENT.

An Objective Structured Clinical Examination (OSCE) is a type of clinical assessment that is used to evaluate a student's clinical skills and knowledge. OSCE stations are typically set up in a simulated clinical environment and students are asked to perform a specific task, such as taking a history, performing a physical exam, or making a diagnosis.

Each station is timed and typically short (5-15 minutes) and students are scored on their performance by a trained examiner. OSCE assessments are designed to be objective and fair and they can be used to assess a wide range of clinical skills. OSCE assessments are also relatively quick and efficient, which makes them a good option for large-scale assessments.

As an educator the most resistance from students will come when they feel that they are not prepared. Most medical students welcome the opportunity to practice OSCE techniques. Students are most eager to practice in the run up to an OSCE examination and the educator can take advantage of this by timing their sessions.

Although creating a complete new clinical scenario is complex and time consuming it is easier to create a large number of informal practice topics. These can be taking a history, performing an examination, reviewing results and explaining a medical issue. The students can then run through many topics in an informal way.

Although the terminology may be foreign for instance 'data gathering, technical and assessment skills, clinical management skills and interpersonal skills' all OSCE examinations test the same areas. These are actually only describing areas of a consultation i.e. history, examination, management, advice etc.

The student needs to be able to choose the correct skills to employ for the scenario they are presented with. It is this need to choose that makes an OSCE difficult, being able to work out what is going on and what is required. In practice a student who is unable to identify cues and change their focus will fail the examination.

This is unnecessary for a teaching episode and the educator should avoid rigid application of the marking schedule. The students should be encouraged to make mistakes and try out different approaches. The purpose of informal OSCEs is to develop the clinical skills as well as pass the formal OSCE.

Running an informal OSCE type session.

OSCEs are a useful learning tool as well as their assessment roles. Students often are keen to learn in this way because the issues are closer to those that they will experience in real life. The educator should avoid strict rules or playing unhelpful patients unless that is the purpose of the scenario.

The students often are highly motivated to learn although may vary on which role they feel comfortable with. By involving them as patients as well as doctors they have the chance to experiment with the format. This flexibility aids learning and should be encouraged with 'that was great but do not do it in a real OSCE'.

1. Choose the right number of students. The ideal number of students is more than 3 because this gives the chance for students to take different roles and rest. There should be less than 7 or each student will not get sufficient time to participate. Where the educator has more than 7 they should break up the group into smaller groups.

2. Prepare the students. Each student should be given a list of topics that they will be the patient for. A 'patient' will start the scenario by describing their situation. The 'doctor' then proceeds as they would in that situation asking questions, examining or explaining.

3. Allow the students to volunteer for the role that they feel comfortable with and allow them to observe if they prefer. Some students will need time to get used to the format of the session and understand what is expected of them.

4. Set the timer. After an appropriate time for the level of the student (typically 15 minutes for preclinical, 10 minutes for clinical and 5 minutes for postgraduate) the student playing the role of the patient gives the answer or hidden detail. Students first starting this exercise are often too self-conscious to absorb more feedback than this.

5. Provide feedback. Where a group request more feedback then they can have an observer who assesses the doctor's skills in their plan of action, their ability to create a rapport and ability to communicate. A good 'doctor' would be organised in their questions and how they work through the material, they would establish and maintain a rapport despite any challenges and would use clear and appropriate explanations.

6. Conclusions. End the session by thanking the students for their active participation, explain that it is good to make mistakes because that helps with learning and encourage them to continue the learning activity with their friends.

Authenticity of the patient profile is of greater importance than accuracy of the clinical scenario. The students need to feel that they are interacting with a real person. They are used to patients getting the medicine wrong or presenting in the wrong way. Students find it harder to work with fake patients because real patients do not behave that way.

The patient template

There are two key documents for a clinical scenario for an OSCE. The patient template and the clinical template. The first is everything about the patient, the second is everything about their current illness. The reason why these are separated is because the patient template can be reused saving time and reducing actor stress.

The key document for a clinical scenario for an OSCE is a patient template containing the full biographical details, all past medical history. The social history should be written out in full and include the family history. The patient template should also have the patient's health beliefs and notes on personality.

The patient template contains the full clinical history and is what a doctor would write if they asked every question and wrote every answer in the patient's own words. As the patient template is the basis of the actor's responses it is essential it is complete. It is challenging to have to add details that have been missed during the testing phase.

Once a patient template is written it can be used to address different learning outcomes. The choice of clinical scenario will depend on the needs of the student and the curriculum. There are many scenarios that are difficult to achieve within the OSCE setting although adjustments can be made. A 'parent' can give a history for a child, findings of an intimate examination can be given on a card.

The clinical template

The clinical template contains the history of presenting complaint or problem in detail, test results, differential diagnoses. The educator should work with the actor to identify the words that the actor would use to describe their problems and the ideas and concerns that the patient would have.

The examination findings should be written on cards unless the actor will simulate them. The responses to management choices and what questions the patient will ask should be included in the template.

To create a clinical template the educator should start with a clinical problem including the diagnosis, the information needed to solve the problem and rule out other illnesses and any psychosocial issues that need to be addressed.

This information can be listed under headings such as data gathering, technical and assessment skills, clinical management skills and interpersonal skills. It can be easier to use the more familiar headings of history, examination, investigations, treatment, referral and advice.

This information can be written in the patient's own words rather than medical language. This makes it easier for the actor to show difficulties with understanding. The scenario itself runs differently each time but following a similar pattern. The educator may wish to identify specific end points which will give rise to responses.

The best OSCEs are puzzles to be solved because the student gets the reward of solving the puzzle even if they do not tick all the boxes. To increase the challenge a clinical dilemma can be included or an ethical choice. The clinical scenario can be changed to include new guidelines or change in medical knowledge.

Running an OSCE station.

The effectiveness of the OSCE station will depend upon the talent of the actor, their understanding and preparation. Sufficient time and practice should be allocated with repeated testing and changes made to address feedback. There is a temptation to fix a case by removing or adding to the patient template however this is artificial and creates further problems.

There are two ways to fix a case that is not working, the first is to change the presentation to a different clinical problem. The same patient will present with different problems, so this is authentic. The second is to use the case for students who are less or more advanced that the group planned.

The marking of an OSCE station is based upon whether the student has completed all the steps. This can be source of debate particularly if the student has used a creative and effective method that did not follow the expected path. Having some flexibility in the marking schedule is against the need for an objective, reliable and valid test.

This problem is solved by giving more time for practice and experiment. There is a phenomenon that although different doctors appear to use very different approaches to the consultation the techniques that they use become closer to each other with experience. They may vary in terms of style but because they are competent they rarely vary significantly in terms of basic skills.

An educator can be patient with students trying different approaches because they will learn what works best. Whilst the educator may have to mark down if the student makes a dangerous or upsetting mistake these are rarer than omitting an important step. Students using creative approaches can be encouraged even if they would not get marks in the formal OSCE. As students advance they will become more reliable in completing necessary steps and will more often achieve desired results.

The educator may feel concerned that a group of students are continuing to use a method that will not get them marks in the OSCE. The educator can discuss with the group which method they think is better and ask questions to clarify the weaknesses of their approach.

It is important not to suggest that the educator is critical of the approach but should describe what they are doing and what the examiners expect in a neutral way. If the educator is unclear why they are using the approach then asking for an explanation can lead to progress.

Creating an OSCE station.

OSCEs need several elements to be successful, this ranges from the two templates (patient and clinical scenarios), training of the actor, identifying clinical actions, marking schedules and testing. These are listed below and apart from the clinical scenarios rely upon the educator's previous skills.

The educator will have written a full history of the patient, helped train in medical matters, identified learning objectives and assessed performance. They will not be familiar with creation of a clinical scenario and should practice this skill. Writing 5-10 clinical scenarios will give the necessary level of experience to have confidence in this skill.

1. Create a detailed template of the patient. This should include the patient's age, gender, medical history, social history and any other relevant information.

2. Train the actor on the template. This will help to ensure that the actor is able to accurately and consistently portray the character they are playing.

3. Choose a clinical scenario for that patient. The scenario should be relevant to the patient's medical history and should be challenging enough to test the student's knowledge and skills.

4. Train the actor on the scenario. This will help to ensure that the actor is able to accurately and consistently portray the scenario.

5. Identify the key steps in the scenario. These are the steps that the student must complete in order to successfully complete the scenario.

6. Test the scenario to calibrate difficulty. This will help to ensure that the scenario is challenging enough to test the student's knowledge and skills, but not so challenging that it is impossible to complete.

7. Mark steps as necessary and desired. This will help to ensure that the student is aware of the steps that they must complete in order to successfully complete the scenario and which are optional.

Once an actor has a detailed template they can play that patient whatever the clinical scenario is decided. This reduces the time taken for an actor to learn the scenario and allows them to provide several scenarios. As each scenario is provided as a series of steps the actor can react more naturally to the student.

The key steps for the clinical scenario should be written as bullet points with each objective and a short description. This allows the actor to quickly identify what is required, look at the description for clarification and avoid extraneous information.

Designing a formal OSCE session.

In any one OSCE session it is important to get a good range of skills. This keeps the interest of the students and provides more challenge than a session just on examination skills. Whether the assessment is formative or summative the formal OSCE process should be followed. The students need to be certain that the feedback and marking is valid.

In contrast with the informal OSCE where the purpose is education the formal OSCE is assessment. The students want to know how good their performance is compared with their peers and the examination pass mark. They need this information to focus their studies on the correct issues and allow them to dedicate the correct amount of time for this task.

- Choose the right clinical skills to assess. Not all clinical skills are created equal. Some skills are more important than others and some skills are more difficult to assess than others. When designing an OSCE assessment, it is important to choose a list of the right clinical skills to assess.

- Create a realistic and challenging environment. The OSCE environment should be as realistic as possible. This will help to ensure that students are able to transfer their skills to the real world. However, the environment should also be challenging. This will help to ensure that students are not able to simply memorise the answers to the questions.
- Create a variety of stations. No one station can assess all of the clinical skills that a student needs to know. When designing an OSCE, it is important to create a variety of stations that assess different clinical skills.
- Use a variety of assessment methods. OSCE assessments can be used to assess a variety of skills, including knowledge, comprehension, application, analysis, synthesis and evaluation. When possible, use a variety of assessment methods to assess each skill.
- Train the examiners. Examiners must be trained to use the scoring rubric and to provide feedback to students. This training is essential to ensure that the assessment is fair and accurate.
- Pilot test the OSCE. It is important to pilot test the OSCE before it is administered to students. This will help to identify any problems with the stations or the scoring rubric.
- Provide feedback to students. Students should be provided with feedback on their performance. This feedback can help students to identify their strengths and weaknesses and to improve their clinical skills. The feedback should be structured to best assist students to improve their performance.

Feedback in OSCEs is more valuable than other examinations where the students can do self-tests. They therefore value clear actionable information from OSCE particularly if this type of assessment is restricted in availability. The feedback should be highly structured with marks and comments.

An example of good feedback is as follows – subject Obs and Gynae, score 38%, comment, the student struggled with knowledge and clinical skills but had good rapport. Subject clinical medicine, score 78%, comment the student had excellent knowledge of the subject and adequate clinical skills and rapport. The student can then focus on both knowledge and clinical skills in Obs and Gynae.

Advantages of using OSCE

The advantages of the OSCE examination are highly dependent upon the skills of the educators who run them. The educators should therefore self-rate their OSCE sessions and ask others to rate them on objectivity, validity, reliability and efficiency and comprehensiveness. Other criteria to consider are artificiality, stress and skill level as these can affect performance.

These rating scores will help the educators to identify problems more rapidly and make the required changes to address them. No OSCE examination will be perfect but having a reasonable idea of the weaknesses will allow adjustments during the examination. If a scenario is known to have a high skill and stress level then a student who is struggling could be offered more help.

Here are some of the advantages of using OSCE type clinical assessment:

- Objectivity: OSCE assessments are designed to be objective and fair. This is because students are assessed on their performance in a standardised setting and they are scored by trained examiners who are using a standardised scoring rubric.

- Validity: OSCE assessments are valid measures of clinical skills. This is because they are designed to assess the same skills that are used in the real world.

- Reliability: OSCE assessments are reliable measures of clinical skills. The stations are standardised as they all use the same criteria. This means that students are likely to receive the same score if they take the same OSCE assessment multiple times.

- Efficiency: OSCE assessments are efficient measures of clinical skills. This is because they can be administered to large groups of students in a relatively short amount of time.

- Comprehensiveness: OSCE assessments are more comprehensive than traditional clinical assessments, as they can assess a wider range of clinical skills. This is because OSCE stations can be designed to assess a variety of skills, such as history taking, physical exam, diagnosis and communication.

The more often students can practice this exam the more likely that they are to develop insight. This is valuable for the student as they can focus their learning efforts but is also useful for the educators who may be unaware of their gaps. Where many students have the same gaps then it may be necessary to put on extra teaching in those areas.

Disadvantages of using OSCE

The first three disadvantages artificiality, stress and skill level are modifiable and therefore should be monitored. They are more sensitive to changes than the other criteria so are a good way of checking for problems. The students will also have strong views which can be easily collected.

Here are some of the disadvantages of using OSCE type clinical assessment:

- Artificiality: OSCE stations can be artificial, as they do not take place in a real-world clinical setting. This can make it difficult for students to transfer their skills to the real world.
- Skill level: OSCE assessments can be more challenging for students who are not yet proficient in the clinical skills being assessed. This is because students are only given a short amount of time to complete each station.

- Stress: OSCE assessments can be stressful for students. This is because they are being evaluated on their performance in a simulated clinical environment.

- Cost: OSCE assessments can be expensive to administer. This is because they require simulated patients (actors) trained examiners, standardised equipment and a simulated clinical environment.

- Time: OSCE assessments can be time-consuming to administer. This is because each student must complete a series of stations and each station is typically timed and has their own examiner.

- Investment: New clinical scenarios are complex to create as they require a standardised scoring rubric, training for the actors and repeated testing. New scenarios are constantly required to ensure that the students do not learn the answers.

The cost, time commitment and investment required can be decreased substantially by separating the patient details from the clinical scenario. They can also be reduced by giving students more access to informal OSCE training. The effectiveness can be increased by improving feedback quality. Using these techniques can overcome the disadvantages of OSCEs.

Conclusions.

In conclusion, the Objective Structured Clinical Examination (OSCE) is a valuable and widely used assessment method for evaluating students' clinical skills and knowledge. OSCE assessments offer several advantages, including objectivity, validity, reliability, efficiency and comprehensiveness. They provide a standardised and fair evaluation of students' performance in a simulated clinical environment. OSCEs are particularly useful for assessing skills such as history taking, physical examination, diagnosis and communication.

However, there are also disadvantages to consider. OSCE assessments can be costly to implement due to the need for trained examiners, simulated patients, standardised equipment and a simulated clinical setting. They can also be time-consuming for both students and examiners. Additionally, the artificiality of the OSCE stations may pose challenges in transferring acquired skills to real-world clinical practice. Furthermore, the creation of new clinical scenarios and ongoing investment in training and testing can be demanding.

To mitigate some of these challenges, educators can conduct informal OSCE sessions for practice and skill development, encouraging students to explore different approaches and learn from their mistakes. It is important to create realistic and challenging environments, use a variety of assessment methods and provide constructive feedback to students to facilitate their learning and improvement.

Despite the limitations, OSCE type clinical assessments remain a valuable tool in medical education, providing a standardised and objective evaluation of students' clinical skills. By understanding the advantages and challenges associated with OSCEs, educators can effectively incorporate this assessment method into their teaching and learning strategies to help prepare future healthcare professionals.

Top tips.

Provide a number of opportunities for informal OSCE sessions where the students are list of topics for roles as patients or doctors.

Create a detailed template for each patient including biographical details, medical and social history and health beliefs so they can be used in multiple clinical scenarios.

Provide structured and actionable feedback to students to help them identify strengths and weaknesses and improve their clinical skills.

Chapter 10: PRECLINICAL EDUCATION.

Preclinical education is the first two years of medical school, during which students learn the basic sciences of medicine that form the foundation of clinical medicine. These subjects include anatomy, physiology, biochemistry, pharmacology and microbiology although each have subdivisions.

In addition to the basic sciences, preclinical education also includes courses in medical ethics, communication and professionalism. These courses help students to develop the skills they need to be effective communicators and to provide compassionate care to their patients.

Understanding of the scientific basis of medicine allows the student to use reasoning and evidence to understand the clinical practice of medicine. Without this basis a doctor will have difficulty with the art of clinical practice.

A doctor who is able to think critically will be able to evaluate the evidence and make the best decision for their patient, even when there is no clear-cut answer. Pattern recognition is easier when the doctor can see the underlying mechanisms of disease.

The pre-clinical curriculum and teaching materials can take years to develop. Much of the course is technical and constantly developing. From an educational point of view there is little novel as lectures are used to deliver the bulk of the material. The practical is an exception to this rule.

The first task of a medical educator is to explain why these subjects are necessary to the student and their future career. Students will only engage fully if they see that it is necessary and useful to do so. The student needs to be able to imagine situations where this knowledge will be called upon.

The medical importance of anatomy.

Anatomy is the study of the structure of the human body. It is a fundamental science that is essential for many healthcare professions, including medicine, nursing, physical therapy and occupational therapy. Anatomy provides the foundation for understanding how the body works and how it can be treated when it is not working properly.

Here are some of the reasons why anatomy is still an important subject:

- Clinical examination: Even in the age of advanced medical imaging, clinical examination is still an essential part of the diagnostic process. A doctor's ability to understand anatomy is essential for making sense of the findings of the new technologies. For example, a doctor who is familiar with the anatomy of the skin can use a dermatoscope to identify skin lesions that may be a sign of cancer.

- 3D imaging: 3D imaging can be a valuable tool for clinicians, but it is not always necessary or practical. For example, it would be impractical to perform a 3D scan on every patient who has abdominal pain. The failure of the number of radiology staff to keep up with demand indicates that all doctors (even generalists) will have increasingly to interpret their own imaging with assistance from AI.

- Functional problems: There are many illnesses that do not show up on imaging. Functional problems are diagnosed clinically and there may not be a test to confirm them. Clinical review requires careful examination to look for changes that indicate that the problem is functional rather than structural. For example, a patient with chronic fatigue may not have any obvious physical findings. However, the doctor may be able to identify changes in the patient's gait or posture that suggest a problem with the nervous system.

- Surgery: Surgeons also require the ability to think in 3 dimensions and to recognise the organs by sight. This skill is arguably of greater importance with the advent of laparoscopic surgery. Laparoscopic surgery is a minimally invasive procedure that is performed through small incisions in the abdomen. This type of surgery requires surgeons to have a clear understanding of the anatomy of the abdomen and to be able to visualise the body in 3 dimensions.

- Developmental issues: Developmental issues are often best understood by reference to the anatomy of the embryo. Although many genetic advances have been made, it is still difficult to predict the effects of abnormal genes on anatomy. Often the doctor will need to use clinical judgment when assessing a developmental disease.

- Histology: Histology is the anatomy of the cell and has led to substantial advances in the treatment of inflammatory disease and cancer. The patterns of different cells and the way that they interact with each other can provide important information about the nature of the disease present. Advances in detection of cells in the blood stream (liquid biopsies) may increase the amount of knowledge that doctors require about histology in their practice.

- Physical therapy: The skills of a physical therapist in relieving muscular skeletal pain depends upon their ability to see what is happening to the patient's anatomy. Mobilisation and massage are more effective when based upon clinical reasoning. Pain conditions become more common as patients become elderly and doctors may need to provide treatments based on anatomy rather than drugs.

- Geriatrics: The elderly often suffer from metabolic and degenerative changes and have disordered anatomy that can confuse diagnosis. They have increasingly survived previous illnesses which leaves scar tissue or missing organs. Understanding how their anatomy can change their pattern of symptoms can help improve the accuracy of diagnosis.

The student who understands anatomy well will be able to detect clinical signs that others miss, identify disease at an earlier stage, understand the significance of investigations and stay at the forefront of medicine. As healthcare continues to evolve, the importance of understanding anatomy is only likely to increase.

The student needs to develop their abilities to visualise, basically the ability to create a three-dimension representation. Students can vary in their ability to see in this way and those who have the skills should be identified. The educator can suggest that they consider careers like surgery and pathology.

How Physiology Explains Our Behaviour, Health and Disease

Physiology is the study of the normal function of living organisms. It is a broad field that encompasses the study of cells, tissues, organs and organ systems. Physiology is important in medicine because it provides a foundation for understanding how the body works and how diseases disrupt normal function.

All doctors need to understand physiology as there are few areas of medicine that have not been changed by physiology. Even psychiatry, where there are few physiological tests, is increasingly being understood as functional MRI yields insights. Treatments are increasingly being understood by their physiological mechanisms.

- Pathology: Physiology is the basis of pathology, which is the study of disease. By understanding how the body is supposed to function, doctors can better understand how diseases disrupt that function. It is difficult to make sense of disease processes without reference to the underlying cause of those diseases.

- Tests. Physiology is the basis of many tests such as blood tests and scans like echocardiograms. The normal function of the organ is described in terms of the measurements and compared with the patient's values. These measures can identify dysfunction at a stage where treatment is still effective.
- Risk factors. The routine monitoring of physiological values has changed the nature of many diseases. For instance, measuring blood pressure has led to complex understanding of the effects of high blood pressure before disease processes become present.
- Targets. As physiological understanding of the way that normal functioning can be modified has advanced, many new drug treatments have become available. These allow manipulation of the body's functions through targeting pathways and receptors in the body.
- Individualised care. Treatment regimens are often based upon the physiological values of the individual. The choice of treatments can change rapidly if the patient's response is problematic. During hospital admission the patient can be monitored many times a day and any change can lead to changes in the treatment.
- Neurophysiology and behaviour. The boundaries between our understanding of neurones and the behaviour of the whole brain are shrinking. AI models are helping close the gap further by identifying emergent properties. Neurophysiologists are using these insights to study human intelligence.
- Physiology can be used to improve performance and allow people to train more effectively and with less risk of injury. There is interest in whether the physiology of ageing can be altered so that people can go beyond health.

Although students may not be interested in becoming scientists and doing research they need to keep up with the developments in physiological understanding. Two years of preparation can only equip students with a superficial knowledge about physiological advances.

Physiology is an important field of study that provides a foundation for understanding how the body works and how diseases disrupt normal function. Physiology is used in medicine to diagnose diseases, develop treatments and monitor patients. As our understanding of physiology continues to grow, we will be able to develop even more effective treatments for diseases and improve the quality of life for patients.

Cell biology and biochemistry

Cell biology and biochemistry are two closely related fields of science that study the structure, function and chemistry of cells. Cell biology is the study of the structure and function of cells at the subcellular level, while biochemistry is the study of the chemistry of living things. Although there is overlap with physiology there are differences between macroscopic and microscopic functions.

Cell biology looks at cell structure and function, cell signalling, cell growth and division, cell death and cell metabolism. Cell biology and biochemistry are essential for understanding how cells work and how they interact with each other. Physiology in contrast looks at the systems within the body or brain.

For healthcare professionals, a knowledge of cell biology allows them to understand the following areas of medical practice:

- Ageing, healing and regeneration: Advances in our understanding of ageing, healing and regeneration will require cell biology concepts and the ability to manipulate cells in order to repair or replace damaged tissues.
- Immunological diseases: Conquering immunological diseases is likely to come from better understanding of the biology of individual immune cells and how they interact with each other.
- Cancer: Cancer is a cell biology disease where the normal processes of development and control are lost. By understanding how cells grow and divide, we can develop new treatments that target cancer cells without harming healthy cells.
- Drug development: Most drugs work on receptors on cells or part of the metabolism of cells. Further understanding of cell biology will allow development of better targeted and tolerated drugs.
- Neurological diseases: Neurological diseases are commonly caused by the interactions of cells in the brain. By understanding how these cells function, we can develop new treatments for diseases like Alzheimer's and Parkinson's.
- Protein folding: Protein folding is a complex process that is essential for the function of many proteins. By understanding how proteins fold, we can develop new drugs that target specific proteins.
- Pathogen-cell interactions: The interaction between pathogens and cells is complex. Cell biology has allowed us to study this interaction in detail, which has led to the development of new vaccines and treatments for infectious diseases.
- Reproductive biology: Reproductive biology has been only possible due to the understanding of the functions of the gametes and early

embryo development. This knowledge has allowed us to develop assisted reproductive technologies, such as in vitro fertilisation.

- Ethics: Cell biology is driving many of the greatest ethical dilemmas facing medicine from reversing ageing to use of human embryos in research, from vaccines to gene editing. Doctors will be on the front-line helping patients making choices about their own lives.

Cell biology is not always taught as a separate subject but promises to be an integral part of the future doctor's understanding of medicine. As an educator it is important to recognise that students may find the area overwhelming and be put off by the complexity of the terminology. They struggle to see how the abstract concepts of cell biology relate to the real world of clinical medicine.

The problem is that cell biology is at the heart of most of the most interesting areas of medicine. Even generalists will need to overcome their reluctance and discuss these issues with their patients so that their patients can make difficult decisions. Discussions about ethics are also unattractive to students so case studies may be a better approach.

Discussing the latest research in cell biology will help students to see how cell biology is constantly evolving. The research shows that new treatments are moving away from pharmacological approaches. The old-fashioned small molecules acting on receptors will remain important. The new cell biology treatments such as RNA, antibodies, immunotherapy is only the start of a change.

Cell biology is not always taught as a separate subject, but it is becoming increasingly important for medical students to have a strong understanding of the field. This is because cell biology is at the heart of many of the most important medical advances. For example, cell biology research has led to the development of new treatments for cancer, heart disease and other diseases.

Educators who teach cell biology to medical students face a number of challenges. Students may find the field overwhelming and be put off by the complexity of the terminology. Students may struggle to see how the abstract concepts of cell biology relate to the real world of clinical medicine. Discussions about ethics are also unattractive to students.

There are a number of strategies that educators can use to overcome these challenges. One strategy is to use case studies to help students see how cell biology concepts apply to real-world patients. Another strategy is to focus on the latest research in cell biology. This will help students to see how cell biology is constantly evolving and how it is being used to develop new treatments.

Pharmacology.

Students are generally interested in pharmacology because they can imagine themselves treating patients by prescribing medication. They can struggle with aspects such as pharmacokinetics and drug classes but this can be overcome by finding real world problems to apply the knowledge to.

In general students have the following objectives from their study and are self-motivated to work through the list. This does not mean that they wish to achieve a deeper understanding. They only want to be able to tick each drug off a list until they reach the end.

This means that they will generally avoid learning more than one or two examples of even clinically important drug classes. They will often struggle to identify the mechanism by which the drug exerts its action and the target of the drug in the body. They may have a one-to-one memory for drugs and their clinical actions.

This is a common fallacy and creates issues in clinical practice. A diagnosis of depression means prescribing an anti-depressant, pain and a pain killer, infection and an antibiotic. Antidepressants do not cure depression, painkiller do not kill pain and antibiotics do not work on (most) infections. The educator should check whether the students have this fallacy and ask them to explain the reasoning.

It is worthwhile discussing the following objectives with the students. The educator can understand if any students want to go beyond this limited understanding. They may be able to stimulate a greater level of engagement by making further points.

- To understand how drugs work. Pharmacology is the study of how drugs interact with the body. By learning about pharmacology, students can gain a better understanding of how drugs work and how they can be used to treat diseases.
- To learn about the side effects of drugs. All drugs have side effects and some of these side effects can be serious. By learning about pharmacology, students can learn about the potential side effects of drugs and how to minimise these risks.
- To learn about drug interactions. When two or more drugs are taken together, they can interact with each other in unexpected ways. By learning about pharmacology, students can learn about the potential drug interactions and how to avoid them.
- To learn about the safe and effective use of drugs. Drugs should only be used under the supervision of a doctor. By learning about pharmacology, students can learn how to use drugs safely and effectively.

There are three further points that might make a difference to some students' interest in the subject. The best argument is that doctor's primary treatment for almost all diseases is currently medication. Of all the sciences this is the one that has the most clinical orientation and will be used in almost every consultation. Pharmacology will not become superseded in the near future.

- To learn about the development of new drugs. Pharmacology is a rapidly evolving field. By learning about pharmacology, students can stay up-to-date on the latest research in drug development and learn about new drugs that are being developed to treat diseases.
- Normal treatment. Drugs remain the usual way that doctors help their patients and this means that a doctor who understands the intricacies of pharmacology will be able to better weigh up the choices when there is no clear answer.
- To learn about the history of pharmacology. Pharmacology is a relatively young science, but it has a long and rich history. By learning about the history of pharmacology, students can gain a better understanding of how the field has evolved over time.

The future of pharmacology in areas such as mental health is exciting. There are already many molecules which are poorly understood and have great potential to be repurposed. Design of new molecules to influence the multitude of targets in areas such as oncology and immunology is substantially easier with AI help.

Some doctors will work for the drug industry building clinical trials and bringing new drugs to market. Without their work the current rapid clinical progress would slow. They are criticised for developing 'me too' drugs but the educator can point out that often more effective drugs are initially a variation on a previous version.

The Worlds of Microbiology.

Microbiology is a vast field that is too complex for a medical student to get more than a sense of those organisms that cause disease. There are millions of different types of microorganisms, each with its own unique properties and capabilities. Each organism has its own biological mechanisms and could be the subject of a lifetime's study.

For the student microbiology remains the last great frontier where an individual can carve out their own place in history. Students may safely develop interest in narrow areas of in microbiology if they have support. The educator should be aware that encouraging interest in this area may distract their studies from medicine.

Old foes such as TB have adapted faster than new treatments have become available. This may change with new technologies such as DNA sequencing and protein folding. These technologies have the potential to open up microbiology to AI methods. It is safer to give the following reasons to study than risk a doctor leaving to study this area.

- To understand how diseases are caused. Microorganisms have extraordinary variability and only a very few cause disease. The specific changes that these organisms have made to evade human defence systems are complex and provide new insights into how our immune system works.
- To develop new drug treatments for diseases. Microbiologists are developing new drugs to treat diseases caused by microorganisms. In recent years, there have been major advances in the development of new antibiotics and antiviral drugs. These advances have made it possible to treat diseases that were once fatal.
- To develop new vaccines. Vaccines are one of the most effective ways to prevent disease. Microbiologists are constantly working to develop new vaccines against a variety of diseases, including COVID, influenza, pneumonia and HIV/AIDS.
- To improve public health. Microorganisms can also cause foodborne illness, waterborne illness and respiratory infections. By studying microbiology, students can learn about the ways in which microorganisms can spread disease and how to prevent the spread of disease.
- To understand the human microbiome. The human microbiome is the collection of microorganisms that live on and in the human body. These microorganisms play a role in a variety of human health conditions, including obesity, diabetes and autoimmune diseases. Microbiologists are working to understand the role of the microbiome in human health and to develop new treatments for diseases that are affected by the microbiome.

The classical teaching of microbiology was slides, laboratories and lectures. With AI and genetics the teaching of microbiology has become exciting and cutting edge. The importance of the microbiome to health has brought functional nutritionists into the spotlight. The links with diseases as diverse as cancer and depression mean that few students will avoid the effects of these advances.

Microbiology has developed a reputation for odd and bizarre theories with candida, Lyme disease and dysbiosis being notable examples. The initial theory of ME being due to an infection has gained support from the experiences of Long Covid. Colonisation of cancers and persistent infections in the blood are of unknown significance.

Many students will prefer to not engage with these findings as they cause cognitive dissonance and resistance from colleagues. The controversies about immunisation, public health policies and social restrictions during outbreaks add to this reluctance. Even significant breakthroughs such as H Pylori in the pathogenesis of stomach ulcers were initially greeted with scepticism.

The educator can address many of these concerns using materials from the humanities and models from anthropology, psychology and sociology. The same prejudices arose when dealing with HIV as with syphilis a century before. Susan Sontag's Illness as Metaphor and AIDS and Its Metaphors is a key text.

It is important to stress the relative ignorance in microbiology when compared with other aspects of medicine. With shot gun genomics science is starting to scratch the surface of the promise of microbiology. The concepts are still primitive and this is the real reason that there is so much mystery around the subject. We just do not know.

Practicals.

Lab work is a large part of many sciences but for medical students it is only one part of the range of learning experiences. The main difficulties are preparing the necessary ingredients and then bringing them together in the recipe. Cooking has many similarities and can be used as a model for improving practicals.

The key problem in practicals is the cognitive load, there are often too many steps for the student to be able to hold in their heads. They will be unfamiliar with many of the steps and the purpose of the experiment. The experiment booklet should deal with these issues.

The information should be provided as a simple list, a short explanation and then a more comprehensive discussion. The list should contain sub-lists so that the information is tiered, the key elements provided first and then those elements broken down into parts. Visually this should be easy to refer to so that the student can find what then need with a glance.

- Outcome. The desired outcome should be specified as a series of objectives and an explanation of what they will add up to. Pre-lab video of the experiment is effective.
- Ingredients. This is a list of all the equipment and materials that will be required and should include pictures when appropriate. Pre-lab opportunity to handle the ingredients can be helpful.

- Recipe. This is a list of the steps that the student must take and the order that they should be taken. They should include the key element and each element broken down. Where the list is too long removing some steps can ensure that it completed on time.
- Glossary. This is a list of any unfamiliar words or concepts and includes a detailed description of any new equipment that will be used. Although this will be far more detailed than needed to complete the practical it is useful background reading.
- FAQ. Although glossary and FAQ both cover similar areas it is worth having them as separate sections. The language used in each can then be different, glossary is a technically correct and detailed list and the FAQ is a more narrative discussion of the problems that the student may face.
- Support. It is worthwhile listing the sorts of issues where support from the educator is appropriate. This reduces questions that are in the experiment booklet and increases the chance that a student who needs help will receive it.
- Writing up. The more detailed the format for writing up the less likely that the students will borrow a colleague's work and copy it. This is generally the least useful part of the practical because only those with good understand will be able to reflect during writing up.
- Post lab activities. There is a tendency to use writing up as a post lab activity but the evidence for this being useful is limited. It is better to provide a pre-written format which can be filled in and then ask for a short reflection or arrange a debrief.
- Safety. It is important to spell out each of the dangers in the experiment and what steps are needed to prevent them. Avoid a separate 'safety talk' as this gives the impression that it is an added step rather than integrated.

The practical is a highly work intensive activity for both students and educator. The value depends upon the cognitive load being optimised for each student. Having an organised approach to managing cognitive load can ensure that each student has the right level of load. The advanced student can read and re-read the whole experiment booklet. The basic student can complete the task.

Conclusions.

Preclinical education plays a crucial role in the medical school curriculum as it provides students with the foundational knowledge and skills necessary for their future careers as doctors. The subjects covered in preclinical education, including anatomy, physiology, biochemistry, pharmacology and microbiology, form the basis of understanding the scientific principles underlying clinical medicine.

Anatomy is important for clinical examination, 3D imaging, identifying functional problems, surgical procedures, understanding developmental issues, histology, physical therapy and geriatrics. It allows doctors to detect clinical signs, identify diseases early and interpret imaging results accurately.

Physiology explains the behaviour, health and disease processes of the human body. It helps in understanding pathology, conducting tests, identifying risk factors, developing targeted treatments, individualising patient care and studying neurophysiology and behaviour. Physiology is constantly evolving and staying updated with the latest research is essential.

Cell biology and biochemistry provide insights into areas that have not previously been understood. Although students may find cell biology complex, incorporating case studies and discussing the latest research can help them see the relevance and application of this field in clinical medicine.

Pharmacology allows students to understand how drugs work, learn about their side effects and interactions and ensure safe and effective use. It is crucial for doctors as medication remains a primary treatment for most diseases. Knowledge of pharmacology helps doctors make informed decisions and stay up-to-date with new drug developments.

Microbiology is a vast and complex field that offers students the opportunity to explore various organisms and their properties. While it can be a distraction from the core medical curriculum, developing a specific interest in microbiology can be beneficial for those interested in this field's research and potential advancements in understanding and treating infectious diseases.

Microbiology also represents an area of great ignorance and irrational beliefs. The science has not got the necessary answers to dispel the beliefs. In fact, some of the 'medical facts' have now been proven incorrect. Without the brightest and the best solving the mysteries of microbiology progress will continue to lag behind other areas of medicine.

Overall, preclinical education provides medical students with a strong foundation in basic sciences and prepares them to apply this knowledge in clinical practice. Understanding these subjects is essential for effective patient care, critical thinking and staying at the forefront of medical advancements.

Top tips.

Stay Updated: The educator should ensure that they stay up-to-date with the latest advancements and research in these fields to demonstrate their importance.

Keep Students Engaged: Encourage case studies and discussions on the latest research to help students see the real-world applications of these subjects.

Focus on Clinical Relevance: Highlight how these subjects directly impact patient care, critical thinking and decision-making in medical practice.

Chapter 11: CLINICAL TEACHING.

Clinical teaching is the process of teaching medical students about the diagnosis and treatment of diseases. Clinical teaching with a patient present can take place in the GP clinic or hospital. This represents a different type of learning from the student's previous experiences. Teaching medical students about the care of patients in a clinical setting is the gold standard.

Clinical teaching can take place in a variety of settings, including the classroom, the laboratory and the clinic. Bedside education is unique and powerful type of teaching as it is highly engaging, gives the opportunity to test a wide range of skills and identify the personal qualities of the student.

Bedside teaching has several advantages over other forms of clinical teaching. First, it allows students and residents to see patients in real-world settings and learn how to apply their knowledge to the care of actual patients. Second, bedside teaching provides students and residents with the opportunity to interact with patients and learn about their experiences with illness. Third, bedside teaching can help students and residents develop their communication skills and learn how to interact with patients and their families in a sensitive and compassionate way.

Interactions with patients cause students several difficulties that are not found in other learning episodes. Students may struggle to ask the right question or gather the right information, they may fail to integrate that information into a coherent plan and they may not manage the interpersonal aspects of the interaction.

Students need to know what is expected of them in clinical teaching so they require an accessible policy document. Educators should be prepared to intervene when students are slow to learn these skills. Educators must ensure that learning episodes are of high quality and deliver the learning objectives.

Clinical teaching policy document.

Clinical teaching policy is a set of guidelines that govern the way that medical students are taught in clinical settings. These policies are designed to ensure that students receive a high-quality education while also protecting the rights of patients.

In the past clinical teaching policy documents have been dry and filed away with students unaware of their contents. In modern clinical teaching it is essential that the student engages with the policy document and follows the guidelines. This ensures that both the student and the patient are protected from being exposed to harm.

Development of the policy document should be in conjunction with student representatives and nursing staff as well as the educators. The utility of a document is limited to whether it is used and referred to during practice. This document should be explicitly designed to be referred to during practice as a resource.

The document should be written as a guide to support students get more out of their clinical attachments. It should include a list of clinical specialties that the student will be rotated through and key objectives for each speciality. There should be no more than three objectives as this is a summary not an exhaustive list.

The students should be encouraged to include the dates of each attachment and any comments that they wish to share about the attachment. They can list any learning gaps that they have identified as a 'to do' list and then tick them off when they are attained.

The document should include standard phrases for use when for instance approaching a patient, asking for consent and discussing privacy issues. The student can amend these phrases to reflect their own style and record their version in their document.

- Recording an opt out. If a patient has withheld consent, it is important to respect their wishes. Students should be able to determine if a patient has declined to participate in clinical teaching without having to approach the patient.
- Introduction. The standard introduction is to state the student's name, that they are a medical student and that they would like to ask a few questions. The student should ask the patient if they happy for the student to proceed.
- Consent. Consent is more than an agreement to have speak to the student. The student should set out their objectives and their purpose and any examination that might be necessary so that the patient can properly understand what is required.
- Part assessment. At this stage the patient may only agree to part of the assessment. There should be a phrase used to thank and accept the limitation.
- Information sharing. Even if a patient has agreed to participate, students should be respectful of their privacy and should not disclose any personal information about the patient without their consent.
- Privacy. Another important aspect of clinical teaching policy is the management of patient privacy. Where the patient is in a public area

such as a ward with other patients then the student or educator should check that the patient is happy to speak in that environment.

- Discussions with others. Patients have the right to expect that their privacy will be respected and students should avoiding discussing patient information in public areas and using only the patient's first name or initials when referring to them in class.
- Workload. Clinical teaching policy also addresses the issue of student workload. Medical students are required to complete a significant amount of clinical training and clinical teaching can be a demanding experience. There should be guidance as to how to raise concerns if workload is excessive.
- Student safety. Clinical teaching policy must address the issue of student safety. Students are at risk of exposure to infectious diseases and other hazards such as violence in clinical settings. The document should list appropriate steps such as PPE and security and how to raise concerns.
- Supervision of students involves having systems where concerns about students are reported to the educator. Students should know when and how to self-report problems so that they can be dealt with promptly and thoroughly.
- The use of technology, such as looking up diagnoses and communicate on a mobile device, should be encouraged to support student learning. However, it is important to ensure that students are using technology in a safe and responsible way. They should be aware that some patients may consider the behaviour to be rude. Also the patient may want to know what the student is looking up which can lead to difficult conversations.
- Evaluation of students must be integrated with a clinical attachment so that a student is not expected to self-learn all the time. This means that students should be regularly evaluated on their ability to assess patients, consider clinical management and on their interpersonal skills. Students should be aware of what evaluations are expected and to raise concerns if it is inadequate.
- Remediation is necessary for students who make slower progress towards the targets. The students should be encouraged to self-identify if they are having problems and raise this with the educator. Clear guidance of what is expected at each stage of the course and what is available can help ensure that needs are addressed.

The policy document should be read and signed by the educator and the student together and become the student's property. The policy will become individualised for each student as it included amendments to policies to reflect their style. Also, restrictions in the document can be removed to reflect students improving skills.

Medical schools are becoming increasingly diverse and clinical teaching policy should be sensitive to the needs of all students. For example, students with disabilities may require accommodations to participate fully in clinical teaching.

The policy document must remain a practical document and should not include sensitive details such as complaints or patient logs. The policy document will contain general information about student safety and workload so that the student can raise issues in these areas with reference to the document.

Where a student is finding it difficult to get the necessary level of evaluation then the document explains how the student can raise this with the educator. Typically this will involve the educator arranging a special session where any outstanding assessments can be made.

Clinical teaching policy documents are an important tool for ensuring that medical students receive a high-quality education while also protecting the rights of patients. By providing students with a personalised document that grows with their experience they have access to guidance to ensure that they continue to understand what is expected of them.

Providing high quality clinical teaching.

Clinical teaching can be improved by identifying the key learning objectives and then working out which require the patient to be present. This can lead to a simplified task when seeing a patient, reducing the stress on the patient and increasing the value of the interaction. For patients who are likely to have many student contacts this can improve their experience.

The length of the teaching session may vary depending on the availability of patients, the time constraints on the students or the educator and emotional demands in the cases. There should be time before and after the clinical teaching for the students to ask questions and receive feedback.

There may be facts that the educator wishes to teach, such as associated problems and similar conditions. If these can be taught without the patient present, then they should be left out of the patient contact. Patient histories, examinations and their experiences and understanding are essential material which can only be achieved through patient contact.

Although an educator should have a list of all the aspects that they wish to teach on their topic this is not a practical way of arranging clinical teaching. The educator should instead consider all the patients that they have access to and the opportunities that they offer. Based on that list they can take the following steps to arrange a high-quality teaching session.

- Choose patients who are appropriate for teaching. Not all patients are appropriate for teaching. Some patients may be too sick or too unstable to participate in teaching activities. Others may have a language barrier or other communication difficulties. It is important to choose patients who are likely to benefit from teaching and who can participate in a meaningful way.

- Prepare the patient for the teaching session. Before you bring a student to see a patient, be sure to prepare the patient. Explain to the patient what the teaching session will involve and what is expected of them. Get the patient's consent to participate in the teaching session.

- Involve the patient in the teaching session. Once you are at the bedside, be sure to involve the patient in the teaching session. Ask the patient questions about their medical history and their current condition. Let the patient know what you are doing and why you are doing it. This will help the patient feel more comfortable and involved in the teaching process.

- Be respectful of the patient's privacy. When you are teaching at the bedside, it is important to be respectful of the patient's privacy. Do not discuss the patient's medical condition in front of other patients or staff members. If you need to discuss the patient's condition with someone else, do so outside of the patient's room.

- Debrief with the student after the teaching session. After the teaching session, take some time to debrief with the student. Discuss what the student learned and how they felt about the experience. This will help the student to reflect on their learning and to identify areas where they need further development.

- Record the teaching. Each teaching session should be recorded as a contact. This is usually in the student's clinical teaching document as part of the debriefing. A separate written report may need to be given to the clinical lead or the nurses if any problems arise during teaching. In rare occasions the educator may need to make a record in the clinical record of a patient.

The educators own clinical and organisational skills are on show with clinical teaching at the bed side. The students will model behaviours like enthusiasm and passion and will be aware how well the patient is treated. Making records is an important part of this process.

Clarity and conciseness increase the ability of the students to understand what they are being taught. Varying the way that the learning points are explained can improve understanding. Feedback from the students can be used to improve engagement with the deeper aspects of the learning episode.

Remediation for slower students.

Remediation is a necessary part of the training for students who are making slower progress. These students may require additional support to diagnose and address their needs. This is because in clinical skills, if a student stops making progress in one area, it can prevent them from progressing generally.

Where these problems arise because of known difficulties, students may be offered this support proactively. Often, these accommodations are made to ensure that a disabled student does not fall behind in the first place. An otherwise excellent student may require considerable support if the skill required falls within their area of disability.

Often, students are making slower progress due to personal issues or unrecognised difficulties. In these cases, the educator should attempt to diagnose the problem before offering support. By understanding the specific reasons why a student is struggling, educators can provide more targeted support that is more likely to be effective.

This support should be arranged in a way that is sensitive to the needs of the students and does not make them feel stigmatised. It is important to explain to the student that requiring support does not mean that they will have problems as a doctor. Helping the student to feel understood and that other students have had the same problems are also helpful.

There are several approaches that can be used when managing slow learning. The task itself can simplified or presented differently, the student can be helped to develop insight and can be given more support.

Change the task.

- Change the task order. If a student is struggling with a particular task, try teaching them a different task first. Once they have mastered the easier task, they may be able to return to the more difficult task with a fresh perspective.
- Break down tasks into smaller steps. Slow learners may have difficulty understanding complex concepts or procedures. Breaking down tasks into smaller, more manageable steps can help them to succeed.

- Remedial materials. Materials can be specifically designed to help students that are having difficulties. These materials provide a different approach to the subject and sometimes are so successful that they are used for all students.
- Extend the time limits. It is important to be patient and encouraging with slow learners. They may need more time to learn than their peers, but they can still reach the targets if given longer time to reach them.
- Provide opportunities for enrichment. Slow learners may need additional opportunities for enrichment beyond the regular curriculum. This can be arranging attachments with areas not typically included in the clinical attachments.
- Increase teaching opportunities. It is also important to provide opportunities for students to practice what they have learned. In clinical training a common problem is that the student simply has not seen enough patients. Arranging teaching sessions where the educators arranges the student to see patients can speed up learning.
- Using a variety of teaching methods. Not all students learn in the same way. Some students learn best by seeing, while others learn best by hearing or doing. Using a variety of teaching methods can help to reach all students, including slow learners.

Develop insight.

- Reflective learning. For important topics such as communication skills and consent the learner may need to provide reflections of their own experiences. This can help them translate what they have learned to the clinical situation.
- Asking questions. Often the problem is that the student has not asked the right questions to understand the topic. The educator can help by asking interesting questions and with practice the student will learn how to do the same.
- Encourage students to use self-assessment tools. Self-assessment tools can help students to identify their strengths and weaknesses and to set goals for improvement. They can also help students learn to explain their strengths and weaknesses to their teachers.
- Provide appropriate feedback and reinforcement. Slow learners often need different feedback and reinforcement to their peers. The learner may be paying attention to a different part of the task and need their individual approach recognised.
- Using Technology. There are many technologies available to assist students who are having problems. For example, LLMs can be used

to provide more detailed explanations of the reasoning behind how to answer questions.

Increased support.

- Provide emotional support. Many students can overcome their problems with emotional support. They may need to talk about their difficulties or giving verbal praise can help them gain insight into their own problems.
- Have robust systems of supervision and encourage self-reporting of problems but also regular meetings between the educator and the staff, or through patient surveys. The educator is then responsible ensuring that any concerns that are raised are investigated promptly and thoroughly.
- Use cooperative learning activities. Cooperative learning activities can help slow learners to learn from their peers and to develop social skills.
- Small group instruction: Small group instruction can also be effective for slow learners. Where the topic is recognised to be challenging there may be several students who are all struggling, learning together can be an effective use of resources.
- Individualised instruction. All students can improve their performance significantly when they have one to one teaching as the educator can identify and help the student with their learning objectives, increase teaching opportunities and feedback.

These steps will ensure that the students have variety of approaches that will suit their individual needs. The educator should empower slow learners to identify their own needs as this will build self reliance. Signposting may be needed to specialist resources where the problem appears to be psychological or require more complex assessment.

Positive reinforcement when students attempt these methods themselves can reduce the burden on the educator to provide the solutions. The student will learn to understand their difficulties and find their own solutions. The educator can assist the slow learner as they develop a plan to address their problems.

Remediation is a necessary part of the training for students who are making slower progress. There are many steps that educators can take to help students and early intervention can prevent the need for more complex and expensive intervention later. It is better to catch a problem early and address it before it becomes a bigger problem.

Conclusion

Clinical teaching is a vital component of medical education, providing students with the opportunity to learn and apply their knowledge in real-world patient care settings. Bedside teaching, in particular, offers unique advantages by allowing students to interact with patients, develop communication skills and understand the complexities of patient care.

To ensure effective clinical teaching, it is essential to have a well-defined clinical teaching policy document that outlines expectations, addresses patient rights and privacy and provides guidance on safety, workload, evaluation and remediation. The policy document should be a practical resource that students can refer to during their clinical attachments, allowing for personalised learning and continuous improvement.

Additionally, educators play a crucial role in providing high-quality clinical teaching by selecting appropriate patients, involving patients in the teaching process, respecting patient privacy and offering feedback and debriefing sessions to students. These experiences allow the educator to assess skills and diagnose deficiencies.

Remediation strategies should be in place to support slower learners, considering their individual needs and providing targeted support. By implementing these measures, medical schools can ensure that clinical teaching is effective, student-centered and aligned with patient safety and rights, ultimately preparing future doctors to provide quality care.

Top tips.

Educators should have a check list of learning objectives so that they make use of any clinical teaching opportunities that arise during clinical practice.

Clinical teaching policy documents should include each of the clinical specialties, key objectives for each specialty and space for students to record learning gaps.

Slow learners can benefit from having tasks altered if they are getting stuck, help to develop insight into their learning patterns and support when trying difficult tasks.

Chapter 12: CLINICAL ROTATIONS.

Clinical rotations extend medical education from the years medical school when they were learning science and clinical skills. They are an apprenticeship that allows the doctors to develop specialist skills. The doctor learns to apply the knowledge they have learned in the classroom and the clinical skills to treat real-world patients.

During clinical rotations, trainees work alongside experienced physicians and other healthcare professionals, learning how to diagnose and treat a variety of medical conditions. Unlike medical student attachments the trainee doctor is part of the team and contributes to the work in the department. They have the chance to experience what it is like to work in that area and must learn rapidly to become useful. Their learning goes beyond clinical skills into the complex management of illness.

Much of the teaching is provided by the medical team rather than medical educators. The educator's role becomes monitoring that the trainee is progressing as expected, they are being properly supervised, they are gathering the correct evidence of experience and they are engaged with the process of education.

This can make it harder for the educator to keep in touch with the trainee and get feedback. The interactions with educators become appraisal meetings and personal development plans rather than delivering the teaching themselves. Appraisal evidence of continuing professional development is usually in the form of a portfolio. It is essential for educators to be aware of doctors who struggle with creating portfolio evidence and offer additional teaching.

Enhancing learning in clinical rotations.

Although knowledge examinations dominate the doctor in training's learning focus there are things that the educator can do to enhance their learning skills. The educator can use Continuing professional development (CPD) and appraisal to help doctors create portfolios. Encouraging the doctor to add reflections can enhance their self-learning and make the portfolios more valuable.

Many doctors have many years of evidence from appraisals and may in future be able to have this processed automatically by an AI system. Encourage the creation of personal development plans that include cross roles such as management, education, politics etc. This evidence may be useful to doctors who wish to practice abroad or change careers.

The educator can help the doctor in training get the most out of their clinical rotations by highlighting the benefits and challenges of clinical rotations. Helping the doctor find their strengths and weaknesses can ensure that they take and make learning opportunities as part of their training. This list can be used to develop a personal development plan.

- Learning from experienced clinicians: Trainees have the opportunity to learn from experienced physicians and other healthcare professionals. This can help them develop their clinical skills and knowledge. Who can the doctor learn from?

- Practicing clinical skills: Trainees can practice their clinical skills and learn new skills under the supervision of experienced clinicians. This can help them develop their confidence and competence. What skills does the doctor need to learn?

- Learning about the healthcare system: Trainees learn about the different types of healthcare providers, the roles of nurses, pharmacists and other healthcare professionals and the importance of teamwork in providing care to patients. What teamwork objectives does the doctor have?

- Developing a professional identity: Clinical rotations can help trainees develop a professional identity. They learn about the expectations of physicians and the importance of professionalism. What areas of conflict between personal characters and expectations does the doctor have?

- Learning about a speciality. They provide trainees with the opportunity to apply their knowledge to a specific area clinical practice. During clinical rotations, trainees work alongside physicians and other healthcare professionals experienced in a specialist area. What learning objectives does the doctor have during attachment?

- Clinical complexity. Trainees are often faced with difficult cases and complex medical decisions. This is a challenging but rewarding experience as they can learn from some of the best clinicians in the world. What plan do they have to learn about complex cases?

- Relevant experience. If a doctor is working in the area that they want to specialise then every patient will be relevant to their progress meaning that their learning is as rapid as possible. How can they optimise their learning from multiple cases?

- Routine work is often managed by more junior staff or allied professionals allowing the doctor to focus on the problems relevant to their level. Teaching of routine tasks can help polish understanding of the basic skills.

- Fellowship training: This is a type of advanced training that doctors may undertake after completing specialty training. Fellowship training is typically focused on a particular subspecialty of medicine and provides opportunities to develop unusual skills.

- Clinical rotations can provide opportunities for doctors to develop other skills such as teaching or mentoring. Encouraging doctors to take on these roles when they are established can improve engagement and their own learning. What other skills does the doctor want to gain?

The doctor can be helped to prepare for the aspects of the job which will decrease the effectiveness of the training. These aspects may slow the doctor's progress by making learning more difficult. Taking steps to avoid the pitfalls can prevent the doctor from having to undergo remediation.

The psychological aspects of training are as important as the learning objectives. The doctor should be prepared so that they are able to deal with the emotions that their work will evoke. This can mean taking part time or job share work in order to maintain a balance. Accepting functional restrictions is important to success.

- Long hours: Clinical rotations can be long and demanding. Trainees may work long hours and be on call at night and on weekends. How sensitive is the doctor to overwork, do they need to limit the workload for their own safety.

- Stressful environment: Clinical rotations can be a stressful environment. Trainees may be faced with difficult cases and complex medical decisions. Will they fit into the jobs that they are considering? Will they need to take steps to ensure that they are not drawn into dysfunctional departments?

- Emotional toll: Clinical rotations can take an emotional toll on trainees. They may see patients who are sick or dying and they may feel the pressure to make the right decisions. What sort of ethical issues will conflict with the doctor's core beliefs? Can the doctor manage these, or do they need adjustments?

- There may not be specific training on important areas such as ethics or regulations and the doctor may need to arrange this training themselves. What are the learning needs and how will the doctor address them?

- All practitioners face complaints and referrals to their regulators which require time and new skills to address. The doctors may not have enough time or support to properly learn from these experiences. What support will the doctor need when faced with a complaint?

- CPD can become a tick box exercise where the doctor collects enough points rather than focuses on their learning needs. How does the doctor feel about CPD? Do they feel that a personal development plan can help them?

- After a few years in a particular specialist area much work will be routine and the department may not have enough of a particular type of case to develop expertise leading to stalling of progress. What options are available for developing knowledge and skills?

Clinical rotations provide trainees with the opportunity to learn from experienced clinicians, practice their clinical skills and learn about the healthcare system. However, clinical rotations can also be challenging, as they can be long and demanding, stressful and emotionally toll-taking. Educators can help trainees get the most out of their clinical rotations by highlighting the benefits and challenges, helping them find their strengths and weaknesses and encouraging them to create personal development plans.

Asking questions can help the doctor enhance their learning experience and keep a good work life balance. The educator should see the appraisal as a key opportunity to help doctors develop their careers. They should also be aware of that all doctors need support to ensure that their functional restrictions are addressed.

Knowledge examinations.

Knowledge examinations need to be based upon best educational practice. Educators are often involved in the creation and development of knowledge examinations. They should advocate for knowledge examinations to meet the needs of doctors, patients and healthcare system in general.

Doctors are often required to take knowledge examinations so that they can be registered as specialists with their regulator. In the USA specialists have to repeat their board examinations to confirm they have retained sufficient knowledge of medical topics after specific periods of time. This has been resisted in the UK with self-regulation being the preferred method of monitoring clinical skills for senior doctors.

Junior doctors will sit a series of examinations before they are permitted to advance in their training. These examinations test various elements of the knowledge, skills and attitudes that are required to practice independently. In the UK they are generally run by the Royal Colleges but increasingly regulators are getting involved with doctor's training.

The GMC in the UK is developing a single examination that doctors from other countries and local medical students will need to pass to practice in the UK. It is clear that regulators will need to employ increasing numbers of educators if they intend to be involved with these functions. Regulators will need to use evidence based methods but be responsive to public concerns.

The current structure of knowledge examinations in clinical medicine is that there are general examinations for each group of specialities, general medicine, paediatrics, obs and gynae, general practice, general surgery, psychiatry, radiology and so on. Passing these examinations ensures that the doctor has the basic skills to work as specialist doctor.

There are then specialist examinations for areas of surgery or medicine that require subspecialist training such as cardiothoracic, learning difficulties and neuroradiology. These examinations are usually arranged hierarchically so that the doctor can only progress to the next examination after passing the previous one.

The standard of these examinations is often very high and they can act as a selection process to determine which doctors can progress. There is an increasing development of posts for doctors whose progress has culminated. These are experienced and talented doctors who are capable but unable to progress to consultant level.

Educators need to ensure that the knowledge examinations reflect clinical needs rather than the political aims of the college. This means that there must be a process to challenge the curriculum where it appears to promote an agenda. There must be involvement of the doctors who are to take the examinations as well as patient groups.

The results of the examinations should be analysed to check for bias or discrimination. There must be reasonable adjustments for doctors with disabilities or illness. There should be independent scrutiny of the process by an examination inspector with regular reports on progress.

The objectives of the examination should be stated clearly and in a form that makes sense. It is not useful to say that the examination to check the standard of the doctors. It is better to say that the examination is to check whether the doctor can manage all the tasks that they will be expected to do as registrar or consultant.

Educators should therefore apply these questions to the following list of advantages and disadvantages for their profession. What is the objective of the profession? What evidence is available for the advantages? What evidence is available for the disadvantages? Can improvements be made?

Advantages

- Knowledge examinations rely upon committees of specialists to precisely define the necessary knowledge and skills to practice in a particular specialty.

- Sitting practice papers can be formative as they help to identify areas where healthcare professionals need additional training or education.

- The examinations give the doctor a target that they can focus on as the next step in their career progression which can improve their motivation.

- Examinations reduce the amount of work that doctors have to do to identify what they need to learn to be successful in their career.

- Ambitious doctors can use knowledge examinations as a way of demonstrating their hard work and talent. This makes it easier for them to progress in their careers and to achieve their professional goals.

- Passing the examinations can be a rite of passage increasing the cohesion of the specialty and mutual respect. This can help to create a sense of community among healthcare professionals and to promote collaboration.

- Knowledge examinations make continuing education and learning an integral part of a healthcare professionals career progress. This can help to ensure that healthcare professionals are up-to-date on the latest medical knowledge.

- They can also help to protect the public by defining the standards necessary for qualified healthcare professionals are providing care. Any gaps identified by regulators can be used to improve the curriculum.

Disadvantages

- Knowledge examinations can be expensive to develop and administer and time-consuming and that burden largely falls upon the individual healthcare professional. This can be a barrier to some healthcare professionals who may not be able to afford the cost of the examination or the time it takes to prepare for it.

- Knowledge examinations may not be sufficient to assess the skills and abilities that are necessary so the doctor may face many hurdles. For example, an examination may not be able to assess a healthcare professional's ability to make decisions under pressure or to communicate effectively with patients.

- They may also be set at too high a standard so that certain groups are excluded from progressing despite being adequate candidates. For example, an examination may be set at a level that is too difficult for healthcare professionals who are from minority groups or who have disabilities.

- Doctors who are not making progress may choose to leave the profession or the country instead of continuing to struggle. This can cause of loss of talented and expensively trained professionals and gaps in the workforce increasing others workload.

- Some doctors will develop illnesses such as mental health problems and the examination structure may be too stressful and anxiety provoking. Reasonable adjustments to allow doctors who develop disabilities show their skills in other ways may be necessary under equality legislation.

- Those in the specialty who have passed the examination can feel that they are better at the job than those that have not. This can lead to a sense of elitism and can make it difficult for healthcare professionals who have not passed the examination to be accepted into the specialty.

- These examinations tend to favour those doctors who are good at those examinations as they are not perfect tests of performance. For example, an examination may favour those doctors who are good at taking tests or who are good at memorising information.

- The curriculum may not be well aligned with the needs of the specialty and can be influenced by factors such as personal interest of one of the committee or politics.

An educator can use the information from impaired doctors investigated by the regulator to identify problems with the examination system. This type of information will be more available as the regulators become more involved in decisions about what should include in specialist training.

The decisions as to what should be included in the curriculum should be informed by educational theory. Arguments that are based on other considerations such as perceived importance of a subject should be subject to scrutiny. The educator can provide a fair analysis of the optimal assessment for each topic.

Where political issues appear to be present then the educator should raise this as an issue. Where patient care is compromised by political choices the educator may not be able to prevent this from happening but can flag their concerns in line with regulator guidance.

Educators have the necessary tools to present unbiased evidence of the choices available to the committee responsible for the knowledge examination. They should avoid discussing the merits of a particular topic but indicate where knowledge examinations might not be the best way of assessing that topic.

Patient involvement is generally required in medical decision making and the educator should arrange feedback to be available even if this is not part of the formal structure of the committee. This feedback should be provided in way that best fits the committees dynamics and learning needs of those on the committee.

General practice.

The following is an analysis of the RCGP examination in the UK. It is based on my experience rather than based upon analysis of written evidence and is a personal opinion. It is provided to help the educator understand the importance of what is included in their analysis. The RCGP is arguably one of the best college examinations and substantial efforts have been made to improve it over the last few years.

What is the objective of the profession?

The objective of the RCGP examination is to provide a professional group that has the knowledge and skills to provide safe clinical care. This means that GPs must be able to use the biopsychosocial model to assess their patients, be able to use a large range of modalities to intervene and to use psychosocial progress to monitor their progress. Score 7 out of 10.

What evidence is available for the advantages?

There is moderate to good evidence that the examinations are determined by a small group of doctors without support from patients or grass root doctors, that practice papers only partly cover the necessary skills, that the RCGP examination is highly regarded for its educational experience, that learning to the exam is a useful guide, that ambitious doctors favour other examinations, that doctors with the RCGP have low level feelings of community, that the exam signifies an end to learning for many GPs, that the exam has a mildly protective effect on the public. Score 6 out of 10.

What evidence is available for the disadvantages?

The evidence is moderate and shows that the RCGP is somewhat inaccessible for some doctors, it does not help GPs to survive in practice, it is set at exactly the right level, few doctors leave the profession or country because of the RCGP but they are predominantly international medical graduates, that the system makes some adjustments for those with disabilities but they are insufficient, GPs do not have any sense of elitism in fact they suffer from low self-confidence, the RCGP exam does not favour those who are good at exams but does discriminate on cultural grounds and the curriculum is well aligned with the needs of the profession. Score 8 out of 10.

Can improvements be made?

Better evidence should be provided on several aspects such as the knowledge and skills that are missing, the involvement of broad range of views into the curriculum.

Have either additional optional examinations or permission to repeat examinations regularly to allow GPs to demonstrate ongoing high performance.

Change to the cultural aspects of the marking schedules in particular the clinical skills examinations.

Investigate whether the examination is contributing to poor self-confidence and high attrition rate of GPs in current practice.

Conclusions.

In conclusion, clinical rotations play a crucial role in the education and development of doctors. These apprenticeships allow doctors to apply their knowledge and clinical skills to real-world patient care under the guidance of experienced physicians and healthcare professionals. Clinical rotations offer numerous benefits, including the opportunity to learn from seasoned clinicians, practice and develop clinical skills, gain relevant experience in a specific specialty and navigate the complexities of patient management.

However, clinical rotations also present challenges. Trainees may face long hours, a stressful environment and emotional strain due to the nature of their work. Additionally, there may be gaps in training on important topics such as ethics or regulations and addressing complaints or referrals can require additional time and skills.

Educators play a vital role in enhancing learning during clinical rotations. They can facilitate the creation of portfolios through continuing professional development (CPD) and appraisal, encouraging reflection and self-learning. Educators can also help trainees identify their strengths and weaknesses, make the most of learning opportunities and create personal development plans that encompass various aspects of their professional growth.

Educators are involved in the creation and use of knowledge examinations. These examinations can provide a standardised assessment of knowledge and skills, motivate doctors to progress in their careers and ensure continuing education. However, they can be costly, time-consuming and may not fully assess critical skills and abilities. They may also set standards that exclude certain groups or favour those who excel in test-taking rather than overall performance.

Educators can contribute to the improvement of knowledge examinations by providing unbiased evidence and analysis, identifying issues in the examination system and advocating for fair assessments aligned with educational theory. They can also ensure patient involvement in decision-making and provide feedback to the examination committees.

In summary, clinical rotations offer valuable learning experiences for doctors, allowing them to acquire essential skills, knowledge and a professional identity. Educators play a vital role in maximising the benefits of clinical rotations and knowledge examinations by supporting trainees, facilitating self-learning and advocating for fair and effective assessment methods. By addressing the challenges and promoting the benefits of clinical rotations, educators contribute to the development of competent and well-rounded healthcare professionals.

Top tips.

Clinical Rotations are an opportunity to develop a specialised knowledge, learn complex skills and demonstrate that learning with professional examinations.

Encourage doctors to create portfolios documenting their Continuing Professional Development (CPD) with reflections for self-learning and appraisal.

Include approaches that monitor the doctor's approach to complaints and other feedback, work life balance and the emotional toll from working hours and intensity.

Chapter 13: TEAMWORK SKILLS

The key areas to explore when teaching about teamwork is the student's own personality and skills, the ways that they can contribute to the team's task and their responsibility in the management of an effective team. These three elements help the student understand their natural role in groups. For many students this will reflect what they already know about themselves.

Teamwork is a foreign concept to those medical students who have been used to learning in isolation. They may be slow to understand why teamwork is necessary and may resist the idea, preferring to master the skills themselves and take over. However, with a logical approach, they can be empowered to learn the theories quickly, although they will need prolonged training to put them into practice.

These students will feel unhappy with the idea that have to rely upon other members of the team preferring instead to do the tasks themselves. Helping them to see their strength and weaknesses and how others can contribute can break down this barrier to becoming involved. Part of their reluctance is that they have had experiences of being excluded from groups and their skills being disregarded.

For those students who have natural skills in teamwork, it is important to provide them with sufficient challenge so that they remain engaged and feel that there are things that they can learn. This group may consider the theories to be an unnecessary distraction and may instead want to focus on the practical examples. Making them responsible for including the whole group can reduce the burden on the educator.

These students will quickly see the potential and be disappointed that they do not have the resource of a team for all their problems. They will need to understand that teams are expensive and time consuming so can only be justified when the task is both important and a team is necessary. They can apply their skills to form informal groups utilising their colleagues.

Some educators may instead prefer to split the group into two and provide tailored teaching to each group. The high and low performing teams can be taught at their own pace. Others may use the differences of performance to stimulate conversations. Both those who prefer to work on their own and those who like teams have much to offer a team.

Methods for teaching teamwork.

Teamwork is essential for success in the healthcare field. Doctors and other healthcare professionals must be able to work effectively with others in order to provide the best possible care for their patients.

By incorporating teamwork into the curriculum, using simulation exercises, providing feedback and modelling teamwork behaviour, educators can help medical students and doctors develop the skills they need to work effectively as a team.

There are many different ways to teach teamwork skills to medical students and doctors. Some common methods include:

- Simulation exercises: Simulation exercises can provide students with the opportunity to practice teamwork skills in a safe and controlled environment. For example, students might be given a scenario in which they need to work together to diagnose and treat a patient.
- Role-playing: Role-playing can help students to develop their communication and interpersonal skills. For example, students might be asked to role-play a paramedic and a nurse who are working together to care for a patient.
- Feedback: Providing students with feedback on their teamwork skills can help them to improve their performance. For example, an educator might give students feedback on their communication skills, their ability to work with others and their ability to resolve conflict.
- Creating opportunities for students to work together: Educators can create opportunities for students to work together by assigning group projects and by providing opportunities for students to collaborate with other healthcare professionals in clinical settings.
- Celebrating teamwork successes: Educators can celebrate teamwork successes by recognising students who have demonstrated teamwork skills. This can help to motivate students to continue to develop their teamwork skills.
- Incorporating teamwork into the curriculum. Teamwork should be a core component of the medical school curriculum. This means that students should have opportunities to learn and practice teamwork skills throughout their training.
- Modelling teamwork behaviour. Educators should model teamwork behaviour themselves. This means being willing to share leadership, listen to others and compromise.

- Create a culture of teamwork. Educators can create a culture of teamwork by emphasising the importance of teamwork in the classroom and clinical settings. They can also do this by rewarding students for demonstrating teamwork skills.

- Provide opportunities for students to work with a variety of healthcare professionals. This will help students learn how to work with different personalities and perspectives.

- Encourage students to reflect on their teamwork experiences. This will help students identify areas where they can improve their teamwork skills.

Educators should see teamwork as a key skill and integrate it into curriculum. This means that the educator should consider how to include teamwork elements whenever possible. These methods can be difficult to apply to individual learning experiences because teamwork is a skill.

The learning process itself is the task which the educator uses to build teamwork. This means that the educator will be giving feedback on the effectiveness of the learning. Educators may not be comfortable with admitting that despite poor quality learning materials and a failed plan the students teamwork skills led to a good result.

The ability to reflect on what has happened and provide insight improves teamwork learning. The students can disentangle their own feelings from the process and see what they did well or could do better. Explaining to a student that their contribution was excellent but that it took some time for the other students to recognise it will encourage them in the future.

Teamwork models.

Although individual teamwork skills are relatively easy to learn it is better to show the students how to put the skills together using a model as an example. This allows them to identity the patterns in teamwork and how the skills interact. The following models are various approaches to understanding teamwork as a concept.

The educator should focus on how to make the learning actionable in a team situation. For instance, ask a student how they think they should behave and then model that behaviour to try out different approaches. Explain the normal features of team behaviour, what roles people take and how they can solve the problems that groups can face.

All the models consider aspects of how to combine different skills sets with communication and goal setting. They consider how to address conflict constructively and identify trust as a key element in engagement. The

Team Behaviours

There are 5 team behaviours and these core elements need maintenance for the group to run smoothy. It is important for at least some of the team members to own these behaviours. They can then take step in when there are problems and address the issue. The students can be asked to self-rate themselves in each area on a five point scale from weak to strong.

- Communication: Teams need to be able to communicate effectively in order to function well. This includes being able to share information, ideas and feedback.
- Cooperation: Teams need to be able to cooperate in order to achieve their goals. This means being willing to work together and to put the needs of the team ahead of individual needs.
- Conflict: Conflict is a normal part of team life. However, it is important to be able to manage conflict effectively in order to prevent it from derailing the team.
- Decision-making: Teams need to be able to make decisions in order to move forward. This means being able to reach consensus, compromise and make decisions that are in the best interests of the team.
- Leadership: Teams need to have leaders who can provide direction, motivation and support. Leaders can be formal or informal and they can emerge from within the team or be appointed by a manager.

Ideally a different person would facilitate communication, another negotiate for agreement, another work with anyone who gets upset, another run the decision making system and another lead. The model does ignore a critical member of the group. One group member needs to be responsible for finding solutions.

Although the overall purpose of the team is to find solutions most group will stall without a person who finds solutions. This is because it can be difficult to get the person with ideas to speak up. They will not have a complete understanding of their solution and be unable to phrase it in a way that others can understand.

The person who can understand the solution can listen to the ideas and bring them together. They are as much part of the group as any other team player. Their role is to listen to and understand the ideas and find solutions within them. This process of explaining what the team is saying is a critical team behaviour.

The solution finding involves spotting and explain other peoples' ideas. A common mistake is to rely upon an individual to come up with ideas. This will not work if they do not have the solution themselves. The other mistake is for the plant to understand but not explain. Typically, the plant will give a contrary view rather than summarise the other person's idea.

The DISC Model

The DISC Model is a behaviour-based personality test that can be used to understand the different ways that people interact with each other. The model identifies four different personality types: Dominance, Influence, Steadiness and Compliance. Each personality type has its own strengths and weaknesses.

> Dominance: Assertive, decisive and good at taking charge.
>
> Influence: Outgoing, enthusiastic and good at building relationships.
>
> Steadiness: Patient, cooperative and good at listening to others.
>
> Compliance: Conscientious, detail-oriented and good at following instructions.

The DISC Model is a way of getting the students to consider their roles within groups. It suggests that dominance will be good in leadership, influence will good cooperation and conflict, steadiness will be good at communication and compliance will be good at decision making. The model is limited and not sufficiently complex to be useful in teamwork generally but is easy to use.

The Myers-Briggs Type Indicator (MBTI)

The MBTI is a personality test that divides people into 16 different personality types. The MBTI can be used to help teams understand the different ways that people think and work and to help them build teams that are more effective.

The MBTI is not without its critics, who argue that it is not a reliable or valid measure of personality. However, the MBTI is widely used in organisations and it can be a helpful tool for understanding the different ways that people think and work.

This builds on the DISC model and gives each student some sense of where they fit into groups using a more complex analysis. The MBTI should be used as a game to help students think about their type. The educator should focus on its limitations and lack of actionable information.

The Belbin Team Roles Model

This model identifies nine different team roles that people can play, each with its own strengths and weaknesses. The nine roles are:

Plant

- Creative, innovative and good at generating new ideas and understanding and assessing other people's ideas.

- Often seen as the 'ideas' person' but can be seen as theoretical and somewhat detached from the practicalities of the team's work.

- May need to be encouraged to focus on the team's goals and to develop their ideas into workable solutions.

Shaper

- Dynamic, outgoing and good at driving the team forward.

- They are often seen as the "leader" of the team and they are typically good at motivating and inspiring others.

- Can be seen as too forceful or aggressive by some people.

- May need to learn to be more diplomatic and to listen to other people's ideas.

Resource Investigator

- Extroverted, enthusiastic and good at networking.

- They are often seen as the "connector" on the team and they are typically good at finding new opportunities and resources.

- May need to learn to focus on the team's goals and to be more organised.

Coordinator

- Calm, organised and good at keeping the team on track and can be seen as somewhat controlling or bureaucratic.

- They are often seen as the "manager" of the team and they are typically good at delegating tasks and ensuring that the team stays on schedule.

- May need to learn to delegate more responsibility and to be more open to new ideas.

Teamworker

- Cooperative, supportive and good at building relationships but are too conflict-avoidant or indecisive.

- They are often seen as the "glue" that holds the team together and they are typically good at resolving conflicts and building consensus.

- May need to learn to assert themselves more and to take on leadership roles.

Implementer

- Practical, reliable and good at turning ideas into action but can be seen as somewhat inflexible by some people.

- They are often seen as the "doer" on the team and they are typically good at taking ideas and making them a reality.

- May need to learn to be more open to new ideas and to be more creative.

Specialist

- Expert in a particular field and good at providing technical knowledge and expertise but can be seen as somewhat narrow-minded by some people.

- They are often seen as the "expert" on the team and they are typically good at providing technical advice and guidance.

- May need to learn to be more flexible and to be more willing to share their knowledge with others.

Monitor Evaluator

- Critical, analytical and good at evaluating the team's performance but can be seen as somewhat negative and critical by some people.

- They are often seen as the "judge" on the team and they are typically good at providing objective feedback and insights.

- May need to learn to be more positive and to be more supportive of the team's efforts.

Completer Finisher

- Conscientious, detail-oriented and good at ensuring that tasks are completed on time and to a high standard and can be seen as somewhat obsessive by some people.

- They are often seen as the "devil's advocate" on the team and they are typically good at ensuring that the team's work is of the highest quality.

- May need to learn to delegate more responsibility and to be more relaxed about small mistakes.

These roles go further than the team behaviours noted above. They present a more complex system where specialist knowledge, evaluation, planning, delegation and resource management is included. Students will often recognise their pattern of skills and see themselves in the roles.

The weakness of the model is that most teams will not require this array of skills. Students who can take on a difficult role will never have the chance to use it because the problem is too simple. Even in training it is not likely that the scenario will be sufficiently sophisticated to require all these skills.

Belbin Team Roles Model gives students an insight into how they should use their skillset if called upon to do so. Analysis of the roles shows that each will have their moment to contribute. Most roles will be passive for most of the time. It is as important to keep quiet as to act at the right time.

The plant should help others understand all ideas not just their own, shapers should chose the right moment to motivate and inspire others and lead the group, the resource investigator should wait until the team needs their input, the coordinator should allow teams to form and storm before trying to get them to perform, the Teamworker should take a lead early on and then handover when cohesion is achieved, the implementer should wait until the options have been explored before implementing, the specialist should share their knowledge early rather than criticising later, the monitor evaluator should summarise what has happened when the team is ready, completer finishers should not try to micromanage the process.

The Belbin Model indicates that for most of the time team members will be focused on the team behaviours of communication, conflict management, cooperation, decisions, leadership and solution finding. They will only step up to higher roles when they are needed. Educators can help students see the difference between normal and exceptional team tasks and their roles in each.

Tuckman's stages of team development:

This model describes the four stages that teams typically go through as they develop:

Forming: This is the initial stage, where team members are getting to know each other and forming their first impressions.

Storming: This is the second stage, where team members may disagree or conflict with each other as they try to establish roles and responsibilities.

Norming: This is the third stage, where team members begin to work together more effectively and develop trust and cooperation.

Performing: This is the fourth stage, where the team is fully functional and working towards its goals.

This is one of the time-based models and it is essential to understand when team roles become active. It can be used as a neutral shorthand to communicate why the team member needs to wait. The team member may not be recognise what stage the team is in but will know that their role is not active until later.

Another use of this model is to understand how groups transit between one stage and the next. An educator could ask a student to imagine that they are in a group at a particular stage and how they could use their skills to move the group to the next stage. This task will help the students to become more aware of the different stages in team building.

The Wheelan model

The Wheelan model is a theory of team development. It identifies five stages of team development:

Stage I: Dependency and Inclusion. In this stage, team members are dependent on the team leader and are focused on inclusion in the team.

Stage II: Counter-dependency and Fight. In this stage, team members begin to challenge the team leader and each other.

Stage III: Trust and Structure. In this stage, team members begin to trust each other and develop a structure for working together.

Stage IV: Work and Productivity. In this stage, team members are focused on the work that they are doing and are productive.

Stage V: Interpersonal Camaraderie and Maturation. In this stage, team members are close and supportive of each other and have a high level of trust.

The educator could ask the students to compare the Wheelan Model and the Tuckerman stages. Would they act differently in the stages described in one model compared with the other? The advantage of the Wheelan Model is that it explains the team dynamics in more detail which is actionable.

When the team is dependent on the leader it is important to have more than one person providing that support. When they are in conflict the groups resources should be focused on increased cohesion. When they are developing a structure the group should have access to ideas and support.

Poole and Roth Model

The Poole and Roth model is a framework for understanding and managing team decision-making. The model identifies four stages of team decision-making: orientation, conflict, emergence and reinforcement.

> Orientation is the stage where team members get to know each other and the task that they are working on. Team members share their ideas and opinions and they begin to develop a shared understanding of the task.

> Conflict is the stage where team members share their ideas and opinions and they work to resolve any disagreements. Team members may disagree about the best way to approach the task, or they may disagree about the best solution to the problem.

> Emergence is the stage where the team reaches a decision. Team members may reach a consensus, or they may reach a compromise.

> Reinforcement is the stage where the team implements the decision and evaluates its effectiveness. Team members monitor the results of the decision and they make adjustments as needed.

The educator can use this model to reinforce the work from the Wheelan Model and the Tuckerman stages. The additional insight from this model is that the group's tasks at each stage is spelled out in more detail. Their needs are clearer and the team roles can be compared with these needs. Communication may be difficult in the first stage and both solution finding and conflict management in the second. Improving cooperation in the third and decisions and leadership in the fourth.

Lencioni's model:

Lencioni model explains five dysfunctions that can prevent teams from being effective:

> Absence of trust: Team members may not trust each other if they do not feel comfortable sharing their thoughts and ideas.

> Fear of conflict: Team members may avoid conflict out of fear of hurting each other's feelings or damaging the team's morale.

Lack of commitment: Team members may not be committed to the team's goals if they do not feel like they have a voice in decision-making.

Avoidance of accountability: Team members may avoid accountability for their actions if they do not feel like they are held to the same standards as other team members.

Inattention to results: Team members may not be focused on achieving results if they are more concerned with their own individual needs than the team's overall goals.

This model can be applied to any dysfunctional team but is generally only considered at the performing stage. It allows the team to analyse what is going wrong and try to fix it. The problems often appear to be intractable because the causes are usually external to the group.

The team members may be micromanaged by their superiors, they may be concerned that the task does not align with their views or that others are unhappy with the task. They may feel that some members of the team are going to sabotage or report back to the seniors.

Healthcare has a reputation for highly dysfunctional teams so this model may generate interest in the students. The educator can use the student's experiences to achieve a deeper understanding of the model. Understand the links between dysfunctional groups and external pressures is vital to successful team work.

GRPI model:

This model focuses on the four key components of teamwork:

Goals: Team members need to have a clear understanding of the team's goals in order to work effectively together.

Roles: Team members need to know what their roles and responsibilities are in order to contribute to the team's success.

Procedures: Team members need to know how the team will make decisions and resolve conflict in order to function smoothly.

Interpersonal relationships: Team members need to have positive interpersonal relationships to work effectively together.

This model brings together many of the ideas in previous models by identifying the ingredients of a good team. It can be used to audit progress rapidly and ensure that all the team members are on the same page. If one team member is unsure of the goals, roles or who they make decisions this can be addressed.

Asking the group to rate their relationship with all the other members of the group can feel uncomfortable. If one member of the group dislikes another member this can only be addressed if the member speaks about it. Usually the feeling is mutual and both can be helped to resolve the tension.

This type of team maintenance needs to be built into any team's processes but often is neglected. It is not uncommon for a team member to remain unsure of what the goals were even after the process. Where different members have different ideas of how the decisions will be made this can lead to prolonged conflict.

T7 model:

This model identifies seven factors that contribute to team effectiveness:

Talent: The team has the right mix of skills and experience.

Task: The team has a clear and challenging task.

Teaming: The team has a positive and productive working environment.

Thrust: The team has a sense of urgency and commitment.

Trust: The team members trust each other.

Training: The team members have the skills and knowledge they need to be effective.

Time: The team has enough time to develop and grow.

The T7 model is useful for managers who need to understand why a team is failing. They can ask the team leader which of the factors are causing the problem. This information can help the manager decide to allow the team more time, give them more support or further team members or close the team down.

Jehn Model

The Jehn model is a framework for understanding and managing conflict in teams. The model identifies three types of conflict that can occur in teams: task conflict, relationship conflict and process conflict.

Task conflict is focused on the work that the team is doing. It can be productive if it leads to better ideas and solutions. However, it can also be destructive if it leads to arguments, hostility and decreased productivity.

Relationship conflict is focused on the personal relationships between team members. It can be destructive if it leads to resentment, distrust and decreased morale. However, it can also be productive if it leads to increased understanding and empathy.

Process conflict is focused on the way that the team is working together. It can be productive if it leads to improved communication, coordination and decision-making. However, it can also be destructive if it leads to confusion, chaos and decreased productivity.

The Jehn Model is another management tool that can assist with determining what interventions are appropriate. The manager may not be able to shut the team down and must try to fix the problems. This is complex and will be costly in terms of time and effort.

Task conflict can be resolved easily by the manager deciding as to the way forward. Relationship conflict can often be resolved by moving a team member onto a different task. This can cause other problems such as the feeling of scapegoating and resentment. Process conflict can be managed by adding an additional team member with the correct skills.

Team Performance Model

The Katzenbach and Smith model defines a team as "a small number of people with complementary skills who are committed to a common purpose, performance goals and working relationships for which they hold themselves mutually accountable."

It identifies four key factors that contribute to team performance:

Team structure: The team's structure includes its size, composition and roles and responsibilities.

Team process: The team's process includes how it makes decisions, solves problems and manages conflict.

Team climate: The team's climate includes its level of trust, cooperation and support.

Team member skills: The team's members' skills include their technical skills, interpersonal skills and decision-making skills.

When choosing to build a team this model provides a useful structure. By answering the four questions the manager has a plan as to create the ideal team for the goals. A task that requires many team members with different skills where the climate and processes are controlled will have a different structure to a more informal task.

The Johari Window Model

This model is a tool for understanding how well we know ourselves and how well others know us. The model is divided into four quadrants:

> The Open Area: This is the area where we know ourselves and others know us.
>
> The Blind Area: This is the area where we don't know ourselves but others do.
>
> The Hidden Area: This is the area where we know ourselves but others don't.
>
> The Unknown Area: This is the area where we don't know ourselves and others don't.

The Johari Window Model describes a technique for improving well performing teams. It asks the team members to understand their own blind spots and hidden areas and become more open and honest. This model describes how people share information with others and how they perceive themselves and others to build stronger relationships.

The educator can discuss with the students what types of teams would require this model and what the risks of this level of sharing would be. The students should understand the high degree of trust that is required and that the environment should feel safe. In healthcare this might be present in counselling groups or family work.

Further study on teamwork.

The teamwork models provide a good grounding on the theory of teamwork. The practice of teamwork is learned from direct experience in team situations. The educator will not always be present for these situations and the students will need to take the role of educator.

Getting students to shout out what is happening when doing group work can prepare them to provide feedback to each other. The educator can use the methods at the start of this chapter to create experiences. The educator can arrange short sessions to discuss those or other teamwork experiences.

Without an integrated curriculum the understanding of teamwork may fade and the students may focus on other aspects. It is therefore important to focus on the key aspects of teamwork; the Belbin roles, the 5 (or 6) team behaviours and the process which a team goes through.

Conclusions.

In conclusion, teamwork skills are crucial in the field of healthcare as they contribute to the overall success and effectiveness of medical professionals in providing optimal patient care. Educators play a vital role in teaching and developing these skills in medical students, recognising that further training may be necessary for those aspiring to pursue management or leadership roles.

To effectively teach teamwork skills, educators should discuss the applications of teamwork theory in healthcare, helping students understand the broader context and principles underlying effective teamwork. By grounding their understanding in these principles, students can make connections more easily and apply their knowledge across different contexts, using a single model as a basis for their experiences.

It is important to acknowledge that teamwork may be a foreign concept to some medical students accustomed to individual learning. Some students may resist the idea, preferring to rely solely on their individual skills. However, with a logical and systematic approach, students can be empowered to learn teamwork theories quickly, although putting them into practice will require prolonged training.

For students who already possess natural teamwork skills, it is essential to provide them with sufficient challenges to keep them engaged and motivated to further develop their abilities. Educators can achieve this by creating opportunities for practical examples and tailored teaching approaches that cater to the diverse needs of different learners.

Various methods can be employed to teach teamwork skills, including simulation exercises, role-playing, providing feedback, emphasising the importance of teamwork, creating collaborative opportunities, celebrating teamwork successes, incorporating teamwork into the curriculum and modelling teamwork behaviour. These strategies help students develop effective communication, cooperation, conflict resolution, decision-making and leadership skills necessary for successful teamwork.

To understand and apply teamwork skills effectively, students can benefit from utilising different models and frameworks. The DISC Model, Myers-Briggs Type Indicator (MBTI), Belbin Team Roles Model, Tuckman's stages of team development, Wheelan model, Poole and Roth Model, Lencioni's model, GRPI model, T7 model and Jehn Model provide valuable insights into individual and team behaviour, stages of team development, decision-making processes, dysfunctions, conflict management and key components of team effectiveness. Each model offers unique perspectives and can help students identify their strengths, weaknesses and preferred roles within a team.

By using these models, educators can guide students in understanding how different personalities, behaviours and stages of team development impact teamwork. This knowledge enables students to recognise and address challenges that may arise in a team setting, fostering collaboration, trust and effective problem-solving.

Ultimately, by integrating teamwork skills into the medical school curriculum and providing opportunities for practice and reflection, educators can empower medical students and doctors to become effective team members. This, in turn, leads to improved patient care and outcomes, as healthcare professionals work together cohesively and efficiently to meet the complex challenges of the healthcare environment.

Top tips.

Show students how an understanding of roles in teams can explain their strengths and weaknesses and encourage others to contribute according to their skills.

Give feedback to students when working in teams so that they can identify their roles and tasks and the stages of group formation.

Incorporate teamwork as a core component of the medical school curriculum to ensure students learn and practice teamwork skills throughout their training.

Chapter 14: SITUATIONAL JUDGEMENT AND ETHICS.

Situational judgement test (SJT) is a type of assessment that measures how people make ethical choices in real-world situations. SJT typically present participants with a series of scenarios and ask them to choose the best course of action. SJT are often used in hiring and promotion decisions, as they can help employers to assess candidates' decision-making skills and ethical judgment in the face of uncertainty.

Ethics is a branch of philosophy that deals with morality and right and wrong. Ethical principles are often used to guide decision-making and they can help people to make choices that are fair, just and respectful of others.

SJ and ethics are closely related, as they both involve making decisions in the face of uncertainty. When faced with a difficult situation, people need to be able to weigh the potential consequences of their actions and make a choice that is both ethical and effective.

Students can learn how to make ethical decisions by reading about ethical dilemmas, participating in role-playing exercises, or simply thinking about how to handle different situations. Thinking and understanding one's own values and beliefs can help guide decisions as can feedback from others.

Situational judgement test (SJT)

The Situational judgement test (SJT) can be studied for by doing practice papers and other steps noted below. The educator's role is to provide ethical theories and other evidence to help the students understand the explanations. The GMC good medical practice provides an underpinning for many decisions.

- Understand the format of the test. SJTs typically present you with a series of scenarios and ask you to rate them. The answers may all be reasonable or poor, what is being tested is the relative strength of the answers.
- Practice with sample SJTs. There are many resources available online that offer sample SJTs. Practicing with these tests will help you get a feel for the format and the types of questions that you can expect to see.
- Review the competencies that are being assessed. SJTs are designed to measure a variety of competencies, such as communication,

teamwork and problem-solving. Review the competencies that are being assessed and make sure that you understand what they mean.

- Read the explanations. The marking schedule will indicate the reasons for the ratings. These can help when choosing between similar answers.
- Think about your experiences. When you are faced with a scenario on an SJT, try to think about how you would handle the situation based on your own experiences. This will help you to make the best decision and to improve your chances of scoring well on the test.

Using a LLM to rate the answers can also help gain insight into the questions. LLMs often consider two answers to be of similar level. The LLM can give pros and cons for each answer. This can reassure the student that their difficulties relate to the not being a clear answer.

A problem at the heart of ethics is that it does not provide answers to the problems. Ethical reasoning gives an approach to thinking about the answers but not the answers themselves. There is always an element of preference and this will change with different cultures and experiences.

There is concern that SJTs are at their heart biased and discriminatory. They assume that professionalism has a single answer and other approaches are incorrect. This one-size-fits-all view of medicine cannot be correct as it is inconsistent with diversity. If medicine is to value all contributions it cannot exclude those who think differently.

Four Principles of Biomedical Ethics.

This ethical model is at the heart of most discussions about ethics in medical settings. Also called Beauchamp's principles it proposes that each principle will conflict with the others and that no one principle trumps the others.

The theory is difficult to apply in clinical practice as it does not give clear answers. In recent years respect for autonomy has become the overriding principle in an attempt to overcome this problem.

- Respect for autonomy: This principle holds that individuals have the right to make their own decisions about their health care, even if those decisions are not what a doctor or other health care provider would recommend.
- Beneficence: This principle holds that health care providers have a duty to do good for their patients. This includes providing care that is effective and that will improve the patient's health.

- Non-maleficence: This principle holds that health care providers have a duty to do no harm to their patients. This includes avoiding treatments that are likely to cause harm, even if the treatment might also be beneficial.
- Justice: This principle holds that health care resources should be distributed fairly. This means that patients should have equal access to care, regardless of their ability to pay.

The principles are a useful starting point but will not on their own allow students to work out the correct answer in an SJT. The theory should be presented as a problem rather than a solution so that the students are engaged to find out real answers to their questions.

An example of a problem that comes out of autonomy is if the patient wants a treatment that the doctor is not offering. If autonomy overrides the others then the doctor should follow the patient's preference. Where there are no good beneficence and non-maleficence arguments this may force doctors to provide treatments that they are unhappy with.

The legal case of Montgomery can be seen simply as an issue of consent but the doctor failed to discuss the caesarean. If the patient had asked for a caesarean and the doctor refused then would the doctor have been in a worse or better situation? The GMC has not provided clear guidance as to the limits of autonomy.

'All patients have the right to be involved in decisions about their treatment and care and be supported to make informed decisions if they are able'. The word involved does not imply that they can request a treatment. *'If after discussion you still consider that the treatment or care would not serve the patient's needs, then you should not provide it'*. The words serve the patient's needs contains a fallacy – it assumes that the doctor understands those needs.

The educator can use the above example or their own experience to illustrate how ethical thinking is developing. The GMC want to avoid the situation where patients tell doctors what treatment they want but also want to give autonomy precedence. The balance between doctor centred and patient centred care will continue to be a challenge in ethics.

GMC good medical practice (2013)

The GMC intended to highlight the four domains safety and quality; communication, partnership and teamwork and maintaining trust however some of these aims were somewhat blurred in the actual document. Many of the statements were less clear than doctors needed to be able to apply them to their practice.

The GMC is currently rewriting Good Medical Practice to incorporate many of the ethical advances that have occurred in the last decade. The general principles are not likely to change and will still include the following seven general areas. It is likely that the desire to create a single document that covered all ethical areas was part of the difficulty.

GMC seven general areas

"1.   Patients' well-being: Good doctors prioritise the care of their patients, staying competent, keeping their knowledge up to date, building good relationships and acting with honesty, integrity and within the law.

2.   Partnership with patients: Good doctors work in partnership with patients, respecting their rights to privacy and dignity. They treat each patient as an individual and strive to provide the best care and treatment tailored to their needs.

3.   Responsibility: It is the doctor's responsibility to be familiar with and follow the guidelines outlined in Good medical practice and the accompanying explanatory guidance. Doctors must use their professional judgment in applying these principles in different situations.

4.   Professional performance: Doctors must be competent in all aspects of their work, continuously update their knowledge and skills and engage in activities that maintain and improve their competence and performance.

5.   Safety and quality: Doctors must work within the limits of their competence, provide a good standard of practice and care, prescribe treatments based on evidence and take steps to ensure patient safety. They should also contribute to quality improvement, actively respond to risks to safety and maintain clear, accurate and legible records.

6.   Communication and teamwork: Effective communication with patients, colleagues and their families is crucial. Doctors must work collaboratively, treat colleagues fairly and with respect and contribute to teaching, training and supporting others. They must also prioritise patient continuity and coordination of care.

7.   Maintaining trust: Doctors must treat patients and colleagues fairly and without discrimination, base treatment decisions on clinical need and respond promptly and honestly to complaints. They should act with honesty, integrity and professionalism and ensure they have adequate insurance or indemnity cover".

The GMC Good Medical Practice 2013 is a good basis for discussions about SJTs as much for what is missing as what has been included. The guidance for specific areas is improving as the GMC develops specific guidance on topics such as consent and confidentiality.

Examples of problems include several in the section on recording consultations. It left it open whether each practitioner having a discussion should make a separate record of that discussion. It was not clear whether a virtual review of a patient was a consultation and should be recorded. It was not clear what elements should be recorded in a consultation.

These problems make the guidance far from satisfactory and leave practitioners having to guess. Students can be encouraged to question the guidelines and offer their own ideas. Educators can explain that this is an evolving field and that there is chance that their ideas may become part of the guidance in the future.

Models For Recording Consultations

The gap between practice and theory can be illustrated by many examples and one of these is models for recording consultations. The educator should choose an example that they are familiar with and can give the students real life experience of the dilemmas. Recording consultations is rarely taught as a specific subject so is not likely to be something that the students have considered in depth.

My model for recording consultations is unsurprisingly my favourite because it has a medical legal approach. The model is designed to be robust against complaints and to demonstrate the highest quality care. It has some elements which prompt the doctor to avoid mistakes and is written so that it is neither patient not doctor centred.

Medical legal approach.

- Clinical assessment: The records should include a detailed description of the patient's symptoms, medical history and any relevant social history. Also include a description of the findings from the physical examination, including any abnormalities.
- Data interpretation: The doctor should read any previous records or other documents available. They should consider whether any biometrics 'obs' would be useful or if recorded by others. Then interpret the findings from the diagnostic tests, such as blood tests, imaging studies and other tests.
- Recording patient involvement: The doctor should record the patient's own words when possible for instance about their goals. Of particular interest is the patient's or carer's health beliefs and

their reactions to the consent process and any preferences. They should also note what the patient was told about follow up.

- Managing red flags: The doctor should document any red flags that were identified during the clinical assessment. Red flags are any signs or symptoms could indicate a more serious problem. They should make the red flag safe by asking more questions, arranging investigations or referring considering what is necessary and proportionate.

The advantages of having a systematic approach to recording a consultation is that it can be adapted to different situations, the doctor will not forget to record essential information such as consent and the doctor will reflect at the end of the consultation to consider whether there is information that they have not considered, or risks that they have not addressed.

This is taken to the extreme with the full medical clerking, the gold standard for diagnosis which is why it is taught at medical school. All doctors should know how to record this model, In practice it is often abbreviated as it can take an hour or two if it includes a full neurological examination.

- The full medical clerking covers the initial complaint, the history of presenting illness, past medical history, family history, social history, medication, allergies, observations and a full multisystem examination, differential diagnoses, management plan including investigations and treatments and advice.

The SOAP assessment is popular but it is more rigid than my model and is somewhat doctor centred as it only involves the patient in the S = subjective section. There is no place to record the patient's consent or their ideas, concerns and expectation.

- SOAP: The SOAP format is a commonly used systematic approach to recording consultations. It stands for Subjective (the patient's chief complaint and history of present illness), Objective (the doctor's findings on physical examination), Assessment (the doctor's diagnosis and plan) and Plan (the doctor's orders).

The CBE (Chief Complaint, Brief History, Examination, Diagnosis and Plan) model has similar limitations as SOAP. The PICOT format is even more rigid and less comprehensive.

Electronic templates such as EMEDS and POMR have substantial problems because they are neither flexible nor comprehensive. They do not include all the necessary records and force the doctor to complete unnecessary sections. They do not have a great reputation for this and other reasons. There is always a compromise between including everything and leaving out something that might be relevant.

- EMEDS (Emergent Medical Data Summary) note: This is a format for recording a consultation in an emergency department setting. It is a more structured format that includes information about the patient's chief complaint, vital signs, physical exam findings, laboratory results and other diagnostic tests. The EMEDS note also includes a section for the doctor's orders and a section for the patient's discharge instructions. The EMEDS note is typically used in emergency departments to quickly and efficiently document patient care.
- Problem-Oriented Medical Record (POMR): The POMR is a structured method of recording patient information that focuses on the patient's problems. The POMR consists of four parts: the database, the problem list, the plan and the progress notes. The database is a collection of all of the information that is known about the patient, including their medical history, physical exam findings, laboratory results and other diagnostic tests. The problem list is a list of all of the patient's medical problems. The plan is the doctor's plan for the patient's care, including medications, tests and follow-up appointments. The progress notes are a record of the patient's care over time.

Record summaries are becoming more popular with models such as AMPS. They are easy to read and use as they contain important information in clear layout. They are not complete records and rely upon the computer records to be prepopulated. The symptoms section often becomes a 'comments' section with any other information recorded there for clarity. This has detrimental effects on the quality of the records as symptoms are often key to diagnosis.

- AMPS: AMPS is a newer format for recording patient consultations. It is a more concise way of recording the patient's assessment, plan, medications and symptoms. It has many of the problems and few of the solutions in other formats.

The educator can use the various models to discuss what the student wants to include in their version of a patient note. The advantages of using a structure compared with developing their own style are interesting topics. Students can be asked to consider how they would defend their medical record in a clinical negligence case and whether using a model would help them.

Asking students to develop their own model record can be useful for engagement. They can then compare their version with the models above. This can help them understand the purpose of the various elements and improve their own record keeping with those models.

Ethical challenges in medicine.

Educators should take students beyond passing the SJT into a deeper look at ethics. Many of the same techniques learned for the SJT can be applied to ethics. Although each ethic issue will present novel aspects there are some common features such as the Beauchamp principles.

The following list is a resource for students and educators who wish to further develop their knowledge in this area. Select a topic and consider an example of the problem from experience. Look for solutions to the problem and what a good result would look like. Ask a student to play devil's advocate and argue alternative views.

- Triage: Triage is the process of prioritising patients for treatment. This can be a difficult decision, as it requires doctors to make judgments about who is most likely to benefit from treatment and who is not.
- Resource allocation: Resource allocation is the process of deciding how to distribute limited resources, such as money, drugs and medical equipment. This can be a difficult decision, as it requires doctors to make judgments about who should receive the limited resources.
- Funding of care. It is generally accepted that those who need healthcare are mostly the groups that can least afford it. This means that there needs to be a system of social redistribution of societies resources. The risk is that this leads to a free for all with the health budget increasing beyond the society's ability to pay and the law of diminishing returns.
- Handing over care. Doctors have a duty to provide care to their patients. However, there are times when a doctor may need to withdraw from a patient's care, such as when the doctor is no longer able to provide the care that the patient needs.
- Patient privacy: Doctors have a duty to protect their patients' privacy. This can be difficult to do in the age of electronic medical records, which are often accessible to a wide range of healthcare professionals. There are old fashioned problems such as lack of a private space when discussing sensitive areas.
- Informed consent: Patients have the right to be informed about their medical condition, the risks and benefits of treatment and alternative treatments. Doctors must obtain informed consent from patients before providing treatment.
- Patient autonomy: Patients have the right to make their own decisions about their care. This can be challenging for doctors, who can see the harm that the patient's risk by their decisions. Patients

can also improve the quality of care by taking a more active role seeking out information.

- Capacity assessment. There is a presumption for capacity but this can be rebutted by age, disease of the mind or brain. This is similar to the rules on insanity where the boundary between understanding right and wrong is blurred. Where a person takes a drug that leads to sedation, anaesthesia or surgical anaesthesia they can be dealt with differently.,

- Screening. There are risks from over investigation and over treatment of abnormal findings on screening tests. This can range of treating the test rather than the patient to invasive and prolonged processes to rule out disease and each test has the risk of psychological harm as well as physical injury.

- Genetic testing: Genetic testing can be used to diagnose diseases, but it can also be used to screen for diseases in people who are not yet symptomatic. This raises ethical concerns about whether people should be tested for diseases that they may never develop and whether the results of genetic testing should be used to discriminate against people.

- Research: Research participants may not gain any advantage but have health risks. Higher ethical standards are imposed upon researchers to reflect that they may cause individuals harm.

- Artificial intelligence in healthcare: Artificial intelligence (AI) is increasingly being used in healthcare to provide a variety of services, such as diagnosing diseases, recommending treatments and monitoring patients. However, AI also raises a number of ethical concerns, such as the potential for bias, the impact on jobs and the question of who should control AI systems.

- Pain management: Doctors must balance the need to relieve pain with the risk of addiction. This can be a difficult decision, especially for patients who are in chronic pain. The disability model provides an approach, that pain management should reduce disability not focus on pain.

- Reproductive decisions. Sterilization, availability of contraception, management of miscarriage, reproductive technologies such as IVF, older mothers, drug and alcohol use in pregnancy, the right to choose, modification of genomes to treat disease, antenatal screening for disease are all areas that have ethical and situational judgement aspects. Other examples are donor eggs and sperm, the creation of embryos for research and the selection of embryos based on their characteristics.

- End-of-life care: End-of-life can be a difficult time for patients and their families and it can raise a number of ethical challenges. For example, doctors may need to decide whether to provide life-prolonging treatment to patients who are dying, or whether to focus on comfort care instead.

- Withholding or withdrawing treatment: Doctors may be faced with the decision to withhold or withdraw treatment from patients who are not benefiting or who have a poor prognosis. This can be a difficult decision, as it involves balancing the patient's right to refuse treatment with the doctor's duty to provide care.

- Assisted suicide and Euthanasia: Assisted suicide is the act of helping a person to commit suicide. Euthanasia is the act of intentionally ending a person's life to relieve suffering. This are both very controversial issues, as there is no clear consensus on whether they can ever be ethical or not. The right to determine one's death vies with societies duty to protect its vulnerable citizens.

- The role of government: The government plays a significant role in healthcare. This includes regulating the healthcare industry, providing funding for healthcare programs and setting healthcare policy. There is a need to find ways to balance the government's role in healthcare with the need for patient autonomy and choice.

- Systems of healthcare: Healthcare is increasingly being treated as a commodity, meaning that it is being bought and sold like any other product. This can lead to patients being treated as customers rather than as people and it can also lead to higher healthcare costs.

- Telehealth: Telehealth is the use of technology to provide healthcare services remotely. This can raise a number of ethical concerns, such as the security of patient data, the quality of care and the doctor-patient relationship.

- Direct-to-consumer advertising: Direct-to-consumer advertising is the promotion of prescription drugs to consumers directly. This can raise a number of ethical concerns, such as the potential for patients to make uninformed decisions about their healthcare and the influence of pharmaceutical companies on doctors' prescribing practices.

- Expectations of healthcare professionals. Healthcare professionals are (mostly) human beings who have flaws and gaps in their skills. Increasing expectations that they should not make mistakes whilst coping with extreme workloads and problems such as workforce crises are unreasonable and unachievable.

- Self-care. Healthcare professionals have a responsibility to maintain their health and wellness. Although resilience is one part being able to step away from situations that are causing them harm is also important.

- Social media. The doctor's professional personality now extends to their online presence and this has advantages in maintaining professional contacts and informing the public but can cause challenges.
- Teaching. All doctors have a responsibility to be involved with education of their colleagues and with this comes the need to ensure that the patients consent to any involvement and that they are protected by supervision.
- Legal obligations. Doctors need to be up to date on the legal frameworks for their professions such as when working with surrogate decision makers. Other areas that doctors may not be fully up to date is writing sick note, death certificate and other legal reports.
- Regulation of healthcare professionals. The balance between having complicated and burdensome processes for patient protection and fairness to the professional in regulation can be difficult to achieve. Removing a doctor from the register is an expensive decision that can impact the availability of doctors. Doctors have a duty to report on each other if they see incompetent or unethical behaviours by colleagues.
- Conflicts of interest: Doctors have position of power over patients and the risk of abuse of power is increased if there are conflicts of interest. Doctors may have financial conflicts of interest which could influence the way that doctors make decisions about their patients' care. One area this can cause problems is the acceptance of gifts.
- Bullying: Bullying is a form of aggressive behaviour that involves a pattern of repeated harmful behaviour. Bullying can occur between healthcare professionals, between patients, or between healthcare professionals and patients.
- Disability discrimination: Patients with disabilities may face discrimination in the healthcare system. For example, they may be denied treatment or they may be treated differently than patients without disabilities.

It is often difficult to find solutions to these problems from first principles and the students may feel they have to learn the answers by rote. The educator should therefore focus on the methodology for finding answers to ethical problems. It is important to focus on the reasoning that the student presents rather than whether that it the correct answer.

There is not likely to be enough time within the curriculum to properly debate all these ethical issues. The students should be encouraged to raise the issues when they occur in practice. If they see a problem that appears to be neglected then they should include the issue in their CPD.

LLMs are good at providing answers and explanations for ethical questions. They focus more on the reasoning and the approaches than finding a correct answer. This helps students explore their own professional values and develop their reasoning skills.

Teaching methods for Situational Judgement tests/Ethics.

Ethics is an area where the content is much greater than the time allocated so it needs to be included when teaching other topics. The educator will need to have discussions with the Obs and Gynae team to ensure that reproductive ethics are not left out.

Elderly medicine is another specialty that deals with ethical dilemmas on an everyday basis. GPs deal with similar issues as they also manage the care of the elderly and may be more open to including these topics. Preparing cases for discussion can make it easier for specialists to be involved.

- Lectures: Lectures can be a good way to introduce students to the basic concepts of SJT and ethics. However, it is important to make sure that lectures are interactive and that students are given opportunities to discuss and debate the concepts that are being presented.
- Case-based learning: This is a teaching method that uses real-world cases to help students apply the concepts they are learning in class. Case-based learning can help students to develop their SJ skills by exposing them to a variety of ethical dilemmas and by requiring them to make decisions about how to best handle these dilemmas.
- Simulation exercises: These are exercises that allow students to practice their skills in a safe and controlled environment. Simulation exercises can be used to teach students about ethical issues, such as how to handle patient confidentiality or how to deal with a patient who is refusing treatment.
- Ethics rounds: These are weekly meetings where students discuss ethical issues that they have encountered in their clinical rotations. Ethics rounds can help students to learn from the experiences of their peers and to develop their own ethical reasoning skills.

It is important not to add in ethics as an extra but integrate the reasoning within the teaching materials. When ethics is a key concept in the topic avoid simplistic requests and think how both sides can be considered. For instance, when discussing miscarriage management the educator can describe the traditional wait and see compared with the active monitoring from an ethical standpoint.

How do people feel about medicalising of miscarriage, do the advantages of emotional support, increased information and discussions outweigh the increased emotional workload it generates. Is it more empowering for a person self-manage their miscarriage or does it leave them feeling overwhelmed and alone?

The educator can then ask the students whether this ethical knowledge will change how they manage the patient. Will the students explain the choice and support the person or persuade them to engage with the early pregnancy clinics? An understanding of ethics can give a doctor a wider range of options and the ability to see alternative points of view.

Conclusions.

Situational judgement tests (SJT) and ethics are closely related as they both involve making decisions in uncertain situations. SJTs are used to assess decision-making skills and ethical judgment, particularly in allocation or selection for jobs. Ethical principles, such as respect for autonomy, beneficence, non-maleficence and justice, guide decision-making and help individuals make ethical and effective choices.

To improve SJT and ethical judgment, individuals can practice making decisions in various situations, engage in role-playing exercises and reflect on their own values and beliefs. Seeking feedback from others can also help improve decision-making skills. It is important to note that the Four Principles of Biomedical Ethics, as proposed by Beauchamp, provide a useful framework for ethical discussions but often do not offer clear solutions in complex situations.

The General Medical Council's (GMC) Good Medical Practice provides guidelines for doctors, emphasising patient well-being, partnership, responsibility, professional performance, safety and quality, communication and teamwork and maintaining trust. While the GMC guidance is a good starting point, it may require further clarification and improvement to address the ethical advances and challenges that have emerged in recent years.

Different models for recording consultations exist, such as a medical legal approach or the full medical clerking. These models provide systematic structures for documenting essential information, ensuring important details are not overlooked. However, electronic templates and rigid formats like

SOAP, CBE and PICOT have limitations and may not capture all relevant information.

Ethical challenges in medicine include triage, resource allocation, funding of care, decisions regarding withholding or withdrawing treatment, handing over care, patient privacy, informed consent, patient autonomy and capacity assessment. These challenges require balancing the rights and well-being of patients with the available resources and ethical principles.

Overall, understanding and developing situational judgment and ethical decision-making skills are crucial for healthcare professionals to navigate complex scenarios and provide quality care while upholding ethical standards. Continuous learning, reflection and considering real-world examples and dilemmas can help healthcare professionals develop their professionalism.

Top tips.

Focus on reasoning: When discussing ethical issues, focus on the reasoning and thought process behind your decisions rather than seeking a "correct" answer.

Competencies. Break down ethical issues into the competencies being assessed: SJTs measure various competencies, such as communication, teamwork and problem-solving.

Opportunities. Ethical challenges are clustered in specialities such as reproduction, psychiatry and elderly medicine but general issues such as writing medical records can be addressed at any time.

Chapter 15: POSTGRADUATE LIFE.

The move from medical student to doctor is more than a transition from lectures and clinical teaching to clinical practice. It is a philosophical change; the doctors have increasing choice as to the subjects of their attention. In medical school students could make small choices such as the topic of their project or elective or whether to spend a year doing an intercalated degree.

As a doctor they need to decide the structure of their future career, where in the country they want to live, whether they want to have a year out. They can get their heads down and study and work hard for their examinations. They can explore non-medical interests or new roles within medical politics or teaching. A mentor is better able to assist than an educator.

Some will have developed learned helplessness because of years of study both at school and medical school. Learned helplessness is a state of mind in which a person believes that they have no control over their circumstances and that their actions will not make a difference. They may need to take time to find out who they are and what they want to do. Others will need to balance their ambitions with a young family or caring roles.

Many doctors will need a mentor to help them make sense of their choices, to reassess their limitations, plan the best way forward and what they would like to do next. This means that many doctors will need to focus on an area of weakness before they can make progress. Mentors can help doctors change their attitudes to stop pretending to be a superhero.

Developing aims as a doctor.

The process of developing aims as a doctor is not significantly different to the process of developing aims in other areas. The doctor will often need support to work through the process as it is more complex than most choices. The mentor is focused upon the emotional aspects of making choices.

- Reflect on your values. What is important to you? What do you believe in? What do you want to achieve in your life? Once you have a good understanding of your values, you can start to develop goals that are aligned with them.
- Consider your skills and interests. What are you good at? What do you enjoy doing? Your skills and interests can help you to narrow down your options and choose goals that are realistic and achievable.

- Set SMART goals. Specific, measurable, achievable, relevant and time-bound goals are more likely to be successful. When setting goals, be sure to specify what you want to achieve, how you will measure your progress and when you want to achieve your goal. Many doctors find making a long list of possible goals is more effective than a to do list.
- Break down large goals into smaller steps. Large goals can seem daunting, so it is helpful to break them down into smaller, more manageable steps. This will make your goals seem more achievable and will help you to stay on track.
- Be flexible and adaptable. Things don't always go according to plan, so it is important to be flexible and adaptable. Be prepared to adjust your goals as needed. See your list as doors that may opened rather than a to do list.
- Celebrate your successes. As you achieve your goals, be sure to celebrate your successes. This will help you to stay motivated and on track.

For some doctors a life coach can help them make sense of these aims. The more complex the doctor's life the more necessary it is to have plans for each part. There is no point in having an amazing career if it is at the expense of having a life.

Many doctors will already have made substantial sacrifices to achieve a medical degree. They may be drawn in by the fallacy that they must keep going because they have already invested so much. The mentor can help the doctor see that other paths are available and as worthy as becoming a consultant.

The mentor can then consider barriers to the doctor's aims, these barriers act a resistance and make it more difficult psychologically to do what is needed to progress. Arranging a meeting with a doctor who has faced the same problems can make them seem more surmountable.

Barriers to a successful career.

The mentor may have an idea of what barriers the doctor is facing, but if not should explore the areas sensitively. Doctors can often follow inappropriate paths which worsens their problems. Also doctors with unconventional approaches can find creating professionalism difficult to manage.

- Cost of education. Medical school is expensive and the cost of tuition and fees has been rising steadily in recent years. The high levels of debt after graduation can make it difficult to accept a lower paid role.

- The cost of professional insurance. Insurance is expensive and it can be a significant financial burden for those who want to work in areas that do not have insurance cover.
- Time commitment. Medical training is a long and demanding program. Students have already spent many years in medical school and need to dedicate further years to post graduate training. Doctors may try to cut corners so that they can have enough time to start a family.
- Lack of academic ability. Medicine is very demanding academically and some people simply do not have the academic ability to achieve their aims. They can change course to an area that they are better able to do and have greater success.
- Stress. The medical profession is a high-stress environment. Doctors are often under pressure through overwork. This can lead to high levels of stress, which can impact both their physical and mental health. Taking a less conventional approach can help them create better balance.
- Physical illness and disability. Some doctors will need to adjust their aims and learn to explain their needs so that reasonable adjustments can be made. They may need reassurance that reasonable adjustments can make disabled doctors more successful than their able-bodied colleagues.
- Burnout. Burnout is a common problem among doctors. It is characterised by feelings of exhaustion, cynicism and detachment from work. Burnout can lead to decreased productivity, increased errors and even early retirement. Once burnout is present the doctor should be encouraged to change career to a more sustainable role.
- Competition. The medical field is very competitive. There are more applicants than there are medical school spots and training programs are also highly competitive. Making progress can be easier and better if the doctor looks for alternatives such as going abroad for experience.
- Hiring discrimination. Doctors who are from underrepresented groups may face discrimination when applying for jobs and advancing in their careers. Having a plan is important as many doctors will not want to involve an employment tribunal.
- Workplace bullying. Bullying is a problem in many workplaces and it can be especially harmful to doctors. Bullying can lead to decreased productivity, increased errors and even suicide. Finding another job is usually a better option than trying to fix the problem. Doctors should not feel that they must solve bullying workplaces although it good practice to tell someone.

- Changing technology. The medical field is constantly changing and doctors need to be able to adapt to new technologies and procedures. There is a risk that any job role will change. E.g. radiologists are likely to change their job role over the next decade or two. Training with AI can help ease that transition.
- Moving abroad. There may be training opportunities from moving abroad at some point in the career. For example, research in the USA, experience in a country with higher demand. Planning can help ensure that maximum benefit is gained.
- Regulations. The medical field is highly regulated. Doctors must comply with many rules and regulations. Some will require assistance to be able to properly prepare their paperwork for job applications or regulatory concerns particularly if they are in a non-standard training scheme.
- Lack of role models. Not everyone has role models who can show them what it is like to be a doctor and inspire them particularly if they want a non-standard career. The mentor may be able to introduce the doctor to a doctor who has had the same path.

The mentor should be able to offer practical advice or signpost where the doctor can find support. It is essential to recognise that doctors are often high maintenance and have greater needs, although will try to be self-sufficient. Doctor's occupational risks are called the five Ds - drugs, drink, depression, divorce and death.

The mentor will not have the specific skills to manage all these problems but must know where to get help. Doctors are more vulnerable because of the challenges that they face as well as often having limited social support outside of medicine. Postgraduate education is wasted if the doctor becomes unwell and is not able to work.

Planning a career.

The question of what the doctor wants to do is not answered by the mechanics of a career, the choice of speciality, examinations to sit and other necessary steps. They may wish to rise to the top, travel the world, use their qualification to join another career or create a portfolio. A doctor has not failed because they leave the world of medicine to become a comedian, nor are they a success if they retire in post.

It is the doctor's identity outside of medicine that is as important to whether their career is successful. A doctor whose mental health is deteriorating or is ambivalent about what they are doing will fail in life and medicine. The mentor needs to under the medical mask and consider who the doctor is and their real needs.

In that regard doctors are no different from other people, they have the same needs for a successful life. It is important as a mentor to check with the doctor that they are not forgetting the keys for resilience. These are necessary for resilience as without them the doctor will be vulnerable. The reverse is not true, even with these present a doctor can still be broken by the system.

- A strong support system. Doctors often deal with a lot of stress and pressure, so it's important to have a strong support system in place. This should include family, friends and colleagues who can help provide a sense of belonging.
- Time for self-care. Doctors need to make time for self-care, which could include exercise, relaxation, or hobbies. Taking care of their own mental and physical health is essential for doctors to be able to provide quality care to their patients.
- A healthy work-life balance. Doctors need to find a healthy work-life balance, which could mean working fewer hours, taking more vacations, or setting boundaries between their work and personal lives.
- A positive attitude. Doctors need to have a positive attitude, even when things are tough. This will help them to stay motivated and to provide the best possible care to their patients.

A holistic approach to planning a career would involve considering all the possible goals. This is more straightforward than planning each goal because it involves creating a list. The list can include initial analysis such as breaking down large goals into smaller, manageable steps. The purpose of the list is to consider what is possible, not to create a to-do list.

Listing all the possible goals provides an overall guide what is available. The doctor then needs to choose the best options to work on. What is best at any particular time depends upon what doors are open. Being open to the opportunities that are available means being flexible and open to adjusting your goals when needed.

Having an overall view also allows the doctor to understand the benefits of individual choices. They will be able to see how to make the most of the opportunities they are offered. They will be one step ahead in understanding realistically what they can gain from a situation.

Conclusions.

Postgraduate life for doctors is a transformative journey that goes beyond the transition from student to professional. It involves a shift in mindset and a series of choices that shape their career and personal life. As doctors navigate this phase, they must consider their values, skills and interests to develop meaningful goals that align with their aspirations. Setting SMART goals and breaking them down into smaller steps can make them more manageable and achievable.

However, doctors may encounter various barriers along their career path, such as sunk costs and high expenses, time commitments, academic challenges, stress, physical illness or disability, burnout, competition, discrimination, workplace bullying, changing technology, the possibility of moving abroad, regulatory complexities and the lack of role models. Mentors play a crucial role in identifying these barriers, offering practical advice and connecting doctors with the appropriate support resources.

It is important to recognise that doctors have unique occupational risks and face higher levels of stress, making their well-being a top priority. A strong support system, time for self-care, a healthy work-life balance and a positive attitude are essential components of a successful and fulfilling career in medicine. The mentor's role extends beyond the professional realm to help doctors maintain their mental health, identify their true needs and foster a sense of self outside of medicine.

Ultimately, the mechanics of a career, such as specialisation choices and examinations, are important, but a doctor's identity and overall well-being are equally vital. By addressing both professional and personal aspects, mentors can guide doctors toward a balanced and rewarding life in medicine. As doctors fulfil their potential and prioritise their holistic development, they can provide the best possible care to their patients and contribute positively to the field of healthcare.

Top tips.

Plan for your career and personal life: List of all the possible goals that you might want achieve in the next decade, making sure you align your goals with your values

Open doors by connecting with mentors, staying updated with changing technology and being open to opportunities.

Maintain a positive mindset by nurturing your identity, having a good work life balance and a supportive network of family, friends and colleagues.

Chapter 16: COMMUNICATION SKILLS

Communication can be considered from many perspectives and is arguably the most complex skill that humans possess. In simple terms communication is about the transmission of information by one person and the receipt of that information by the other person. In practice there are many different types of information that may be transmitted at the same time, the clarity of the transmission and the receipt can be impaired and the emotional responses can be important.

Communication can also be seen as one person trying to reprogram another person's software. This can be resisted by either party, the doctor may have their idea about what is causing the problems and resist the patient's ideas. The reprogramming might fail because the ideas do not link with the patient's ideas.

The skills of communicating are in the personal qualities of the doctor 'professionalism', whether the doctor performs all the necessary tasks, the objectives and the content. This classification has some advantages as it is simple and each of the skills mentioned are trainable.

The educator can teach how to behave in a professional way, the order of tasks in a consultation, what objectives the doctor wants to achieve and techniques that can be used. These different approaches then can be combined to provide the doctor with a comprehensive approach.

Personal qualities of a professional.

Doctors need to be able to communicate effectively with patients, colleagues and other healthcare professionals to provide quality care. Doctors who have developed useful personal qualities are more likely to be effective because they are able to evoke positive responses in the other person. Here are some of the key communication skills that doctors need written as personal qualities:

- Empathy: Doctors need to be able to empathise with patients to build trust and rapport. This means understanding and acknowledging patients' feelings and concerns. It may take time for the patient to open up and share their concerns. Patients may be feeling anxious or stressed when they see a doctor, so attending to their emotional needs and understanding their feelings and concerns can help with communication.

- Respect: Doctors need to treat patients with respect, regardless of their age, race, ethnicity, or socioeconomic status. This means being polite, considerate and non-judgmental. It also means being sensitive to patients' cultural beliefs and practices. Doctors should involve patients in decision-making about their care. This includes discussing treatment options, risks and benefits and the patient's preferences.

- Honesty: Doctors need to be honest with patients about their diagnosis, prognosis and treatment options. This means being truthful and avoiding sugar-coating the truth. Doctors need to be able to answer patient questions in a clear and concise way. They should also be able to provide additional information or resources if the patient needs them. Doctors should give feedback to patients about their progress and about any changes in their treatment plan. This helps to ensure that the patient is understanding and following the doctor's instructions. This can be difficult, but it is essential for building trust and ensuring that patients make informed decisions about their care.

- Professionalism: Doctors need to manage any situation calmly and professionally. They should maintain confidentiality and behave in a way that gives rise to trust. Doctors need to communicate in a professional manner, even in difficult situations. Doctors need to conduct themselves in a professional manner at all times. This means being respectful of patients, colleagues and other healthcare professionals. It also means being mindful of the ethical and legal implications of their actions.

The student will find it difficult to make these points actionable in their consultations. The problem is that the list is more of a series of aspirations than a guide to how to perform these. We will return to professionalism in more detail but at this point it is worth focusing on the link between professionalism and outcome.

A doctor who appears to have empathy will create a deeper emotional impression and achieve greater trust and engagement. Respecting others helps the doctor engage with those who have different life experiences. This can improve the chance of the patient complying with the treatment. Honesty has direct impacts on the patient attention to what is being said as well as improving the doctor's reputation.

Having the ability to use these professional qualities means that the doctor has a larger range of options to draw from. These qualities increase the emotional risk to the doctor as well as chance that the patient will take offence. Removing barriers to communication comes with benefits and burdens.

The tasks that are required in a consultation.

Communication skills can also be written as tasks that the doctor must perform to have effective communication. The doctor can work through the task list and when they have completed the list they will have done what is required. The problem with the list is that the doctor may attempt to perform a task but not succeed.

- Build rapport with patients: Doctors need to build rapport with their patients to get them to trust them and to be open with them about their medical history and symptoms. This can be done by being friendly, approachable and empathetic.

- Gather information from patients: Doctors need to be able to gather information from patients to make accurate diagnoses and to develop appropriate treatment plans. This includes asking open-ended questions, listening attentively and observing the patient's body language.

- Explain medical conditions and treatments to patients: Doctors need to be able to explain medical conditions and treatments to patients in a way that they can understand. This includes using clear language, avoiding jargon and being patient and understanding.

- Involve patients in decision-making: Doctors need to involve patients in decision-making about their care. This includes discussing treatment options, risks and benefits and the patient's preferences. Patient centred care is more likely to lead to a treatment plan that meets their needs.

- Involve the Team: Doctors need to be able to involve their team in the care of patients. Writing good medical records and discussions are examples of this. This is important for ensuring that patients receive coordinated and consistent information.

- Make effective use of technology: Technology can be a valuable tool for communication. Doctors can use technology to send patient education materials, make records and find useful information.

- Provide emotional support: Doctors may need to provide emotional support to patients who are facing difficult medical challenges. This can be done by listening to the patient, offering words of encouragement and helping the patient to develop coping mechanisms.

This way of describing the elements of communication is practical and task oriented. It makes communication look like a recipe to be followed and ignores that these activities occur simultaneously. The consultation rarely follows this neat order and usually jumps back and forth.

Medical students are often drawn to this model because it more closely aligns with their view of their role. They are attracted to the neutral nature of the tasks, the list does not state how they should achieve them. The student can use the method that feels most aligned with their views.

Objectives to achieve in a consultation.

A third way of explaining communication is to consider objectives of the communication, what the doctor wants to achieve by their communication. This approach is sometimes called the meeting of minds. The doctor is focused on the patient's experience of the communication rather than their check list. They can then use effective techniques to deal with problems in the communication.

- Active listening: Doctors need to be able to listen actively to patients in order to understand their concerns and needs. This means paying attention to what patients are saying, asking clarifying questions and showing empathy. One way to practice active listening is to repeat back what the patient has said in your own words. This shows that you have been listening and that you understand what they are saying.

- Clear and concise communication: Doctors need to be able to communicate clearly and concisely with patients, colleagues and other healthcare professionals. This means using language that is easy to understand and avoiding jargon. If you are not sure what the patient is saying, ask clarifying questions. This will help you to better achieve effective communication. Avoid using jargon or technical terms that the patient may not understand.

- Ideas, concerns and expectations (ICE). Doctors need to understand their patient's views and feelings to ensure that they are not missing emotional elements to the communication. The doctors should recognise the emotional factors are at least as important as cognitive factors for patient compliance and satisfaction.

- Timely. Doctors need to choose the right moment to share insights, sensitive information and bad news. They need to prepare the situation by choosing the correct location for the communication, that they have prepared the patient and relatives for the information and that the patient is emotionally available to the conversation.

- Confidentiality: Doctors need to keep patient information confidential but also to use that information effectively. This means not discussing patients' medical information with anyone who is not authorised to receive it. Equally doctors need to be able to communicate effectively with other healthcare professionals, such as nurses, pharmacists and other doctors. This is important for ensuring that patients receive coordinated and consistent care.

This model is difficult to apply to consultations because it appears to state the obvious. All students want to listen actively, communicate clearly and timely, understand what the patient thinks is important and keep it confidential. The model does not really explain how to achieve these goals.

As a diagnostic tool it can be applied to help students make sense of what they are doing wrong. They represent different focuses for attention so that the student can be too involved in listening to pick up cues. They can be too keen to communicate clearly to choose the right moment.

The educator can help the student maintain balance between these competing demands on their attention. They can help them take the time to understand the patient's point of view more fully before they give advice. This model can also be used by students to self evaluate their own communication skills.

Techniques of the communication.

A fourth way of understanding communication is to consider what is being communicated and the best methods for achieving this. Although the various communication elements are arranged in a logical order, they are not a task list. The doctor choses the correct element to deal with what is happening at that point of the consultation.

The doctor may start with discussing treatments and then move to cues and then to data gathering. This reflects observed behaviour by doctor in consultation with real life patients. The doctor should use the correct approach to deal with each element of the consultation when it arises rather than trying to follow an order.

- Establish rapport with the patient and allow the patient to say what they have prepared without interruption.
- Data gathering. Ask the patient questions about their illness, general health and lifestyle to understand the pattern of problems causing them to be unwell.

- Cues. Be alert to any cues that the patient gives that there may be sensitive information that they are finding difficult to share.
- Summarise what the patient has said and check that the doctor has fully understood what has been said.
- Describe the findings on examination and what these findings mean about the person's health.
- Treatment plan. Discuss the next steps for tests, referral or treatment and the rationale behind the recommendations and any alternative approaches.
- Education: Share any educational information that the patient needs to understand how they can manage their condition, prevent worsening and prognosis.
- Providing support. Attend to the patient's emotional language and give them time to process or problem solve their responses.
- Safety netting: Recommend a plan for monitoring and review and any safety netting issues such as worsening advice.
- Housekeeping. Ensure that the medical records are complete and the doctor has addressed all the issues in the consultation.

Each technique has a communication flow, the patient says their problem, they give background details, they use hints that there is more information and any emotions. The doctor describes what they have understood, findings on examination, what treatment they suggest, general education on the condition, advice on emotional consequences, plan for future care and writing notes.

The consultation moves from a patient centred to a doctor centred focus. The flow of information is largely controlled by the doctor and the technique is designed to maximise information flow. The techniques are aligned with the tasks but there is an important difference. The techniques are more explicit as to what the student should do and how they should do it.

This means that the student can learn to apply these techniques more effectively than the other ways of explaining the consultation. The techniques also more closely map the pattern of a medical consultation so involve less new learning. The focus on the technique means that there are many actionable elements.

The educator can show how the four ways of explaining the consultation can be used together. Personal qualities can improve outcomes as can keeping the consultation focused and on task. Having objectives that the doctor can check off can help them identify if they have missed something. Choosing the right technique means that they use the right approach to perform each task or objective.

Models.

There are many different communication skills models and the educator should choose a variety of the more popular models to discuss their strengths and weaknesses. One approach to teaching about models is to describe the model and ask the students to give their ideas about what insight the model gives them.

They can then discuss how useful that insight is and whether it can be applied to real life situations in any way. This approach is good at balancing a realistic view of the model with good engagement. The students can help each other spot the key learning point to maintain flow of the learning experience.

The Interpersonal Communication Model

The Interpersonal Communication Model is a communication model that views communication as a process that involves three elements: the sender, the message and the receiver. The model also emphasises the importance of context, which is the environment in which communication takes place.

> The sender is the person who initiates the communication process. The message is the information that the sender wants to convey to the receiver. The receiver is the person who receives the message from the sender. The context is the environment in which the communication takes place. The context can include factors such as the physical setting, the relationship between the sender and receiver and the culture in which the communication is taking place.

The Interpersonal Communication Model is a useful tool for understanding how communication works. It can help us to identify the different elements involved in communication and to understand how these elements interact with each other. The model can also help us to identify potential problems with communication and to develop strategies for improving communication.

The insight from the Interpersonal Communication Model is that in an audience different people will get different messages depending on the previous relationship they have with the speaker, their belief systems and their perception of the forum where the talk is occurring.

The Johari Window

The Johari Window: It is a four-quadrant model that shows how much information we share about ourselves with others. The quadrants are:

Open: This quadrant contains information that we know about ourselves and that others know about us.

Blind: This quadrant contains information that others know about us but that we do not know about ourselves.

Hidden: This quadrant contains information that we know about ourselves but that we do not share with others.

Unknown: This quadrant contains information that neither we nor others know about us.

The insight here is that we do not share all the information we have and as a doctor we should be aware that we know things about the person that they are blind to. Also there are hidden things that the person indicate they want to share by using cues. This means that a doctor must be careful when sharing information that they could assume the person knows and that they should pick up cues rather than believe that they know all the answers.

The Transactional Analysis Model

The Transactional Analysis Model: It is a model of communication that focuses on the roles that people play in relationships. The three main roles are:

Parent: This role is characterised by a nurturing and caring attitude.

Adult: This role is characterised by a rational and objective attitude.

Child: This role is characterised by a playful and spontaneous attitude.

The insight is that we can play different roles and there is a risk that the doctor will take on a parent role 'paternalistic' which would force the patient into the role of a child. This means that doctors should be careful to remain in adult role even if their patients try to behave like parents or children.

The Gricean maxims

The Gricean maxims are a set of four principles that govern effective communication. These principles are:

Quantity: Make your contribution as informative as is required for the current purpose of the exchange.

Quality: Do not say what you believe to be false.

Relation: Be relevant.

Manner: Be clear, brief and orderly.

The insight in the Gricean maxims is that being able to communicate in a clear, informative, truthful and relevant way is more effective. It can used to practice specific communication tasks such as common explanations.

The PACE model

The PACE model is a four-step process for active listening. This model is designed to help you listen to others with the intent to understand their perspective. The four steps are:

Pay attention: Focus on what the other person is saying and doing.

Ask questions: Clarify anything you don't understand.

Check for understanding: Summarise what you've heard to make sure you're on the same page.

Express empathy: Let the other person know that you understand and appreciate their perspective.

The PACE model insight is that both emotional and cognitive information should be listened to and feedback is important in communication.

The Active Listening Model

The Active Listening Model is a technique for listening effectively that involves paying attention to the speaker's words, body language and tone of voice and then reflecting back what you have heard to ensure understanding.

Pay attention to the speaker: This includes paying attention to the speaker's words, body language and tone of voice.

Reflect back what you have heard: This involves repeating back to the speaker what you have heard them say.

Ask clarifying questions: This involves asking questions to ensure that you have understood the speaker correctly.

Respond appropriately: This involves responding to the speaker in a way that is appropriate to the situation.

The Active Listening Model adds the further insight that body language and tone of voice are part of the message that the patient is giving.

The Non-Verbal Communication Model

The Non-Verbal Communication Model emphasises the importance of nonverbal communication, such as body language, facial expressions and tone of voice, in conveying meaning. Nonverbal communication can be used to reinforce or contradict verbal communication. It can also be used to express emotions, such as anger, sadness, or happiness. Nonverbal communication NVC can be a powerful tool for communication. However, it is important to be aware that nonverbal communication can be misinterpreted. For example, a smile can be interpreted as a sign of happiness or as a sign of nervousness.

The Non-Verbal Communication Model insight is that non-verbal can be inconsistent with verbal information and that can indicate that the patient is putting on a mask but also that interpreting NVC can be difficult.

The YAVIS model

The YAVIS model is a technique for giving feedback. This model is designed to help you give feedback in a way that is both constructive and positive. The four steps of the YAVIS model are:

> You: Start by focusing on the other person's behaviour.

> Are: Use the word "are" to describe the behaviour.

> Valuable: Focus on the positive aspects of the behaviour.

> Inspire: End by inspiring the other person to continue the behaviour.

The YAVIS model has the insight that positive feedback is far more effective than negative feedback. In practice finding something positive to say when asked for feedback will reduce the risk of negative effects.

The IMAGO Dialogue

The IMAGO Dialogue is a process for resolving conflict. This process is designed to help you and the other person understand each other's perspectives and to find common ground. The IMAGO Dialogue process consists of three steps:

> Mirroring: Repeat back to the other person what you've heard them say.

> Empathising: Put yourself in the other person's shoes and try to understand how they're feeling.

Dialogue: Once you've mirrored and empathised, you can begin to have a dialogue about the conflict.

The IMAGO Dialogue insight is that it is difficult to deal with conflict until rapport is established. Feeding back cognitive and emotionally the doctor's understanding of what the person has been saying will make them feel understood or find the cause of the conflict.

The Elaboration Likelihood Model (ELM)

The Elaboration Likelihood Model (ELM) is a model of persuasion that suggests that there are two routes to persuasion: the central route and the peripheral route. The central route is used when people are highly motivated to process information, while the peripheral route is used when people are less motivated.

> When people are highly motivated to process information, they are more likely to carefully consider the arguments presented in a message. They are also more likely to be persuaded by messages that are relevant to their interests and that are supported by strong evidence.

> When people are less motivated to process information, they are more likely to be persuaded by messages that are easy to understand and that contain attractive features, such as humour.

The Elaboration Likelihood Model (ELM) has an insight that doctors need at least two explanations, one that engages the heart and the other that engages the mind. Then can then choose the most appropriate for the situation.

The Social Judgment Theory model.

The Social Judgment Theory (SJT) is a model of persuasion that suggests that people evaluate messages by comparing them to their own attitudes.

> If the message is consistent with their attitudes, they are more likely to be persuaded. If the message is inconsistent with their attitudes, they are less likely to be persuaded.

> The SJT also suggests that people are more likely to be persuaded by messages that are moderate in their position. Messages that are too extreme are likely to be rejected, while messages that are too close to the person's own position are not likely to be persuasive.

The Social Judgment Theory (SJT) has the insight that doctor needs to understand their patient's point of view before choosing an explanation. The explanation should be chosen to be between a moderate position and the patient's point of view to be most effective.

The Theory of Reasoned Action model.

The Theory of Reasoned Action (TRA) is a model of behaviour that suggests that people's intentions to perform a behaviour are determined by their attitudes and beliefs about the behaviour and their perceived norms about the behaviour.

> The TRA suggests that people's attitudes about a behaviour are determined by their beliefs about the consequences of the behaviour. If people believe that the consequences of a behaviour are positive, they are more likely to have a positive attitude towards the behaviour.

> The TRA also suggests that people's perceived norms about a behaviour are determined by their beliefs about what other people think about the behaviour. If people believe that other people think that they should perform a behaviour, they are more likely to intend to perform the behaviour.

The TRA insight is that patients can be persuaded to undertake a behaviour if they believe that the consequences are good and other people think that it is a good idea. In practice this is useful when the patient fears the treatment.

The Theory of Planned Behaviour model

The Theory of Planned Behaviour (TPB) is an extension of the TRA that includes a person's perceived control over the behaviour as a factor in their intentions.

> The TPB suggests that people's perceived control over a behaviour is determined by their beliefs about the resources and opportunities they have to perform the behaviour. If people believe that they have the resources and opportunities to perform a behaviour, they are more likely to intend to perform the behaviour.

The TPB insight is that if a patient can see step by step how they can achieve the goal they are more likely to agree than if it seems too complicated.

The 7 Cs of Communication model.

The 7 Cs of Communication is a model of effective communication that emphasises the importance of being clear, concise, correct, complete, courteous, credible and consistent.

Clear: Communication should be easy to understand.

Concise: Communication should be to the point.

Correct: Communication should be free of errors.

Complete: Communication should provide all of the necessary information.

Courteous: Communication should be respectful and polite.

Credible: Communication should be from a reliable source.

Consistent: Communication should be consistent with other messages.

The insight is that the effectiveness of communication depends on the professional manner of the doctor. Actionable messages are preparing before giving communication and to consider the way it is presented.

The Relational Communication Model

The Relational Communication Model is a way of understanding how communication builds and maintains relationships. It is based on the idea that communication creates a relationship between people and this will influence how they understand what is being said. On a simple level this can be the establishment of rapport with the patient. On a more complex level this can be the combination of all the previous interactions. Any previous experience of how listening, empathy and trust went well or badly will influence the current communication.

The insight is that doctors and patients may come to the consultation with baggage and this may influence how they understand what is being said.

The Ladder of Inference

The Ladder of Inference: This model describes how individuals make assumptions and draw conclusions based on limited information. It highlights the importance of being aware of one's own mental processes and considering alternative interpretations before jumping to conclusions.

The insight in the Ladder of Inference is that the patient may appear to understand something but have missing information. This will alter their responses and it can be difficult to work out why they are reacting as they do.

The Five Love Languages:

The Five Love Languages: Although primarily used in the context of romantic relationships, this model can also be applied to other interpersonal interactions. It suggests that people have different ways of expressing and receiving love, such as through words of affirmation, acts of service, receiving gifts, quality time, or physical touch. Understanding these love languages can enhance communication and deepen connections.

This model has a number of insights relevant to medicine in particular how nurses achieve the impossible when they are caring for very sick or dying patients. The doctor may feel uncomfortable about receiving gifts or hugging a patient as they are personal acts. This model can help them understand where it is appropriate to incorporate a different approach.

The Conflict Resolution Model

The Conflict Resolution Model: This model provides a structured approach to resolving conflicts and reaching mutually satisfactory outcomes. It typically involves steps such as defining the issue, understanding perspectives, generating options, evaluating alternatives and reaching a resolution. It emphasises the importance of active listening, empathy and collaboration.

The insight from the Conflict Resolution Model is that there are specific tasks that can be used when dealing with an angry patient. The doctor does not have to get upset and fight back but can remain professional and use a technique.

The Cultural Dimensions Model

The Cultural Dimensions Model is a framework to understand and compare cultural differences. The model identifies six dimensions of culture:

- Individualism vs. Collectivism: This dimension refers to the degree to which people in a culture value individual or group goals. In individualistic cultures, people are more likely to value their own independence and achievement, while in collectivist cultures, people are more likely to value group harmony and cooperation.

- Power Distance: This dimension refers to the degree to which people in a culture accept that power is distributed unequally. In high-power distance cultures, people are more likely to accept that there is a natural order in which some people are superior to others, while in low-power distance cultures, people are more likely to believe that everyone is equal.

- Uncertainty Avoidance: This dimension refers to the degree to which people in a culture feel uncomfortable with uncertainty and ambiguity. In high-uncertainty avoidance cultures, people are more likely to feel anxious and stressed in situations that are unpredictable or unfamiliar, while in low-uncertainty avoidance cultures, people are more likely to be comfortable with change and ambiguity.

- Masculinity vs. Femininity: This dimension refers to the degree to which a culture values traditionally masculine or feminine traits. In masculine cultures, people are more likely to value assertiveness, competition and material success, while in feminine cultures, people are more likely to value cooperation, compassion and quality of life.

- Long-Term Orientation vs. Short-Term Orientation: This dimension refers to the degree to which a culture values long-term or short-term goals. In long-term oriented cultures, people are more likely to focus on saving and investing for the future, while in short-term oriented cultures, people are more likely to focus on immediate gratification.

The insights in the Cultural Dimensions Model are complex and multiple. The model provides a comprehensive method for analysing a difficult relationship. The 6 areas can be considered against the healthcare professionals experience of the patient and their family. Whilst it does not give direct answers it can provide an explanation of the difficulties and possible ways forward.

The Emotional Intelligence Model

The Emotional Intelligence Model: Emotional intelligence refers to the ability to recognise, understand and manage one's own emotions, as well as empathise with others. This model emphasises the importance of self-awareness, self-regulation, social awareness and relationship management in effective communication and interpersonal relationships.

The insight from the EI model is that some doctors will have less EI and need to use a broader range of tools to ensure effective communication.

Limitation of models.

The educator will want to cover the main communication models and may wish to consider some of the models from general practice. They are useful as a basis for discussion of the student or doctor's communication approaches. They are however quite theoretical and difficult to apply to real life situations.

The educator should therefore discuss the limitations of communication models with their students and ask them whether they believe that the criticisms apply. This will help them develop a critical understanding of communication and understand the difficulties of creating a model for communication.

In medicine the topic of communication recurs throughout the professional's career. It is important to elicit long term engagement of the student with communication skills. This is a careful balance between the student feeling that understanding is impossible and making them feel that there is one simple answer. Students need to have their personal journey towards understanding of communication.

- They are not always accurate. Communication skills models are based on research, but they are not always accurate representations of how people actually communicate. For example, some models suggest that people should always be polite and respectful, even when they disagree with someone. However, in some situations, it may be more effective to be direct and honest, even if it means being less polite.

- They can be too general. Communication skills models often focus on general principles of communication and do not provide specific advice for specific situations. For example, a model might suggest that people should always be clear and concise in their communication. However, what is clear and concise in one situation may not be clear and concise in another situation.

- They can be difficult to apply. Communication skills models can be difficult to apply, especially in high-pressure situations. For example, a person might know that they should be listening actively during a conversation, but they might find it difficult to do so when they are feeling stressed or anxious.

- The complexity of human communication. Human communication is a complex process that involves several factors, including verbal and nonverbal communication, context, culture and individual differences. Communication models are often unable to capture the full complexity of human communication.

- The limitations of language. Language is a limited tool for communication. It can be difficult to express complex ideas or emotions in words. Communication models that rely on language are therefore limited in their ability to capture the full range of human communication.

- The subjective nature of communication. Communication is a subjective process. The meaning of a message is not always clear or shared by all parties involved in the communication. Communication models that assume that the meaning of a message is objective are therefore limited in their ability to capture the full reality of human communication.

- They are based on assumptions: Communication models are based on assumptions about how communication works. These assumptions may not always be accurate. For example, the Transactional Model assumes that communication is a two-way street. However, this is not always the case. In some cases, communication may be one-way, such as when a teacher lectures to a class.

- They are simplified: Communication models are usually simplified representations of a complex process as a result, they can be misleading. For example, the Interpersonal Communication Model suggests that communication is a linear process. However, communication is actually a complex, nonlinear process.

The theory of communication is complex and it is difficult for the educator to help students to engage with the subject matter. Communicating feels very different from the theory and it can be difficult to diagnose what has gone wrong. Analysis of communication is not straightforward, even experts disagree as to classification.

The 4-step approach to communication (professionalism, tasks, objectives and techniques) can provide a structure for students to link their learning. It is practical and is tailored for doctors rather than other communication situations. The principles are general enough for another professional group such as managers to adapt the approach to their work.

Conclusions.

Communication skills are vital for doctors to effectively interact with patients, colleagues and other healthcare professionals. Successful communication requires a combination of personal qualities, performing specific tasks, setting clear objectives and using the write techniques.

Doctors' personal qualities play a crucial role in establishing trust and rapport with patients. Empathy, respect, honesty and professionalism are key qualities that contribute to effective communication. By understanding patients' emotions and concerns, doctors can provide the necessary support and create a supportive environment.

Performing tasks such as building rapport, gathering information, explaining medical conditions, involving patients in decision-making and utilising technology facilitate effective communication. These tasks ensure that patients receive comprehensive care, understand their conditions and treatment options and actively participate in their healthcare decisions.

Setting clear objectives helps doctors focus on the desired outcomes of communication. Active listening, clear and concise communication, understanding patients' ideas, concerns and expectations, timely sharing of information and maintaining confidentiality contribute to achieving these objectives.

The techniques used by doctors include establishing rapport, data gathering, recognising cues, summarising information, describing findings, discussing treatment plans, providing education and support, ensuring safety netting and managing administrative aspects. These techniques are actionable and can be used to improve communication.

While communication models provide frameworks for understanding and improving communication skills, they have limitations. Models can be inaccurate, too general, difficult to apply, fail to capture the complexity of human communication and rely on assumptions and simplifications. Each model can provide insights into aspects of communication.

There are numerous communication models available, each with its strengths and weaknesses. Educators can select popular models to stimulate discussions and encourage students to reflect on the insights provided by the models and their applicability to real-life situations.

In the field of medicine, communication skills are essential throughout a professional's career. Recognising the personal journey towards understanding effective communication and emphasising the importance of continuous learning and adaptation is crucial.

By continually honing their communication skills, doctors can enhance patient satisfaction, improve healthcare outcomes and build strong professional relationships. Effective communication is not a one-size-fits-all approach but a dynamic and evolving process that requires ongoing effort, self-reflection and empathy.

Top Tips.

Break down the consultation into a series of tasks, build rapport, gather information, explain, involve and support to keep the consultation organised.

Monitor progress with objectives, listen activity, communicate clearly, understand patients concerns, choose the right moment to explain and keep confidential.

Choose the right technique. Patient speaks without interruption, closed questions for data gathering, respond to cues, provide a summary, form a treatment plan, explain with illness model and record consultation.

Chapter 17: PREPARING LECTURES

Lectures are a traditional teaching method that involves a lecturer presenting information to a group of students. Lectures are a structured and often engaging learning experience for students and can be effective in transmitting factual information, but they can also be passive and disengaging for students.

The quality of lectures can dramatically impact the quality of the learning that occurs. A well designed and prepared lecture can achieve high quality learning outcomes. A poor quality lecture can be confusing and lead to disengagement with the topic.

When preparing a lecture, the educator should expect to put aside several hours to work on the various elements. This time commitment is necessary if the educator wants to provide the best possible learning experience. Much of the time is spent working out what to leave out and how to explain the learning objectives more simply.

Planning the lecture depends upon the learning objectives which are the heart of the lecture. The learning objective determine which concepts, processes and story that the educator wants to give. This means that it is important to conduct thorough research even on familiar topics.

The rough draft is used to translate the outline of the lecture into an audio-visual experience. It identifies all the work that will be required to achieve the desired results. The design and production of the visuals and improving the lecture can then be worked on.

Planning the lecture.

Preparing lectures requires careful planning and execution. Here are some tips for preparing effective lectures:

- Choose the learning objectives. A lecture cannot cover every element of a subject and at most can make three main learning objectives. Consider which learning objectives are best dealt with in a lecture so that you can focus on them.
- Do your research. Once you have chosen a topic, it is important to do your research. Even if you have a good understanding of the material there are always advances and new material you may be questioned on.
- Create an outline. Once you have done your research, it is a good idea to create an outline for your lecture. The outline should be

structured to include each of the main points in a logical way and a discussion around them including any evidence or examples you wish to use.

- Leave out irrelevant information. Where content does not contribute to the learning objectives, it is vague or complicated then it should be left out. The presumption should be to leave out material unless it contributes to the learning objectives rather than include everything that might be relevant.
- Practice your delivery. Once you have created an outline, it is important to practice your delivery. This will help you to become comfortable with the material and to ensure that you are able to present it in a clear and engaging way.
- Use visuals. Visuals can be a great way to engage your audience and to help them to understand the material. You can use slides, handouts, or even props to illustrate your points.
- Be prepared to answer questions. It is always a good idea to be prepared to answer questions from your audience. Where there is a common question or new advance preparing an answer will make them clear and concise.
- Be enthusiastic. The most important thing is to be enthusiastic about your topic. Explaining why the topic is important will help to get your audience excited about the material and to make the lecture more enjoyable for everyone involved.

The first lecture that an educator creates will lack many of these elements and should be used as an opportunity to practice and learn. There will be a disconnect between the visuals and the lecture content will lack the engaging nature. The educator should continue to work on that lecture until they create a high-quality lecture.

These steps will only allow the educator to produce an adequate lecture. It will perform reasonably and not be too boring. The students will be able to follow the chain of thought and achieve the objectives. To create high quality lecture the educator will take more work and a deeper understanding of the medium.

Rough draft.

Rough draft. The educator should create a rough draft which sets out the steps that the visuals will take to present the information. The purpose of this is to have an overview of the task so that each visual element can be worked on separately.

The rough draft transforms a lecture from an unlinked series of learning points into a complete whole. The slide is used as a foundation for a learning experience. Each slide is worked on until the educator has a series of powerful experiences that they can share. They are then linked into a coherent whole which takes the student through an audiovisual experience.

- Each slide, handout or video should have a tag to make it clear what the purpose of the slide is for. This means that it is easier to orientate and reorder if necessary.
- Start with a strong title. The title of your slide should be clear, concise and attention-grabbing, it may be the same as the tag but not always. It should give the audience a good idea of what the slide is about.
- Use a strong visual. A strong visual can help to engage the audience and make your presentation more memorable. The visual should be relevant to the topic of the slide and it should be large enough for everyone in the audience to see.
- Use a hierarchy of information. The most important information should be at the top of the slide and the less important information should be at the bottom.
- The slide should have text which is clear and concise with no more than three or four lines and ideally a font size of 72 for the title and 36 for the text. The orientation will normally be landscape.
- Use bullets to list your points. Bullets make it easy for your audience to follow your points and to take notes.
- Handouts: Handouts can be a great way to provide students with additional information or resources. The text will be normal size, portrait orientation and should be a summary of all the information rather than the slides.
- Prepare for questions. Anticipate any questions that your audience might have and be prepared to answer them.
- Keep your audience in mind. How will they respond to the material, would activities or assessment improve their engagement and interest.

Each component of the experience needs to be complete on their own but contribute. This means that the slide should be enough to identify the objective and an explanation. The handout should expand upon the slide's points in an accessible way that does not distract. The verbal component should be clear and consistent with the slide.

Use visuals.

Start with a clear purpose. What do you want your visuals to achieve? Do you want to illustrate a concept, provide data, or tell a story? Once you know your purpose, you can start to brainstorm ideas for your visuals. They need to be a hook that links with the objective and engaging to the student.

Finding the right visual can take time and access to resources. Having an idea what the right visual will look like can target the search. The following are suggestions as to the purpose that the right visual will take. They can help decide where to focus the search and make it easier to recognise the visual when it is found.

- Use visuals to emphasise important information: Visuals can be used to emphasise important information and to make sure that your audience remembers it.
- Use visuals to illustrate concepts. Visuals can help to illustrate concepts and make them easier to understand. For example, you could use a flowchart to illustrate a process or a diagram to illustrate a concept.
- Use visuals to explain processes. Visuals can help to explain processes step-by-step. For example, you could use a video to show how to perform a procedure or a series of images to show how something works.
- Use visuals to tell a story. Visuals can be used to tell a story that helps to engage your audience and make your lecture more memorable. When you tell a story with your visuals, make sure that it is clear, concise and relevant to your topic.
- Use visuals to engage your audience. Visuals can help to engage your audience and keep them interested in your presentation. For example, you could use humour, animation, or other eye-catching elements in your visuals.
- Use visuals to support your arguments. Visuals can help to support your arguments and make them more persuasive. For example, you could use statistics or graphs to show the evidence for your claims.

Visuals that emphasise important information are relatively easy to find, a visual for this chapter might say 'keep it simple'. Searching for that phrase would lead to many options. Concepts may be a good choice if there is a visual component such as happy students. Processes can be visually represented as a machine. 'A picture paints a 1000 words' and this can be a story. Evidence can be presented visually as a graph.

With generative AI the need to use pre-prepared visuals is reducing. The educator can draw their own idea or write it as a text and get the AI to improve it. This means that creating visuals will take longer and require more input. The resulting visuals should be more relevant and engaging than copying an artist's work.

Visual tools.

The best visual tool for you will depend on your needs and preferences. If you are looking for a simple and easy-to-use tool, PowerPoint or Google Slides may be a good option. If you need a more powerful tool that can create high-quality visuals, Adobe Illustrator or Adobe Photoshop may be a better choice. Check that the lecture hall has compatible IT and be prepared to change the file type if required.

Whatever you choose make sure that you are familiar with the program and you know how to use it effectively. It is better to use a simple program that you know you can get results than start on a learning curve for a program that you do not know. Technical problems when presenting can generate substantial disruption.

- PowerPoint is a popular and easy-to-use software program that can be used to create a variety of visuals, including slides, charts and graphs.
- Google Slides is a free online presentation tool that offers many of the same features as PowerPoint.
- Canva is a web-based graphic design platform that can be used to create a variety of visuals, including infographics, posters and flyers.
- Adobe Illustrator is a powerful vector graphics software program that can be used to create high-quality visuals.
- Adobe Photoshop is a popular image editing software program that can be used to enhance and edit photographs and images.

These are not universally available so the educator should be able to change to low tech methods such as a whiteboard, chalkboard or a flip chart. A laptop or tablet can be used with a projector. Posters and a laser pointer can be highly effective when in low tech environments.

Other useful tools in a lecture are a copy of the syllabus, a list of frequently asked questions and a textbook. Bringing a microphone and a timer can solve technical difficulties. Being prepared for disaster means that it is much less likely to occur.

Designing visuals

Graphic designers will still be important when creating visuals for lectures. AI is very good at producing art that is attractive and partially relevant. It is not good at adding creative details and improving the relevance based upon further prompts. The educator will need a graphic designer to work on these generated images.

Designing visuals with a graphic designer requires an idea of what you want them to look like. The graphic designer needs to understand the purpose of the visuals and general guidance as to your specific needs. This is much easier if you send AI generated ideas with suggestions as to improvements.

- Keep it visually simple. Visuals should be easy to understand and follow and should not distract from your lecture.
- Use high-quality images: Images should be high-resolution and should be relevant to the topic of your lecture.
- Use animation and transitions: Animation and transitions can be used to add interest to your visuals and to make your lecture more engaging.
- Use colour and imagery. Colour and imagery can help to make your visuals more visually appealing and memorable.
- Use white space to make your slides easy to read. White space is important for readability. It helps to break up the text and to make the slide less cluttered.
- Use visuals to create a sense of flow: Visuals can be used to create a sense of flow in your lecture and to make it easier for your audience to follow along.
- Use visuals to break up your lecture: Visuals can be used to break up your lecture and to make it easier for your audience to follow along.
- Use clear and concise language: The text on your visuals should be easy to read and should not be too long. Avoid using too much text or complex graphics.
- Be consistent. Use the same fonts, colours and styles throughout your visuals. This will help to create a cohesive look.

The design of slides and other visual materials should occur in conjunction with the other aspects of the lecture. An idea of how to explain the concept may change the way the visual needs to work. Having a rough draft can make it easier to add and remove details. Do not allow technical details distract from creating a compelling learning experience.

Improving a lecture.

Once the lecture is planned and the materials and outline are prepared the educator should improve the lecture. This means adding further elements whose purpose is to improve student engagement and provide memory hooks for the learning objectives to be placed upon.

- Start with a hook, the best hooks are short questions or promises, they use strong and specific language and are attention grabbing. For example, 'The secret to giving a lecture that students will actually remember.' 'How to create a lecture that is so engaging that students will beg for more.'
- Use active learning strategies. Active learning strategies involve students in the learning process. This can be done through out of lecture activities such as group work, problem-solving exercises and class discussions.
- Make the lecture interactive. This can be done by asking questions, inviting students to share their thoughts and providing opportunities for students to participate in activities.
- Use humour. Humour can help to make the lecture more engaging and to help students to remember the material. The best humour is also a hook as it links the student to what will be learned.
- End with a summary. This will help students to remember the key points of the lecture. The summary should be action based directing the students to do a task as a result of the information. For example 'Write your lecture, improve the lecture and add great visuals.'

Hooks can be a personal story, a question, a statistic, a quote, a description, a problem, a challenge or a call to arms. If a hook does not work then try a different one or use a story or humour. The hook gives purpose so it is the single most important part of the lecture. Without a hook the students will have to find their own reason for paying attention.

Improving the lecture often involves scrapping a slide and starting again. Educators can feel overwhelmed with the workload of tens of slides in tens of lectures. They can feel that they must prepare other teaching materials and do not have time to create great lectures.

The planning the lecture section is designed to get an adequate lecture that can be delivered. The educator should return to that lecture once they have time to do so and improve it. Once they have written one great lecture and seen the response from students they will not want to give an adequate lecture again.

Conclusions.

Preparing effective lectures requires careful planning and execution. By choosing clear learning objectives, conducting thorough research, creating a well-structured outline and leaving out irrelevant information, educators can provide a focused and engaging learning experience for their students.

Practicing the delivery and using visuals, such as slides, handouts, or props, can further enhance the lecture and help illustrate key concepts. It is important to be prepared to answer questions and to maintain enthusiasm for the topic, as this can greatly impact student engagement.

Creating a rough draft and using visual tools can assist in organising and designing the visuals for the lecture. Keeping visuals visually simple, using high-quality images, animation, transitions and employing consistent design elements can make the visuals more effective and visually appealing.

To improve a lecture further, educators can incorporate hooks at the beginning to grab students' attention, use active learning strategies and interactivity throughout. They can include humour to engage students and aid in memory retention and end with a summary that highlights the key points and encourages students to take action based on the information learned.

Overall, the quality of a lecture can greatly impact the learning outcomes for students. By following these guidelines and continuously striving to improve, educators can create lectures that are engaging, informative and memorable, fostering an effective learning environment.

Top tips.

Identify the main learning objectives of the lecture and communicate them to students at the beginning. Repeat them to link them with further information.

Make it interesting. Hooks starting with a question or a surprising fact. Visual summaries, such as charts, graphs and diagrams. Active learning, asking questions or activities. Tell relevant stories or jokes.

End with a summary and action points. At the end of the lecture, summarise the key points and provide actionable tasks that students can do to reinforce their learning.

Chapter 18: SMALL GROUP TEACHING AND FACILITATION

Small group teaching is a teaching method in which a small group of students (typically 3-10) learn together with the help of a facilitator. The facilitator's role is to guide the discussion, encourage participation and ensure that all students are learning.

Small group teaching has a number of advantages over traditional lecture-based teaching. It allows for more active learning, individualised attention and collaboration and teamwork. Students learn to work together to solve problems and to share their ideas.

It is an expensive approach to learning and may not be necessary for all students and all learning. It is important to consider the fit between the needs of the students and the type of learning that is chosen. A topic with a high fact burden that needs to be understood passively would not be a good fit for the student's learning needs.

Small group teaching can provide unique assessment opportunities. It is essential when planning a small group teaching session to build in assessment tools. These tools range from an assessment of team roles to flexibility of thinking and diagnosis of problems with learning.

Small group teaching also has a remedial role, it allows the educator to offer more intensive assistance. The group can provide a structure for individuals learning so that they can grasp difficult concepts. The group is essential when teaching complex interpersonal skills such as teambuilding.

When planning teaching a topic the educator should consider all options against their objectives. The correct teaching method to achieve the objectives can be modified if for instance a group is having difficulties emotionally or in learning. Small group teaching should not be the default.

Factors favouring Small Group Teaching

A group that requires individualised instruction with opportunities to practice their skills, emotional and learning support will benefit from small group teaching. They will have increased social skills, self esteem and can be monitored more intensely by the educator. They will learn to collaborate in their learning and have increased motivation.

- Increased individualised instruction: In a small group setting, the teacher can provide more individualised instruction to each student.

This can help students to learn at their own pace and to address any areas where they may be struggling.

- More opportunities for practice: In a small group setting, students have more opportunities to practice what they are learning. This can help them to solidify their understanding of the material and to develop their skills.

- More positive learning environment: Small group settings can often be more positive and supportive learning environments than large lecture halls. This can help students to feel more comfortable and engaged in their learning.

- Active learning. Small group teaching promotes active learning. Students are more likely to be engaged and involved in the learning process when they are working with other students and the facilitator. This can help students to better understand the material and to develop their critical thinking and problem-solving skills.

- Increased social skills: Small groups can help students to develop their social skills. they must learn to communicate effectively, listen to each other's ideas and consider different perspectives.

- Improved self-esteem: Small groups can help students to improve their self-esteem. They can learn that their contribution is useful and respected.

- Build relationships between students and the facilitator: In a small group setting, students have more opportunities to get to know the facilitator and the facilitator can better monitor individual student progress.

- Collaboration: Small group teaching can help students to develop their collaboration skills. When students work together to solve a problem, they must learn to communicate effectively, listen to each other's ideas and consider different perspectives.

- Increase motivation and engagement: Small group teaching can help to increase student motivation and engagement in the learning process. Students are more likely to be motivated to learn when they are working in a small group setting and when they feel like they are part of a community of learners.

Working in small groups is a learned skill and the educator may need to focus on housekeeping activities particularly with an inexperienced group. The educator will need to develop specific learning materials and analysis of individual students needs. This preparation may not reusable as it will not apply to a different group.

The educator should have a full range of supportive materials available even if they are not used. This ensures that the small group teaching is not disrupted by lack of direction. Where remedial work is required this can be extensive. Other students should not be left to fill the gaps in the preparation.

Roles for a facilitator.

The educator is responsible for facilitating the small group work. The preparations should be sufficient so that the facilitator can concentrate on these tasks. It is very challenging to both facilitate and teach at the same time. The educator should focus on the following tasks when facilitating.

- Manage the discussion: The facilitator should manage the discussion to ensure that it remains on track and that all students have a chance to participate. This can be done by keeping the discussion moving, by redirecting the discussion when necessary and by summarising the discussion periodically.
- Provide feedback: The facilitator should provide feedback to students throughout the discussion. This can be done by asking clarifying questions, by summarising students' contributions and by providing positive feedback.
- Summarise the discussion: At the end of the discussion, the facilitator should summarise the key points that were discussed. This can help students to solidify their understanding of the material and to identify any areas where they need further clarification.

Facilitation can be achieved by different styles of interaction in small group teaching. The facilitator can be a guide, a coach, a mentor, or a mediator. The style of facilitator's role will vary depending on the specific needs of the group and the learning objective.

There is some overlap between guide, a coach, a mentor, or a mediator but it is helpful to consider them separately. Identifying the style of help that a group requires and providing the correct facilitation requires experience. An educator will need training in these various approaches so that they are proficient.

- Guide: Guides can be helpful for people who are new to a particular area or who are facing a difficult challenge. A guide is someone who leads or directs someone or something. A guide can help the group to set goals, develop strategies for achieving those goals and overcome obstacles.
- Coach: Coaches can help people to reach their full potential, both personally and professionally. Coaching can be helpful for group who are looking to improve their performance in a particular area,

such as understanding or clinical skills. They can identify gaps in the knowledge or diagnose problems and give insight.

- Mentor: A mentor is someone who provides guidance and support when practicing skills. This can be advice, support and encouragement when the student is roleplaying or talking to a patient. The type of support is more informal and collaborative in nature.
- Mediator: A mediator is a neutral third party who helps two or more people to resolve a conflict. Mediators are impartial and do not take sides. Mediators typically have training in conflict resolution and mediation. Mediators are trained to listen to both sides of a conflict, identify the underlying issues and help the parties to reach a mutually agreeable solution.

When facilitating the educator is part of the group rather than a teacher. This can be challenging for some educators who lapse into teaching mode. The transition between 'sage on the stage' to 'guide by the side' takes practice and experience to achieve well. The educator may need to explain the difference between these roles.

Running a small group.

Ensuring that the small group runs smoothly involves some simple steps. Preparing the teaching materials is more complex than for other sorts of teaching. The educator needs to be prepared for the group discussion taking a different approach to the topic. The educator will be busy with the facilitator role and should avoid trying to teach to fill gaps.

- Teaching materials: Small groups need a good summary of the topic, clear instructions as to what their task is, reference materials that are easy to use during the discussion and further learning.
- Be prepared: Before the group meets, make sure you have a clear plan for the discussion. This will help you keep the discussion on track and ensure that all students have a chance to participate.
- Set clear expectations: At the beginning of the session, the facilitator should clearly explain the expectations for student participation. This includes things like the ground rules, the desired outcomes and the roles and responsibilities of each group member.
- Create a positive learning environment: The facilitator should create a positive and supportive learning environment where students feel comfortable sharing their ideas and asking questions. This can be done by being welcoming and encouraging, by using active listening skills and by providing positive feedback.

- Encourage participation: The facilitator should encourage all students to participate in the discussion. This can be done by calling on students by name, round-robin discussion, by asking open-ended questions and by summarising the discussion periodically to ensure that everyone is on the same page.
- Be an active listener: When students are talking, listen carefully and ask clarifying questions. This will help you to understand their perspectives and to ensure that they are understood by the rest of the group.
- Be patient: It takes time for students to get used to working in small groups. Be patient and understanding and help them to learn how to participate effectively.

There is a risk that the small group will misunderstand the topic and discuss incorrect ideas. The educator should avoid trying to correct the group and should instead focus on facilitating the discussion. A common problem with increasing participation is that it increases the risk of disruption from individuals who have issues.

The educator may feel conflicted between helping the group manage the disruption and correcting the incorrect ideas. The priority in small groups is to ensure that the group does not become dysfunctional. By creating a positive learning environment the group can actively listen to each person's contribution and clarify inconsistencies.

Often the teaching materials will be used to challenge an incorrect idea or another student will question the idea. Learning is a journey and the process of active listening will ensure that all students participate. Being patient can help the group address the incorrect idea more thoroughly and effectively than challenging them.

Disruptive Elements

There will often be disruptive elements in small groups which can negate some of the advantages. Asking these individuals to not be part of small groups, setting ground rules and managing their behaviour are all useful.

The first step should be to use social pressure from the group to reduce the disruption and its effects. This allows the group to learn self-management behaviours and to become independent of the facilitator. These methods feel less personal to the individual as they place responsibility with group rather than the individual.

- Talk to the whole group. If the disruptive behaviour is affecting the entire group, it can be helpful to talk to the group as a whole about the importance of respectful communication and collaboration.

- Encourage group members to speak up. If someone is being disruptive, it can be helpful to encourage other group members to speak up and say something. This can help to create a sense of accountability and make it more likely that the disruptive behaviour will stop.

- Provide training on conflict resolution. If disruptive behaviour is a recurring problem, it may be helpful to provide training on conflict resolution to group members. This can help them to learn how to effectively deal with conflict in a constructive way.

When the disruptive behaviour occurs during the session and social pressures are ineffective then further steps will be needed. The educator will need to address the behaviour directly to prevent the learning from being halted.

- Address the behaviour immediately. Don't wait for the disruption to escalate before taking action. The sooner you address the behaviour, the easier it will be to resolve.
- Be direct and assertive. Don't beat around the bush. State the behaviour that is unacceptable and explain why it is a problem.
- Be respectful. Even though the behaviour is unacceptable, it is important to be respectful of the person who is exhibiting the behaviour. Remember that they may not be aware that their behaviour is disruptive.
- Be specific. Don't just say, "You're being disruptive." Instead, be specific about what the person is doing that is disruptive. For example, you could say, "You're interrupting other people when they're speaking."
- Offer a solution. Once you've addressed the behaviour, offer a solution. For example, you could say, "Please wait until someone is finished speaking before you say anything."
- Follow through. If the behaviour continues, you need to follow through with the consequences that you have outlined. This may mean speaking to the person again, or it may mean taking further action, such as removing them from the group.

There is a difference between those who disrupt the group but are not contributing to the group aims and those who disrupt the group with ideas. The latter person is called a plant and they need special management in a small group. The group needs to learn to understand how to manage and respect the contribution of the plant.

Managing the Plant.

The Plant role in Belbin's Team Roles Model is a creative, innovative and good at generating new ideas. They are often seen as the "idea person" on the team and they are able to come up with new and innovative solutions to problems. Plants are typically free-thinkers and are not afraid to challenge the status quo. They are also good at seeing the big picture and can think outside the box.

However, Plants can also be seen as being aloof and detached from the team. They may be so focused on their own ideas that they may struggle to communicate effectively with the rest of the team. They can also be forgetful and absent-minded, which can lead to problems with completion of tasks.

Plants are both a hidden strength and a great weakness of small group work, their creativity can help and hinder the small group at the same time. They are good at providing new ways of looking at the problems but this disrupts the group through cognitive dissonance.

Cognitive dissonance is a state of discomfort caused by holding two conflicting beliefs, values, or attitudes. It is a normal and common human experience and can increase engagement and motivation. It can also lead to negative consequences, such as denial, rationalisation and aggression.

Where the contributions are unusual then it is worth reflecting whether they can be incorporated into the learning and increase engagement. Many groups contain plants who can see aspects of the problem that the educator have not. The plant's contribution can be creative and inspiring.

- They can provide new perspectives. Plants often come from different backgrounds and experiences than educators, which can give them a unique perspective on a problem.

- They can be creative problem-solvers. Plants are often not afraid to think outside the box, which can lead to new and innovative solutions to problems.

- They can be inspiring role models. Plants can show other students that it is possible to be successful, even if they are different from the majority.

There are general steps that the educator can take to help the plant function well within a small group. The educator can model these steps and encourage others to recognise and support plants and respond to their ideas. They can help reduce resistance by identifying those who dislike cognitive dissonance and help them become more flexible.

- Give them time to warm up. Plants may be shy at first, so give them time to get to know the team and feel comfortable sharing their ideas. They are often slow to get to the point and patience can be worthwhile.

- Be open-minded. Don't dismiss a plant's contribution just because it is different from what you expected. Instead, take the time to understand their perspective and see how it can add value to the group.

- Be supportive. Plants may be hesitant to share their ideas if they feel like they will be judged or ridiculed. Make sure to create a safe and supportive environment where plants feel comfortable sharing their thoughts.

- Collaborate: Build on their ideas so that other group members can understand what the plant is contributing.

- Don't be afraid to challenge them. Plants can sometimes get so caught up in their own ideas that they lose sight of the big picture. Be willing to challenge them to think outside the box and consider other perspectives.

- Be flexible. Be willing to adjust your plans and activities to accommodate the contributions of plants. This may mean changing the way you teach a lesson, or it may simply mean giving plants more time to share their ideas.

- Learning materials: Having prepared materials about the plant and how they can help the group can improve the group's understanding and acceptance of the plant.

These steps can ensure that the facilitator avoids many of the issues with having plants in groups. The plant will feel included in the group and their ideas will be heard. It is possible to go further than this and help the plant develop their skills to a higher level. Plants have the capacity to develop high level skills if they can overcome their problems.

Developing the Plant.

Plants have specific problems which they need help with such as finding it difficult to communicate their ideas, they often have low self confidence as their ideas can be shouted down and may have less developed social skills. There are general steps that can help the plant become integrated with the group.

- Opportunities to lead. Plants can often be shy and hesitant to speak up in class, but they may be more comfortable taking on a leadership role in a smaller group setting. Consider giving plants the opportunity to lead small group discussions, or to work on projects with a small team of students.

- Provide plants with extra support. A plant may struggle to keep up with the material as they have a deeper engagement with the material. They may require one-on-one tutoring or creation of a modified learning plan that is tailored to their individual needs.

- Encourage plants to collaborate with other students. Plants can often benefit from collaborating with other students who struggle with creativity. This can help these other students develop respect for the plant's contribution and both will benefit from the collaboration.

- Celebrate plants' successes. When a plant makes a contribution to the group, be sure to celebrate their success. This will help to boost their confidence and encourage them to continue participating. Other students will understand the role of the plant better.

One-to-one assistance to plants is often necessary so that they can engage more effectively. The plant will often see themselves as disruptive to the group and feel that their ideas are not valuable.

- Name the Plant. Give the student a better understanding of their own identity by giving a name to their situation. Understanding what a plant is and how it can contribute to the functioning of a small group. Plants can play a valuable role in groups by providing different perspectives, asking questions and listening to others.

- Forum. Plants are poor at choosing the forum (right time and place and method) to share their ideas. Whilst it is important for any student to have the right effect plants will need more help. They should not interrupt someone else who is speaking and they should not try to dominate the conversation.

- Social skills. Plants may lack social skills and require help. Students who are struggling to engage in group discussions may also need help developing social skills. This includes learning how to listen to others, how to disagree respectfully and how to build relationships with other group members.

- Scripts. If a plant needs to explain the same insight many times in different situations, practicing may be helpful. Educators using educational techniques can help plants find a clear and concise script that they can use to explain their point.

Each of these strategies can help all students to improve their group skills but plants benefit more than most. This is because other types of student will develop these strategies without help. The plant is dependent on facilitation to ensure that they can overcome their weaknesses.

Plants often prefer to work independently and this allows them to develop their ideas and take risks. Most plants find collaborative work more satisfying because they can bounce their ideas off another person. The ideas generated in collaboration are of a higher standard, contains less errors and are easier to follow.

Small group teaching methods.

Small group teaching methods are the different ways that a session can be structured. They can be based upon opinions in a discussion, solving problems, experiencing and observing role play or coming up with ideas.

The best small group teaching method depends on the specific topic being taught and the needs of the students. However, all facilitators should strive to create a safe and supportive environment where students feel comfortable sharing their ideas.

- Brainstorming: The facilitator poses a question to the group and students generate as many ideas as possible. This can be a helpful way to come up with new ideas or to solve problems.
- Peer support. The group focuses on teambuilding and helping students who are struggling to catch up.
- Problem-solving: The facilitator presents a problem to the group and students work together to find a solution.
- Role-playing: Students take on different roles and act out a scenario. This can be a useful way to explore different perspectives and to learn how to deal with conflict.
- Discussion: The facilitator leads a discussion on a particular topic. Students are encouraged to share their ideas and to challenge each other's thinking.

The educator should make it clear in the teaching materials and the introduction what is expected of the students. Where the group is unfamiliar with the type of activity they may require additional training and specific teaching materials.

The materials should be comprehensive enough so that the students can run the group without assistance. This means that the educator can concentrate on facilitating the group rather than trying to teach the group about the subject.

Brainstorming:

Brainstorming is a group creativity technique by which efforts are made to find a conclusion for a specific problem by gathering a list of ideas spontaneously contributed by its members. The brainstorming method is frequently used in business for new product development, as well as in schools for creative writing.

Brainstorming typically follows a four-step process:

1. Define the problem or topic. The first step is to clearly define the problem or topic that the group is trying to brainstorm about. This will help to focus the group's efforts and generate more relevant ideas.

2. Gather a group of people. The ideal size for a brainstorming group is 6-12 people. A group that is too large can be difficult to manage, while a group that is too small may not generate enough ideas.

3. Set a time limit. Brainstorming sessions typically last for 30-60 minutes. This helps to keep the session focused and prevents the group from getting bogged down in any one idea.

4. Generate ideas. During the brainstorming session, there are four basic rules that should be followed:

   o No criticism. During the brainstorming session, no idea should be criticised or evaluated. This allows people to feel free to share their ideas, even if they seem crazy or unrealistic.

   o Quantity is important. The goal of brainstorming is to generate as many ideas as possible. Don't worry about the quality of the ideas at this stage; just focus on quantity.

   o Build on each other's ideas. Encourage people to build on each other's ideas. This can help to spark new ideas and generate even more creativity.

   o Have fun! Brainstorming should be a fun and relaxed experience. If people are stressed or anxious, they will be less likely to share their ideas.

The educator should give feedback on performance particularly the benefits and limitations. This means recognising when the group has achieved an objective and general feedback. The following are examples of the types of comment that the educator can use.

Brainstorming has a number of benefits, including:

- Increased creativity. You were thinking outside the box and come up with new and innovative ideas.

- Improved problem-solving skills. The group is providing a forum and people are feeling happy to share their ideas and work together to find solutions.

- Increased productivity. You are working collaboratively, focusing your efforts and generating more relevant ideas.

- Improved communication skills. You are getting better at sharing your ideas and working together to achieve a common goal.

Brainstorming is not without its limitations, including:

- Groupthink. There is some Groupthink, you are so focused on reaching consensus that you are failing to consider all of the possible options.

- Free-riding. There is some Free-riding is some people are contributing more ideas than others how can we get everyone's ideas before people feel resentment and frustration.

- Poor facilitation. I am not doing well with facilitating this group which is making it difficult to generate and maintain a high level of creativity.

The above description of brainstorming can help a group get more out their experience. These teaching materials are more helpful than general guidelines as they set out what is required in a specific way. They allow the group to read what is required and find their own way to that outcome.

All small group work is an opportunity for teamwork and providing the group with teaching materials that they can refer can improve this. The person in the group who has read the materials will be able to guide the group into better performance.

Peer support

Peer support is the act of providing emotional, social and practical support to a peer. In the context of small group teaching, peer support can be provided by students to each other. This can be done in a variety of ways, such as:

- Collaborating on assignments. When students work together on assignments, they can learn from each other's strengths and weaknesses. They can produce a piece of work that neither could have managed on their own.

- Helping each other to understand the material. If one student is struggling to understand a concept, another student can often explain it in a way that makes more sense. This can help the struggling student to catch up and to avoid falling behind.

- Providing encouragement. Sometimes, all it takes to help a student succeed is a little bit of encouragement. When students work together, they can offer each other support and motivation. This can help them to stay on track and to reach their goals.

Peer support requires knowledge of each person's roles in the group. They need to understand how to ensure that the group is not dysfunctional. It is important not to leave peer support to a single individual but see it as a group responsibility.

Practicing peer support can be beneficial for all participants as they gain insight into how to ask for help and what can be provided. Educators should be ready to use an opportunity that becomes available rather than trying to artificially construct a situation. This means that the group needs access to appropriate teaching materials in advance.

Problem-solving

Problem-solving is a skill that can be learned and improved with practice. It is a process of identifying a problem, generating solutions and evaluating the effectiveness of those solutions. Problem-solving is an important skill in both personal and professional life.

- Define the problem. It is important to clearly define the problem before you can start to generate solutions. This means being able to identify the specific symptoms of the problem, as well as the underlying causes. Once you have a clear understanding of the problem, you can start to generate possible solutions.

- Generate solutions. There are many different ways to generate solutions to a problem. One common approach is brainstorming. Brainstorming is a process where you generate as many ideas as possible, without judging or criticising any of them. This can be a helpful way to come up with creative solutions to problems.

- Choose a solution. Once you have generated a list of possible solutions, you need to choose one. This involves considering the pros and cons of each solution, as well as the resources that are available. It is also important to consider the feasibility of each solution. Some solutions may be more feasible than others, depending on the resources that are available.

- Implement a solution. Once you have selected a solution, you need to implement it. This may involve making changes to your behaviour, your environment, or your resources. It is important to be patient and persistent when implementing a solution. It may take some time to see results.

- Evaluate the solution. Once you have implemented a solution, you need to evaluate it to see if it has been effective. If the solution is not effective, you may need to go back to try other solutions.

Problem-solving is a skill that can be learned and improved with practice. The ability to create a comprehensive list of solutions can improve the overall performance. Applying this technique to working on a problem alone can be difficult. Students often stop at two or three options and fail to analyse their choices.

Iterative problem solving is a new technique where the students are asked to generate further solutions after they have chosen one. They can often identify a better solution but are reluctant to share it with others. Further iterations can often generate further solutions as the process of defining the initial ideas can leave gaps.

Discussion

Discussion is a technique in which group members share their ideas and perspectives on a particular topic. It works by ensuring that the group understands what each person is saying. It is therefore the ability to listen and clarify rather than giving the most eloquent ideas that is important.

Directions for the group can be to identify new, interesting and novel approaches to the subject. These will include new insights and perspectives, different ways of solving problems and a list of the pros and cons. Focusing on collecting a larger range of opinions rather than finding a single best answer improves this type of learning.

Benefits of discussion include:

- Increased understanding: Discussion can help group members to understand different perspectives on a topic. This can lead to a deeper understanding of the topic and insights.

- Improved problem solving: Discussion can help group members to identify and solve problems. By sharing their ideas, group members can come up with a wider range of solutions than they would be able to come up with on their own.

- Enhanced decision making: Discussion can help group members to make better decisions. By discussing the pros and cons of different options, group members can make a more informed decision.

Tips for conducting a successful discussion include:

- Set a clear goal: Before the discussion begins, it is important to set a clear goal. What is material or has a logical connection to the subject?

- Choose the right participants: The participants in the discussion should be people who have different perspectives on the topic. Identifying gaps can help students fill those gaps.

- Create a safe environment: The participants in the discussion should see the process of discussing pros and cons part of the process not a personal attack on them.

- Encourage participation: The facilitator should encourage all participants to contribute to the discussion. This can be done by asking questions, summarising the discussion and calling on people who have not spoken yet.

- Legal thinking. A technique law that can help discussions is to consider when two diametrically opposed views would be correct. At each extreme the different views are correct and then ask if both views can be right at the same time.

- Be respectful: All participants should be respectful of each other's ideas. This means that it is important to find pros for ideas that you disagree with and cons for ideas that you believe in.

- Summarise the discussion: At the end of the discussion, the facilitator should summarise the main points that were discussed. This can include noting if an area was ignored.

Discussion is not designed to achieve agreement rather it tries to set out the range of different opinions. The value is the breadth of the discussion and listening and understanding other people's viewpoints. The outcome is a clearer view of what the areas of agreements and disagreements are in the subject as a basis for further work.

It can be difficult to assess the richness of a person's understanding of a subject. Small group discussions are the best way to observe students directly and understand their thoughts processes. The educator can use the information from facilitation to inform their assessment of each student's performance.

Role-playing:

Role-playing is a method of teaching where students take on different roles and act out a scenario. This can be a useful way to explore different perspectives, to learn how to deal with conflict and to develop communication skills.

Role playing has experiential value in putting the students into the shoes of the patient. It also has real world elements that allow the student to practice skills such as communication. The key barrier is that students need to behave in a way that they are not comfortable with.

To use role-playing in the classroom, you will need to:

- Choose a scenario that is relevant to the learning objectives. The scenario should be something that the students can relate to and that will help them to learn the desired concepts.
- Assign roles to students. The roles should be distributed fairly and each student should be given a role that they are comfortable with.
- Give students time to prepare for their roles. This will allow them to think about their characters and how they will act in the scenario.
- Set ground rules for the role-playing activity. This will help to ensure that the activity runs smoothly and that everyone feels comfortable.
- Observe the role-playing activity and provide feedback. This will help the students to improve their performance and to learn from the experience.
- Debrief the role-playing activity with students. This will allow the students to reflect on the activity and to discuss what they learned.

The educator should focus on the experiences of taking a role as the students will need to understand their responses. The performance in role play should focus on finding positive comments at least at first. It is better to point out a good aspect of a simulated consultation rather than criticise a poor aspect.

Although OSCEs are the commonest type of role play in medical training there are other approaches that can be useful. Role playing different professionals or the patient explaining an experience to their relatives is also possible. Running a teaching session as the educator can help students gain insight into learning.

Role playing has been gamified and educators can use a Dungeon and Dragons type of approach to role play. The dungeon master takes the adventurers around a hospital where they must solve clinical puzzles.

Playing characters such as an evil goblin manager or a celestial nurse can allow exploration of issues such as the meaning of professionalism.

The educators should provide clear objectives for role play and identity the likely benefits of role-playing for those objectives. The students can be involved in the assessment of the effectiveness of the role play and asked how far the experience achieved the following outcomes.

- Identifying with others: Role-playing can be a great way to put the students in the position of other people and understand their experiences.

- Communication skills: Role-playing can help people to improve their communication skills, as they need to be able to clearly and effectively communicate their thoughts and ideas to others.

- Teamwork skills: Role-playing can help people to learn how to work effectively as a team, as they need to be able to cooperate with others to achieve a common goal.

- Timely Problem-solving: Role-playing can help people to develop their problem-solving skills, as they need to be able to think critically and come up with solutions in real time.

- Creativity: Role-playing can help people to express their creativity, as they are given the freedom to express themselves in any way they see fit. This can help them to come up with new ideas and solutions to problems.

- Empathy. Role-playing allows students to see the world from different perspectives. This can help them to develop empathy for others.

The educator may be disappointed if the students give the task low ratings in these areas. This feedback can help explain low satisfaction and identify what needs to be changed. The greatest problem with medical role playing is that it not actually role play at all.

In the OSCE the doctor plays themselves rather than role plays another person. This reduces the possibility of creative approaches or gaining insight into another person's experience. The dominance of OSCE has led to deskilling of educators in the art of role play. It is better to consider humanities rather than role play for increasing empathy.

Conclusions.

Small group teaching and facilitation offer numerous benefits for both students and educators. Small group settings foster active learning, individualised instruction and increased opportunities for practice. They provide a positive and supportive learning environment that promotes collaboration, critical thinking, problem-solving skills, social skills and self-esteem. Small group teaching also helps students develop their collaboration skills, motivation and engagement in the learning process.

To effectively facilitate small group teaching, the educator must take on various roles such as a guide, coach, mentor, or mediator, depending on the needs of the group and the learning objectives. The facilitator should manage the discussion, provide feedback and summarise key points to ensure productive and meaningful learning experiences.

While small groups can be highly beneficial, there may be disruptive elements that need to be managed. Addressing disruptive behaviour immediately and directly, setting clear expectations and using social pressure from the group can help reduce disruptions. In cases where disruptive behaviour persists, further steps may be necessary, such as conflict resolution training or applying consequences.

Plants, individuals who contribute unique and creative ideas, can be both a hidden strength and a challenge in small groups. Their perspectives and problem-solving abilities can be valuable, but their aloofness and focus on their own ideas may hinder communication and task completion. Educators can manage plants by giving them time to warm up, being open-minded and supportive, challenging their thinking and providing flexibility in plans and activities.

Furthermore, educators can help integrate plants into the group by offering opportunities for leadership, providing extra support, encouraging collaboration with other students and celebrating their successes. One-on-one assistance may be necessary to address the plant's communication difficulties and build their confidence.

Overall, small group teaching and facilitation offer a dynamic and engaging approach to learning, fostering collaboration, critical thinking and problem-solving skills. By effectively managing disruptive elements and supporting the contributions of plants, educators can create a productive and inclusive small group learning environment.

Top tips.

Managing the Plant: Recognise the role of a plant in a small group, which refers to a creative individual who generates innovative ideas but may struggle with communication or task completion and need additional assistance.

Small Group Teaching: Practice all the methods for small group teaching, such as discussions, problem-solving, role-playing and brainstorming until confident in each.

Group performance. Use team building techniques such as setting clear expectations, creating a positive learning environment, encouraging participation, being an active listener and being patient with the group's progress.

Chapter 19: PROBLEM-BASED LEARNING (PBL)

Problem-based learning (PBL) is a student-centered instructional method that promotes active learning and critical thinking through the investigation of real-world problems. PBL is typically used in higher education and help students move towards real life situations.

In PBL, students are presented with a complex problem with an element that can be solved. They then work in small groups to research the problem, identify potential solutions and develop a plan of action. PBL projects typically involve multiple disciplines and require students to use a variety of skills, including critical thinking, problem-solving, communication and collaboration.

PBL is deceptively simple, the educator gives the students a problem and they work in a group to solve the problem. As an educational technique controlling the content and ensuring that the group achieve the learning objectives is more challenging. The learning plan is a critical element of preparation.

- Start simple: When you are first starting out with PBL, it is helpful to start with a simple problem that students can solve in a short amount of time. This will help them to get used to the PBL process.
- Identify a problem that is relevant to your students' interests and experiences.
- Create a learning plan that outlines the key concepts and skills that students will need to learn to solve the problem.
- Learning resources: Students need to have access to resources to solve problems. This could include textbooks, articles, websites, or experts.
- Collaboration: Provide students with opportunities to collaborate with each other and to work with experts in the field.
- Provide feedback: It is important to provide feedback to students on their work. This will help them to improve their problem-solving skills.

PBL has the same elements as other teaching techniques – learning objectives, learning materials, planning, learning experience and assessment. Educators cannot control how students will approach the problem or what solutions they will come up with. This can make PBL feel less controllable and more dependent on the students than other teaching methods.

There is a risk that PBL sessions have insufficient learning resources and the assessment is less effective. Students can find that their contribution is not recognised. They may not receive enough feedback to properly learn from the experiences. Educators need to approach PBL in a structured way.

Practical steps for PBL.

The theory of creating a PBL experience makes it sound straightforward but in practice it can be challenging. The educator may have an idea about the topic they wish to cover but struggle with adding emotion.

The PBL scenario needs to engage the students, it needs to be tailored to their needs and should have control element. The following steps are practical and easy to follow making the creation of a compelling PBL scenario.

- Choose a problem. When choosing a problem the best approach is to find something that evokes emotion. These are typically stress at work, emotional staff, relatives or patients, pay and conditions, medical errors, time constraints, technology, medical emergencies and lack of sleep.
- Make the problem come alive. The clinical details and background and how the doctor feels can put the students in the situation. They can start to see the problem as something that they might face. This takes the problem from being a question of the logical steps to an engaged response. A picture or other evidence to examine can help with this.
- Create a learning plan. Each problem will have its own learning opportunities and these are worth listing. Although the group may not follow the approach that the educator expects having a plan helps when they get stuck. The plan should contain a few words such as "what information is needed" or "who to ask for help" or "what test would help".
- Start with a simple problem. Simple problems are those where the solution is straightforward and obvious. For instance, a doctor might be given too much work and they need to decide which patients they should see and which to leave for a colleague. This example is basically a triage question and an experienced group would find a solution in a few seconds.
- Provide students with resources. With ethical issues having access for instance to guidelines such as Good Medical Practice can show

the group how hard it is to apply theory to practice. The learning resources should be detailed and comprehensive so that they are not relying on the internet.

- Provide opportunities to collaborate. In large projects students should be encouraged to work out systems so that they can collaborate. This may include social media (consider confidentiality), meeting up etc. The LLMs can allow a different sort of collaboration and should be encouraged.
- Provide feedback: The group may require further clues or clarifications to make good progress. The learning materials can also be a good source of feedback. The facilitator can use standard small group work assessment for feedback.
- Summarise the learning steps and the outcomes that the group achieved. This can allow the task to complete within the timescale, the group can see how far they got and reflect on how they missed any important steps.

Educators should ensure that they complete their roles of preparation, providing stimulating materials and observing for problems. The educator should ask for consent before they intervene and should keep quiet when the group is working. They should be careful to avoid interrupting the group even when it is making the wrong direction.

It is tempting to try to help the group reach every goal however they are more likely to be engaged if they feel that may not succeed. The educator should remain within the role of a facilitator and rely upon the learning materials to guide the group. The group will learn more about small group work from seeing how close they got to the learning aims than if they succeed.

Benefits of problem-based learning:

The use of PBL has been increasing and the reasons are that it can solve many of the problems that educators have when teaching medical subjects. The focus on solving problems means that students are better prepared for their work as doctors. It is engaging and enjoyable which reduces learning fatigue.

There are many learning challenges where PBL is unrivalled and others where there is no other reasonable alternative. PBL is relatively cheap compared to some alternative methods but is not free. The cost of creating the learning materials can be high. It is important to consider whether PBL is the best way of achieving the learning objectives.

Other small group teaching methods have similar benefits to PBL without the level of complexity. Where a group is struggling with PBL it is better to use a simpler method. This allows the group to develop their skills sufficiently to ensure that PBL is effective. PBL depends on the group having all the required skills but where they do not the educator must diagnose the problem.

A useful checklist is whether the group is achieving the potential benefits of PBL. If the group is not actively learning or developing critical thinking skills this may require further analysis. Each of the benefits can be broken down into activities that the student must undertake to achieve that benefit.

- Promotes active learning: PBL requires students to actively participate in their own learning by researching, discussing and solving problems.

- Develops critical thinking skills: PBL challenges students to think critically about problems and to come up with creative solutions. They must identify the relevant information, generate hypotheses and evaluate evidence.

- Improves problem-solving skills: PBL helps students to develop the skills they need to solve problems in real-world situations. They learn how to break down problems into smaller steps, identify potential solutions and evaluate the effectiveness of their solutions.

- Improved communication skills: PBL requires students to communicate effectively with each other and with the instructor. They must be able to clearly explain their ideas, listen to the ideas of others and work together to reach a consensus.

- Fosters collaboration: PBL requires students to work together in groups to solve problems. This helps them to develop teamwork and communication skills. They learn how to work together effectively, share ideas and compromise.

- Increases motivation and engagement: PBL can help to increase student motivation and engagement in their learning. Making the task difficult but not impossible can increase student motivation.

- Deeper understanding of material: PBL helps students develop a deeper understanding of the material they are learning. They are not simply memorising facts, but rather they are learning how to apply the material to real-world problems.

The educator can use these benefits as the basis for an assessment. Scoring each benefit out of 10 can give a sense of the strengths and weaknesses of the session. They can then further examine the reasons for weaknesses both on a group and student level. These problems can occur due to insufficient practice in techniques such as discussion, poor quality learning materials or uninteresting problems.

There is a risk that PBL becomes a way of getting groups of students to teach each other the subject. This can occur for instance if the problems are not compelling or the solutions can be found in textbooks. Describing a clinical case as a problem may lead to problems that do not have sufficient challenge.

Ideally PBL would practice techniques that are not achievable in other ways. A PBL with no opportunities to develop for instance critical thinking or negotiation may be better taught as an MCQ. PBL by their nature are dependent on the participants and how they work as a group. Weak students need remedial help not relying on the group to solve their problems.

When not to use PBL.

Although PBL has considerable advantages and is a highly flexible way of generating active knowledge there are times when it should not be used. If, for instance, the students only require passive knowledge of the subject then PBL is not necessary. PBL is not the best approach of teaching passive knowledge.

The medical curriculum is packed with little spare time and PBL needs to justify its place. There are other important subjects which are vying for attention from the students and they may not have enough time to get the most out of this teaching style. PBL should be used appropriately not used as the default learning approach.

- When students lack basic knowledge. PBL is most effective when students have a foundation of basic knowledge in the subject matter. If students do not have this foundation, they may struggle to understand the problem and develop solutions.
- The topic is too complex. If the topic is too complex, it may be difficult for students to work through the problem on their own even with complex learning materials. In this case, it may be better to use a more traditional teaching method, such as lectures or demonstrations to create the necessary knowledge foundations.
- The students are not prepared. If the students are not prepared for PBL for instance because they have not learned other small group techniques, it may be difficult for them to participate effectively. In this case, it may be better to provide them with some preliminary instruction or training.

- The resources are not available. PBL requires access to a variety of resources including learning materials and now just textbooks, journals and computers. If these resources are not available, it may not be possible to use PBL effectively.
- The time is not available. PBL can be time-consuming, especially if the students are not familiar with the method. If there is not enough time to do PBL effectively, it may be better to use a more traditional teaching method. Without assessment and feedback the value of the PBL session is limited.
- When there is a need for a quick learning curve. PBL can be a time-consuming approach to learning. If there is a need for students to learn a large amount of material in a short period of time, PBL will often lead to a short term reduction in performance.
- When there is a need for specific skills. PBL is not always effective for teaching specific skills, such as surgical techniques or diagnostic procedures. In these cases, more traditional teaching methods, such as lectures or demonstrations, may be more effective.
- When students are not motivated. PBL requires students to be self-directed and motivated to learn. If previous PBL sessions have been of poor quality and lacked resources the students will have low motivation.

The university should have a complete list of PBL subjects that have been approved for PBL as not too complex, requiring specific skills or a quick learning curve, that the materials are available and the basic knowledge is provided. Students then can use this resource if they wish to do self-study in their groups.

The advent of LLMs means that students who wish to do PBL on their own can now work collaboratively with AI. Although this should be monitored it may have educational advantages over reading textbooks or watching videos of lectures. Guidance should be provided to ensure that the choice of subject is appropriate.

Conclusions.

Problem-based learning (PBL) is a student-centered instructional method that offers numerous benefits for student learning and development. PBL engages students in active learning, promotes critical thinking and problem-solving skills, improves communication and collaboration and fosters motivation and engagement. By presenting students with real-world problems and challenging them to find solutions, PBL helps prepare them for future academic and professional success.

To implement PBL effectively, educators should carefully select relevant and engaging problems, provide resources and opportunities for collaboration and offer feedback to support student progress. It is important to start with simple problems and gradually increase the complexity as students become more experienced with the PBL process. Educators should also consider the learning objectives and determine whether PBL is the most appropriate teaching method for achieving those objectives.

While PBL has many advantages, there are situations where it may not be the best approach. When students lack basic knowledge, the topic is too complex, or there is a need for specific skills, alternative teaching methods may be more suitable. Additionally, if students are not adequately prepared or motivated for PBL, it may not yield optimal results. It is crucial for educators to assess the context and determine whether PBL aligns with the specific learning needs and constraints.

Ultimately, PBL can be a powerful tool in education, providing students with valuable opportunities to develop essential skills and knowledge. As the field continues to evolve, incorporating new technologies such as AI-powered language models, students can even engage in PBL experiences independently, enhancing their learning experience. By utilising PBL effectively and judiciously, educators can empower students to become active, critical thinkers and problem solvers, equipping them for success in their academic, professional and personal lives.

Top tips.

Use another method. PBL should only be used where there is no other effective alternative. Having a list of topics that are best taught with PBL will help avoid overuse.

Choose an emotional problem: Select problems that evoke emotions in the students or involve dealing with emotions in others such as staff and patients.

Summarise Learning Steps and Outcomes: At the end of the PBL project, summarise the learning steps taken by the students and the outcomes they achieved. This reflection allows students to assess their progress and learn from the experience.

DISTANCE LEARNING IN MEDICAL EDUCATION

Distance learning is a form of education in which students learn online, without being physically present in a classroom. As technology improves the effectiveness of distance learning is increasing. There are still aspects of learning that cannot easily be replicated by distance learning.

Distance learning in medical education is a growing trend. It allows students to learn at their own pace and from anywhere in the world. Educators who are tasked with developing distance learning programs should be aware that the resources required are much greater than face to face.

The educator needs to have access to a large range of educational materials so that they can effectively address the student's needs. Most education is still delivered by the educator speaking to the student. Students need a large choice of materials for each subject so that they can replicate all the learning experiences of face-to-face learning.

Chapter 20: BENEFITS TO DISTANCE LEARNING

The key advantage of distance education is that the learner can integrate their learning with their normal life reducing the investment needed to get an education. With ideal resources the distance learning is almost as good as face-to-face techniques. Many universities have not been able to keep up with the demands for new resources and continue to rely upon traditional techniques.

When creating a distance learning program the educator should focus upon achieving the benefits. The key benefit is increasing access to the educational program. In medicine there are two problems, the first is that doctors are selected from a very limited group of people. This has implications for diversity and the quality of doctors.

The second problem is that there are silos between different health professions so that a qualified doctor would need to undertake full nurse training if they want to change career and vice versa. This is an unnecessary barrier to those who realise that they are in the wrong career. This has implications on retention and job satisfaction.

There are many benefits to distance learning in medical education, including:

- Increased access. Medical studies are restricted to a limited number of people in the world. Increased access to medical studies will ensure that the best people can be selected to become doctors and other health professionals.

- Flexibility: Distance learning can be modulised so that the student can build their own course. The choice of modules can allow students to progress following their interests. Many health professions can study together removing the need for retraining if a student changes direction.

- Convenience: DL eliminates the need for students to commute to campus, which can save time and money. This includes students who live in rural areas or who have other commitments that make it difficult to attend a traditional medical school.

- Access to resources: Distance learning students have access to a wide range of resources, including online textbooks, journals and simulations. This can help them to learn more effectively and to stay up-to-date on the latest medical research.

- Disability friendly: The modular nature of the course allows students to make reasonable adjustments. Students can increase the time that they take to make progress. They can learn in a way that is more suited to their functional restrictions.

Many experts consider that there will be an inflexion point in education within the next few years. They believe that online universities will disrupt the current model leading to most students choosing not to attend in person. Given the social advantages of a university campus it is unlikely that universities will close but any large change will impact university finances.

Allowing students to build their knowledge using modules, high quality resources in a disability friendly way appears to be an obvious move forward. The lower costs of accessing learning from home and joint learning with other health professionals make this superior to the current system. Why would education stand against opening the door to students drawn from a larger pool?

Challenges to distance learning

The key challenges are that universities are not prepared to make these changes. They need to work on a joint curriculum for all healthcare students so that areas of overlap can be identified. They need to develop the substantial resources that distance learning will require. Assessment processes are inadequate to manage these challenges.

The lack of preparedness of universities is only one of the challenges that distance learning must overcome to be the first choice. There are significant organisational problems that have not been addressed making it difficult to interact with peers and educators. Technical difficulties are improving but can still be challenging and the emotional aspects of learning are largely unaddressed.

The challenges to distance learning in medical education include,

- Lack of interaction with peers and faculty: Distance learning can lead to a lack of interaction with peers and faculty. This can make it difficult to get help when needed and to build relationships with other students and faculty.

- Technical difficulties: Distance learning can be susceptible to technical difficulties, such as internet outages or software problems. This can disrupt learning and cause frustration for students.

- Self-discipline: Distance learning requires a lot of self-discipline. Students must be able to stay on track and motivated without the structure of a traditional medical school.

- Isolation: DL can lead to feelings of isolation, especially for students who do not have a strong support network. It is important for students to stay connected with their classmates and professors, either through online forums or in person.

- Lack of social interaction: One of the biggest disadvantages of distance learning is the lack of social interaction. This can be a problem for students who learn best by interacting with others.

- Lack of support: Distance learning students may not have the same level of support as traditional classroom-based students. This can be a problem for students who need help or guidance.

- Lack of skills training: Healthcare roles require substantial skill development and DL is not likely to replace face to face practice. Apprenticeships have been suggested as a way of addressing both shortage of healthcare professionals and a chance to learn skills.

Although all these challenges can be addressed by simple changes such as apprenticeship there appear to be little progress. The promise of distance learning depends upon having a leader who can change the status quo. The idea of a single degree in medical sciences as an entry qualification for further training is strongly resisted.

The suggestion that all health professionals should follow the apprenticeship route is struggling to find support. There are many political and financial barriers to changing the way that medicine is taught. Many teaching hospitals depend on the money that students bring in and apprenticeship would be more based in the community.

It might be more difficult for doctors to keep their elevated status if their training is linked to nurses and pharmacists. Universities will be concerned that their teaching materials are provided by cheaper institutions so they cannot maintain their fees. The students may prefer to study medicine rather than risk becoming another healthcare professional.

Student preparation.

The student may not have undertaken any prolonged self-directed learning and the educator should ensure that they are prepared. This includes things that the student can do such as make plans and things that the educator can offer such as resources, feedback and instructions.

The educator should formally teach how to learn with distance learning. The student will need to learn specific techniques in time and self management. The educator should help support the student making plans as to how they can arrange their learning. Having a practice session where the student tries to use the DL materials can be useful.

Here are some tips for success in distance learning in medical education:

1. Set realistic expectations. Distance learning can be challenging, so it's important to set realistic expectations for yourself. Don't expect to learn everything in the same way you would in a traditional classroom. It may take some time to adjust to the new format.

- Acknowledge that distance learning requires more self-discipline and motivation. You will need to be proactive in managing your time and staying on track with your studies.

- Be realistic about how much time you can commit to studying each week. Don't overload yourself, or you'll risk burnout.

- Build in some flexibility for unexpected events. Things don't always go according to plan, so it's important to have a backup plan in case you need to miss a class or assignment.

2. Be organised. It's important to be organised when you're learning remotely. This means having a quiet place to study, setting aside dedicated time and learning where the online resources such as tutorials, videos and discussion boards can be found.

- Create a study schedule and stick to it as much as possible. This will help you stay on track and avoid procrastination.

- Set up a dedicated workspace in your home. This will help you create a routine and focus on your studies.

- Label everything. This will help you find what you need when you need it.

- Take advantage of online resources. Many universities offer online tutorials, videos and discussion boards that can help you learn the material.

3. Communicate with your instructor and classmates. It's important to communicate with your instructor and classmates regularly. This will help you stay on track and get the support you need. You can communicate with your instructor and classmates through email, discussion boards, or video conferencing.

- Don't be afraid to ask questions. If you're struggling with the material, don't be afraid to reach out to your instructor or classmates for help.

- Contribute to class discussions. This is a great way to stay engaged in the material and learn from your classmates.

- Participate in online activities. Many universities offer online activities such as group projects or simulations that can help you learn the material and collaborate with your classmates.

4. Look after yourself. It's important to take breaks when you're learning remotely. This will help you stay focused and avoid burnout. Get up and move around every 20-30 minutes and take a longer break every hour or two. Reward yourself. When you complete an assignment or reach a goal, reward yourself. This will help you stay motivated and on track.

- Set aside time for self-care. This could include exercise, relaxation, or spending time with loved ones.

- Don't forget to eat healthy and get enough sleep. This will help you stay energised and focused.

- Take breaks when you need them. Don't try to power through when you're feeling burnt out. Take a break, recharge and come back to your studies refreshed.

The session of how to plan distance learning should be as realistic as possible. The students should send emails when communicating with the educator. They should locate the materials online and make a written plan of how they will approach the learning. They should give feedback as to missing learning materials.

Distance Learning Techniques.

There are many different distance learning techniques that can be used in medical education. Educators should use several techniques for each topic to ensure that the students can access an appropriate form of learning. Although the material will be repeated each technique should focus on the material from a different angle.

For instance in a webinar the focus will be on engagement and visual presentation. In an asynchronous discussion forum the focus will be on asking interesting questions and getting the students to think more deeply about the topic. In online courses the focus is on completeness of the material.

Some of the most common techniques include:

- Online courses: Online courses are typically delivered through a learning management system (LMS). Students can access the course materials, such as lectures, readings and activities, at any time and from any location.

- Webinars: Webinars are live online presentations that can be attended by students from anywhere in the world. Webinars are often used to deliver lectures or to provide students with the opportunity to ask questions of an instructor or other experts.

- Asynchronous discussion forums: Asynchronous discussion forums are online forums where students can post questions and comments and where other students and instructors can respond. Asynchronous discussion forums can be a great way for students to collaborate on projects, to get help from their peers and to learn from each other.

- Synchronous chat: Synchronous chat is a real-time online chat that can be used to facilitate discussion between students and instructors. Synchronous chat can be a great way for students to get help from their instructors and to ask questions about the material.

- Simulations: Simulations are interactive educational activities that allow students to practice skills and to learn about concepts in a safe and controlled environment. Simulations can be used to teach a variety of medical skills, such as how to perform a physical exam or how to manage a patient with a particular condition.

- Virtual reality: Virtual reality (VR) is a technology that allows users to experience a simulated environment. VR can be used to teach medical students about anatomy, physiology and other medical concepts.

- Blended learning: Blended learning is a combination of online and traditional learning. This type of learning can be a great option for students who want the flexibility of online learning but also want the support of a traditional classroom. Blended learning programs typically include a combination of online courses, face-to-face classes and online discussion boards.

There will be gaps in the material that the above techniques cannot address. The educator will need to arrange additional learning opportunities to fill these gaps. The educator should still provide materials that allow the students to engage with those gaps. It is as important for the students to understand what they have not learned as what they have.

The educator should maintain a list of the topics so that students can monitor their progress. This should include the gaps with comments so that students are eager to take opportunities that become available. The students can then feedback their experiences so that the educator can learn how to fill those gaps.

Teaching materials for distance learning.

A major barrier to distance learning is the very large number of learning materials necessary. The problem is made more difficult by the need to have different versions of the same material. Many gaps can be partially closed by using several different teaching materials.

If using commercial materials the educator needs to be able to explain exactly where a student can obtain the correct learning materials for each learning objective. This is a complex and time-consuming task and not easy to delegate to AI. The educator then must identify gaps or weaknesses in the materials and write or search for materials to fill them.

As educators are already working full time teaching and performing research this additional burden may take years to complete. Any changes in the curriculum are likely to lead to a further need to find the right materials. This is on top of the need to constantly update and upgrade the materials that are already used.

The solution to the problem is that materials that are used by one institution become available for others. This would save time and expertise in creating the materials. There is a business model for company to provide these materials and keep them updated.

- Personalised learning plans: Personalised learning plans can help students to focus on their individual needs. These plans can be created by the instructor or by the student themselves.
- Textbooks: Textbooks are still a valuable resource for distance learners, even though they may not be the only resource. They can provide students with a comprehensive overview of the material, as well as practice problems and exercises.
- Lecture handouts: Lecture handouts can be a helpful way to provide students with an overview of the material that will be covered in a lecture. They can also be used to provide students with additional information or to clarify concepts that were discussed in the lecture.
- Asynchronous video: Asynchronous video allows students to watch lectures or other content at their own pace. This can be a helpful option for students who have busy schedules or who need more time to digest the material.
- Video lectures: Video lectures are a great way for students to hear from experts in their field and to see concepts being explained

visually. Video lectures can be found on a variety of websites, including YouTube and Khan Academy.

- Online courses: Online courses are becoming increasingly popular, as they offer students the flexibility to learn at their own pace and from anywhere in the world. Online courses can be found on a variety of topics and many of them are offered by accredited universities.

- Podcasts: Podcasts are another great way for students to learn on the go. They can be listened to while commuting, working out, or doing other activities. Podcasts are often produced by universities or other educational organisations and they can cover a wide range of topics.

- Group projects: Group projects can help students to develop their teamwork and communication skills. They can also be a great way for students to apply what they are learning to real-world problems.

- Virtual classrooms: Virtual classrooms are a more interactive way for students to learn. They can participate in live lectures, ask questions and interact with their instructor and classmates in real time.

- Virtual reality: Virtual reality (VR) can be used to create immersive learning experiences. Students can use VR headsets to explore virtual worlds, such as anatomical models or patient surgery.

- Augmented reality: Augmented reality (AR) can be used to overlay digital information onto the real world. Educators can use AR apps to provide commentary when the students are observing.

- Interactive simulations: These can help students to learn by doing. For example, students can use a simulation to practice performing a medical procedure.

- Discussion forums: Discussion forums are a great way for students to interact with each other and with the instructor. They can ask questions, share ideas and get help from their peers. Discussion forums are often a required part of online courses, but they can also be used in conjunction with other teaching materials.

- Learning objects: These are small, self-contained pieces of content that can be used to teach a specific concept. For example, a learning object could be a video lecture, a quiz, or a practice problem.

- WebQuests: These are inquiry-based activities that allow students to explore a topic in depth. WebQuests typically include a set of tasks, resources and a rubric for assessment.

- Wikis: These are collaborative websites that can be used to share information and ideas. Wikis can be used by students to collaborate on projects, to create study guides, or to keep track of their progress.

- Mind maps: These are visual representations of information. Mind maps can be used by students to organise their thoughts, to brainstorm ideas, or to create study guides.
- Quizzes and exams: Quizzes and exams are a way for students to assess their understanding of the material. They can be used to track student progress, to provide feedback and to prepare students for final exams.
- Assessments: Assessments are an important part of any distance learning course. They can help students to measure their progress and to identify areas where they need more help.
- Interactive exercises: Interactive exercises can help students to practice what they are learning. These exercises can be found in a variety of formats, including online quizzes, simulations and games.
- Artificial intelligence: Artificial intelligence (AI) can be used to create personalised learning experiences for students. AI-powered tutors can provide feedback, answer questions and help students stay on track.

The large number of types of teaching materials that can be used for distance learning can be dizzying for educators to start to understand how to use them. Many can be bought from suppliers as ready to go resources although they many do not add much to the student's learning experience.

It is not clear which will be the successful technologies, but I predict that videos and podcasts will dominate. These modalities have a proven track record and have AI support built in. The most popular video lecture on a particular topic can already be found using algorithms on well-known sharing sites. Materials for assessment will continue to be in high demand from students.

Educators should adapt successful approaches they already have used in face-to-face teaching for distance learning. This will reduce the learning curve and play to the educator's strengths. Start with simple modalities such as video or podcast or handouts before attempting to learn more complex modalities.

Funding for DL is highly political and there is little chance at present for a comprehensive DL program. Distance learning requires substantial effort to achieve good results. If engaged with a distance learning project it is better to create one good topic rather than several poor quality topics.

Conclusions.

Distance learning in medical education is a growing trend that offers numerous benefits and challenges. The flexibility, personalisation, convenience, affordability and access to resources provided by distance learning make it an attractive option for students. Additionally, distance learning promotes increased collaboration, engagement and the opportunity to interact with experts from around the world.

However, there are challenges to overcome in implementing effective distance learning in medical education. These challenges include the lack of interaction with peers and faculty, technical difficulties, the need for self-discipline, feelings of isolation, lack of social interaction and potential lack of support. It is crucial for students to set realistic expectations, be organised, communicate effectively and prioritise self-care to succeed in distance learning.

To ensure the success of distance learning, educators must carefully prepare students for self-directed learning and provide the necessary support and resources. The development and availability of appropriate teaching materials for distance learning are essential and educators should be aware of various techniques such as online courses, webinars, asynchronous discussion forums, simulations, virtual reality, blended learning and more.

Student preparation is key and educators should guide students in creating personalised learning plans while addressing the emotional and psychological aspects of distance learning. Collaboration and sharing of teaching materials between institutions can save time and effort in developing resources, ultimately benefiting all involved.

While there is still much to be explored and refined in distance learning, it holds great potential for revolutionising medical education. By addressing the challenges and leveraging effective teaching materials and techniques, distance learning can provide a valuable and accessible educational experience for aspiring medical professionals.

Top tips.

Learning materials. In distance learning the materials must be well prepared, comprehensive and well organised to provide a framework around the learning process. Poor quality materials will damage confidence and motivation.

Multiple methods. Repeating a subject using different methods overcomes blocks in understanding. Online courses, webinars, discussion forums, simulations, virtual reality and blended learning can provide different ways of learning the same material.

Planned communication. Regular contact with peers and the instructor helps stay on track and get the support you need. These resources should provide prompt answers to problems and reflection on the learning plan.

Chapter 21: EDUCATIONAL TECHNOLOGY IN MEDICAL EDUCATION.

Educational technology (EdTech) is the use of technology to improve teaching and learning. EdTech is a rapidly growing field and there are a wide variety of EdTech products and services available. When choosing EdTech products and services, it is important to consider the needs of your students and your teaching goals.

The current problems with EdTech appear intractable apart from a few applications. EdTech cannot be written off yet as technical advances may lead to new solutions. Educators should be aware of the difficulties with developing EdTech and the practical problems with implementing it.

It is difficult to predict the type of EdTech which will transform education. I imagine an app on the phone that learns with the student. It monitors things that the student reads and writes (and maybe what they hear and say). It models the student's own knowledge and predicts what they do and do not know.

The app could then suggest new areas of knowledge based upon recent experience. It could ask questions to deepen learning and understand the learner's approach. The app could even predict when the student is ready to qualify and work independently.

Development difficulties.

Educational technology (EdTech) has the potential to revolutionise education, but its development has been limited by a number of factors.

- Cost is one of the biggest challenges facing EdTech. Developing new EdTech systems is expensive and the market for these systems is often too small to make them profitable which may be changing. For example, there are now online services that can be used to check for plagiarism.
- Lack of specificity is another challenge facing EdTech. Many EdTech systems are designed to be used for a wide range of applications, but this can make them too general to be effective. For example, a video sharing application that is designed for general use may not be as effective for teaching specific skills as a system that is specifically designed for that purpose.
- Assessment is another area where EdTech has struggled. Developing automated systems for creating questions for multiple-

choice tests (MCQs) and other assessments has been difficult. This means that assessments often have to be designed by humans, which can be time-consuming and expensive.

- Engagement: EdTech systems are often better at teaching limited, specific skills than broad knowledge. This is partly because the costs of developing an EdTech system increase with the amount of information that it covers. It is also because students can quickly become bored with repetitive material, even if it is novel. As a result, it can be difficult to keep students engaged with standardised EdTech materials.

- Personalised learning: Personalised learning was one of the initial promises of EdTech, but the technical difficulties of providing sufficient resources have limited its ability to be implemented for normal students. One solution that has been suggested is to use big data analytics to create algorithms that can personalise learning experiences for each student. However, there are still challenges associated with obtaining enough data and developing the artificial intelligence (AI) necessary to make this approach feasible.

Big data analytics is one potential solution to the challenges of personalised learning. Big data analytics can be used to create algorithms that can personalise learning for each student. However, big data analytics is still a developing field and there are a number of challenges that need to be addressed before it can be widely used in EdTech.

MOOCs (Massive open online courses) are one example of how EdTech is overcoming some of its challenges. MOOCs are free, online courses that can be accessed by anyone with an internet connection. This makes them a viable option for students who may not be able to afford traditional education.

Practical Problems with EdTech.

There are currently a number of issues that make using EdTech a problem that the educator should be aware of. Being aware of the problems means that educators can ask the right questions and choose the right solution for their institution.

They need to avoid the common pitfalls and the risk of buying a technology which will never be used. The educator should be able explain the role that this technology will play in the overall programme and which learning problem it solves.

- Cost: Edtech can be expensive to develop and implement especially for schools and universities with limited budgets. This is because it requires specialised skills and resources.
- Technical issues: Edtech can be prone to technical problems. This can disrupt the learning process and frustrate students.
- Lack of quality: Not all edtech is created equal. Some edtech programs are poorly designed and do not meet the needs of students.
- Over-reliance: Edtech can be overused. If it is used as the sole method of instruction, it can lead to students becoming disengaged and bored.
- Lack of qualified instructors: There may be a lack of qualified instructors who are familiar with EdTech. This can make it difficult to implement EdTech effectively.
- Distractions: EdTech can be a distraction for students. This can be a problem if students are not self-directed and do not have the discipline to focus on their work.
- Not be as effective as traditional teaching methods. There is a lack of evidence to support its effectiveness, it may improve student learning, more research is needed on long-term impact of ET on student outcomes. Additionally, the effectiveness of ET may vary depending on the specific learning context and the needs of the students.
- Accuracy: ET systems can be inaccurate, especially when they are not properly developed or maintained. This can lead to students learning inaccurate information, which can have a negative impact on their ability to provide care to patients.
- Bias: ET systems can be biased, especially if they are not designed with diversity and inclusion in mind. This can lead to students learning biased information, which can have a negative impact on their ability to provide care to patients from different backgrounds.
- Privacy: ET systems can collect a lot of data about students, which raises privacy concerns. This data could be used to track students' progress, identify students who are struggling, or even discriminate against students.

There are already many EdTech systems in current use but none of them have reached the threshold. The perfect EdTech system would be universal so that it could be used to teach any subject, self-sustaining and robust. This universality would allow the developer to ensure privacy, bias and cost are addressed.

A universal system will have the flexibility to model any body of knowledge. This means that less effort will be required to train it with accurate, engaging and high-quality knowledge. This concept of the internal structure of EdTech reflecting the knowledge that is being taught may gain more traction with time.

The future of EdTech.

The promise of EdTech may lie in AI but there are questions that need to be asked about the future of EdTech if the current problems can be overcome. EdTech can only cause a paradigm shift if it can address real world learning problems. Small EdTech solutions that addresses a specific issue will never make a big difference.

Students learn by building mental models of their knowledge. They have pattern recognition and develop responses to common problems. EdTech needs to mimic these steps for a chance to compete with the alternatives. The transition would occur if EdTech systems were able to understand what the student has learned.

- The use of EdTech to improve access to medical education. EdTech can be used to provide students with access to high-quality medical education regardless of their location or financial resources. For example, MOOCs can be accessed by anyone with an internet connection.

- The use of EdTech in clinical settings. EdTech can also be used to improve patient care in clinical settings. For example, EdTech can be used to provide patients with educational materials about their condition, to train medical staff on new procedures and to monitor patient progress remotely.

- The role of EdTech in lifelong learning. Medical education is no longer a one-time event that takes place in college or medical school. With the rapid pace of change in the medical field, it is more important than ever for doctors to be lifelong learners. EdTech can play a key role in lifelong learning by providing doctors with access to up-to-date information and resources, as well as opportunities to collaborate with other professionals.

- The ethical considerations of using EdTech in medical education. As with any new technology, there are ethical considerations to be taken into account when using EdTech in medical education. For example, it is important to ensure that students' privacy is protected when using EdTech and that EdTech is not used to discriminate against students.

Students will only accept Big Brother EdTech systems modelling their learning if it is effective. Progress has already been made in predicting what a customer would like to buy next. The same algorithms could be used to predict what a student would like to learn. With further development it is likely that EdTech will be able to predict what the student knows.

Conclusions.

Educational technology (EdTech) holds great potential to transform medical education. It offers numerous advantages such as enhanced accessibility, personalised learning experiences and the ability to overcome traditional educational constraints. However, there are several challenges that need to be addressed for EdTech to reach its full potential.

Cost remains a significant obstacle as developing and implementing EdTech solutions can be expensive, especially for institutions with limited budgets. Additionally, the lack of specificity in many EdTech systems and the difficulty in automating assessments pose challenges in effectively addressing the diverse learning needs of students. Ensuring student engagement and avoiding over-reliance on EdTech are crucial to maintaining a balanced and effective learning environment.

The concept of personalised learning through big data analytics shows promise, but there are still technical and ethical challenges to overcome. The quality and effectiveness of EdTech programs can vary and there is a need for more research to assess their long-term impact on student outcomes. Privacy concerns and the potential for biases in EdTech systems must also be carefully addressed to ensure fair and secure learning environments.

Despite these challenges, there are promising developments such as Massive Open Online Courses (MOOCs) that provide accessible and affordable education opportunities. With careful selection and implementation, EdTech can greatly enhance medical education and improve student learning outcomes.

In conclusion, EdTech has the potential to revolutionise medical education, but its success depends on addressing the practical problems, selecting appropriate solutions and continually evaluating and adapting to meet the specific needs of students and educators. By leveraging the advantages of EdTech while being mindful of its limitations, we can unlock new opportunities for teaching and learning in the medical field.

Top tips.

Avoid using EdTech solutions. Unless EdTech solutions are cheap, adaptable and of proven effectiveness in a difficult to teach area the cost will not be worthwhile.

Recognise EdTech advances. In the future there may be useful developments such as EdTech that can predict what a student wants to learn or can assess a student's knowledge.

Massive Open Online Courses. If an EdTech solution for teaching unlimited numbers of students is found this is likely to be a both cheap and adaptable way of addressing the lack of medical training in developing countries.

Chapter 22: USING LLM IN MEDICAL EDUCATION.

Large language models (LLMs) are a type of artificial intelligence (AI) that can generate human like text. They work by predicting the next word in a sequence and have emergent properties such as answering questions in an informative way. They are trained on massive datasets of text and code and they can learn to perform many kinds of tasks.

LLMs are still under development, but they have the potential to revolutionise the way we interact with computers. They could be used to create more natural and engaging user interfaces, to improve the accuracy of machine translation and to generate more creative and informative content.

Many students are already incorporating LLMs into their studies and some report substantially increased learning speeds. The key advantages are that the learning is under the students control and is responsive to the student's inputs. It can be used for learning, assessment, clinical decisions and research.

Large language models (LLMs) can be used in medical education in a variety of ways, including:

- Personalised learning: LLMs can be used to create personalised learning experiences for students by tailoring the content and difficulty level to each student's individual needs. LLMs automatically provide answers to prompts at the same or higher level of understanding as the prompt itself.

- Adaptive assessment: LLMs can be used to assess student learning in a more adaptive way than traditional assessment methods. This can help to identify areas where students need additional support and provide them with the resources they need to succeed. The LLMs provide constant feedback to the student helping them understand their gaps and how to fill them.

- Clinical decision support: LLMs can be used to provide clinical decision support to doctors and other healthcare professionals. This can help them to make better decisions about patient care and improve patient outcomes. LLMs are good at generating possible choices and empower the doctor to make a holistic assessment.

- Research: LLMs can be used to conduct research during medical education. The unique way that students can interact with LLMs means that they explore the subject in ways that were only available in one-to-one teaching before. LLMs can be used to create contents lists, subheadings, structure the material.

The correct response to powerful new technologies is to consider how to incorporate it into current practice. With the LLM those doctors who learn to harness it power will have better outcomes than those who ignore it or try to get it do everything. Learning to use LLMs is not straightforward or easy and is outside of many doctors' comfort zones.

Educators will on the front line helping even the most senior doctors learn how they can benefit from using LLMs. Training on the use of LLMs will be traumatic for many as it is a complex skill and requires previous IT knowledge. Applying that knowledge to clinical practice will require substantial support from institutions to achieve the promised advantages.

How to work with LLMs.

The basic steps of working with an LLM are no different from working with any new technology. The task needs to be prepared so that the technology can work effectively, different approaches may be needed for it to work properly and the results need to be assessed to check that they meet the goals.

Avoiding the technical aspects of LLMs can help those who are not IT literate to make sense of what they need to do. They should be helped to see the process before introducing the new concepts. Use simple language such as 'what question do you want to ask?' rather than 'what prompt should you use?'.

1. Define the goal. What do you want to achieve by collaborating with an LLM? Do you want to create an essay, learn about a subject or find an answer to the questions in an informative way?

2. Use natural language. LLMs are trained on text data, so it is best to use natural language when interacting with them.

3. Break down the goal into smaller tasks. Once you have a clear goal, break it down into smaller tasks that can be completed in a single iteration. This will make it easier to track your progress and make sure that you are on track.

4. Get feedback. As you iterate on your ideas, get feedback from others. Using an LLM is complex and you will not have all the answers. This feedback can help you to identify areas where you can improve and make sure that you are on the right track.

5. Train the LLM. Once you have a system for achieving the task you need to train the LLM to follow that system. This can be done by providing the LLM with examples of the type of work you want it to produce, prompts or iteration.

6. Iterate. Once the LLM has been trained, you can feed it with its own responses. As you work with the LLM, you will likely identify areas where the answers it gives can be improved. You can then provide parts of the answer to the LLM and see how the responses change.

7. Be patient. Collaboration with an LLM can be a time-consuming process. It can take time to master the techniques. It is important to be patient and persistent as you work towards your goal.

8. Evaluate the results. Once you are satisfied with the results of the collaboration, you can evaluate the work that the LLM has produced. This may identify other tasks you need to complete to improve the outcomes further.

When explaining the LLM it is better to use language that the learner is comfortable with. Explaining that sensitive areas can upset the LLM is easier to accept than saying that the developers have prevented it from answering those types of questions.

It is better to explain that LLMs can get confused and make up answers when trying to help rather than they are unstable and cannot be trusted. Saying that the LLM will not give the full answer first time and the student should iterate on the answers is better than criticising their prompt.

These somewhat anthropomorphic explanations avoid the need for the learner to fully understand the internal programming of the LLMs. The learner develops expectations that are realistic rather than expecting the LLM to work perfectly. With practice the student will get a feel for how the LLM will respond.

Iteration.

Iteration is a process of repeating a series of steps until the desired outcome is achieved. It can be used in collaboration with an LLM to improve the quality of work.

Iteration can be used in a number of ways with an LLM to get different responses.

Iteration is one of the key techniques that the learner uses to obtain the outcomes that they desire. The steps are not complex and a learner does not need to use all the available steps to get good results. As the learner becomes more confident they can explore different types of iteration.

- Ask a question and then refine the question based on the responses from the LLM. This allows the student to work out how the LLM is approaching the question and guide it to the correct issues.
- Give the LLM back part or whole of its answer as prompt for the next iteration. This allows the LLM to refine the points it is making and add further points. The LLM uses both the information in the prompt and the order that information is given to create a further response.
- Bring together parts of several answers and ask the LLM to identify any gaps in the information considered. This allows the LLM to identify areas that have been missed out and offer further comments.
- Create a list of possible options and then ask the LLM to generate information on each. This allows the student to explore the different options and create a summary for easy reference.
- Ask the LLM to improve the generated text. The LLM gives different approaches that the student can use to change the way the text is written. This can help students find a different style or approach to the text.
- Offer the LLM feedback on their generated content. The LLM will then generate further content based upon the previously generated content and the feedback. The feedback can be in the form of suggestions, questions or additional information.
- Start with a hypothesis and can use an LLM to generate different ways to test that hypothesis. This is a way of getting an LLM to collaborate on solving a problem. The LLM can offer arguments for and against the hypothesis.
- Personalising the LLM's response by iterating and asking the LLM to focus on specific topics, areas of interest or tailored to a specific learning style. The LLM can translate the material from one form to another.

Iteration is one of the easiest ways of using an LLM because the student just selects something already there. Iteration increases learning by the student as repeatedly working with the same material in different ways and increases engagement and understanding. Students spend longer in the learning zone because they are spend less time locating information.

Although it is possible to write complex prompts it is much easier to use part of the LLMs reply to a simple prompt. There are times when the LLM will go round in circles and the only way of making progress is to provide a more specific prompt. Small changes in the wording can lead to large changes in the result.

Prompts.

In the context of large language models (LLMs), prompts are short pieces of text that are used to guide the model's output. They can be used to specify the task that the model is supposed to accomplish, provide additional information that the model needs to complete the task, or simply make the task easier for the model to understand.

Prompt engineering is a constantly evolving field as the performance of LLMs can be improved by helping them focus their attention. As LLMs become more powerful, the need for effective prompts will become even more important. Learning how write good prompts involve being aware of the range of possible prompts available and experimenting to see which approach works best.

- Instructional prompts: These prompts tell the LLM what to do. For example, an instructional prompt might say "Summarise this article". The response is more likely to be factual and logical.

- Question prompts: These prompts ask the LLM a question. For example, a question prompt might say "What are the causes of heart disease". The LLM will provide some background information about the causes as well as the facts.

- Creative prompts: These prompts allow the LLM to be creative. For example, a creative prompt might say "Write a scenario of a patient suffering from a disease for a PBL session". This prompt allows the LLM to provide a creative response.

- Data-driven prompts: These prompts provide the LLM with data to work with. For example, a data-driven prompt might say "Given the following text please write a conclusion" or "give a list of possible diagnoses based upon the patient's records". The LLM uses the provided data as well as its training data to make its answer and can provide divergent answers.

- Step by step prompt. A step-by-step prompt is a type of prompt that asks for a series of steps to be taken to complete a task. This type of prompt is often used in technical writing, where it is important to provide clear and concise instructions. It has been discovered to improve LLMs responses and create a more logical sequence of suggestions.

- Multi-step prompts: These prompts ask the LLM to complete a series of steps to achieve a goal. For example, a multi-step prompt might say "Write a plan to create a good teaching session" This type of prompt gives the LLM the opportunity to internally iterate to come to an answer.

- Argumentative prompts: These prompts ask the LLM to take a position on a controversial issue and defend their position. For example, an argumentative prompt might say "Should cosmetic procedures be on the NHS?". This type of prompt is useful when looking for opinions and points of view rather than the right answer.

- Hypothetical prompts: These prompts ask the LLM to imagine a situation that is not real and to describe how they would react. For example, a hypothetical prompt might say "If LLMs developed emotional intelligence how could that improve mental health treatment?". The LLM will provide hypotheses on what might happen based upon different assumptions that could be made.

- Self-reflective prompts: These prompts ask the LLM to reflect on their own understanding. For example, a self-reflective prompt might say "What are the current limitations of LLMs in medical education". The LLM will draw upon their own training on their performance to provide an answer.

- Open-ended prompts: These prompts do not have a specific answer. The LLM is free to generate any response that it feels is appropriate. For example, an open-ended prompt might say "Write a story to illustrate the importance of doctors having communication skills." Allowing the LLM to have free rein means that the output is less predictable and may consider aspects that would otherwise be missed.

- Challenging prompts: These prompts are designed to test the LLM's abilities. For example, a challenging prompt might say "Write a speech that would convince the government that primary care funding is the key to the NHS being effective." LLMs have guardrails and this might prevent them from write persuasive arguments despite the need for this type of response.

- Personalised prompts: These prompts are tailored to the individual user. For example, a personalised prompt might say "Write a letter to this patient explaining more about their cancer diagnosis." Requests about sensitive areas can also be a problem so careful use of personalised prompts is recommended.

LLMs have high performance even when asked conversational prompts using words such as 'improve this, any more examples, which is the weakest area, tell me about'. Providing different styles of prompts can create different answers. LLMs can vary in how well they cope with different approaches but this is within the expertise of prompt engineers.

If a LLM is having difficulty with a particular type of prompt then another LLM may cope better, changing the type of prompt or breaking the prompt into smaller parts can fix the problem. The LLM can be asked to provide a prompt to achieve a specific purpose.

Training the LLM.

Training can be achieved by including in the prompt the desired output. For example providing examples of the type of work you want it to produce, prompts or iteration. When AI specialists talk about training the LLM they mean providing a large body of new data. The model then processes that data so that the outputs more closely match the new data.

There are already AI models available that can be trained by relatively inexperienced IT professionals. In future it is likely that the training process will be simpler and within the expertise of an ordinary person. The problems with training are having access to sufficient data, the requirements are falling but there still needs to enough to teach it all the points.

For the non-specialist having access to a large number of human written documents may be enough. For simpler tasks the LLM may simply need to be shown the format and then will be able to copy the approach with straightforward commands. For those who wish to develop bespoke systems the following may be important.

- Select a Model: There are many different types of LLMs and each type has its own strengths and weaknesses. It is important to select the right type of LLM for the task at hand. The architecture of an LLM can also affect its performance. Some architectures are better suited for certain tasks than others.

- Data cleaning and preparation: LLMs are trained on massive datasets of text and code. However, these datasets can often contain errors or biases. It is important to clean the data before training an LLM to ensure that it is accurate and representative of the real world. It is important to select data that is relevant to the task that the LLM will be used for and will fill gaps in the model.

- Feature engineering: Feature engineering is the process of transforming raw data into features that are more useful for machine learning algorithms. This can be done by extracting features from the data, such as the number of words in a sentence or the sentiment of a text.

- Hyperparameter tuning: LLMs have many (hyper)parameters that can be tuned to improve their performance. This can be done through a process of trial and error or by using a machine learning algorithm.

- Regularisation: Regularisation is a technique that can be used to prevent LLMs from overfitting the training data. Overfitting occurs when an LLM learns the training data too well and is unable to generalise to new data.

- Evaluation: It is important to evaluate the performance of an LLM on a held-out test set. This will help to ensure that the LLM is not overfitting the training data. It is important to monitor its performance over time for instance with attention maps and saliency maps This will help to identify any problems with the LLM and take corrective action.

These tasks are at present outside of the ordinary expertise of educators and should be avoided. Doctors will increasingly need to be able to use this language if they are working with an LLM. Having technical skills in LLM training will allow doctors to engage with their LLM engineers to achieve results more rapidly.

Having an LLM that can generate questions for medical students and doctors in examination preparation is a critical task for educators. Hand designing questions is extraordinarily time consuming. Once this problem is solved, there will be students who are able to learn much of the course simply by answering questions.

Weaknesses of LLMs in Medical Education.

There are many areas that LLMs have which are recognised to be weak. Some like hallucinations arise as an emergent feature from the need to be creative. Others come from deficiencies in the training material such as bias. Blocks are built into the LLM by the developers to prevent it from behaving in ways that are not acceptable.

LLMs currently all fail on three areas – creativity, emotional intelligence and common sense. All LLM generated responses whilst very eloquent have a similar feel and are rarely truly creative. They can appear to understand how someone is feeling but then say something inappropriate and they can make silly mistakes.

Educators cannot control for all the weaknesses of LLMs but this should prevent them from helping students. Educators need to teach their students and the university about the LLMs weaknesses. The first list of issues are those that are best dealt with by helping students stay safe.

- Lack of Creativity: LLMs often struggle with generating truly creative responses. While they can provide eloquent and coherent text, their outputs can lack originality and novelty, limiting their ability to engage learners in innovative ways.
- Emotional Intelligence: LLMs may appear to understand emotions but can often fail to respond appropriately. Their lack of emotional intelligence can result in inappropriate or insensitive remarks, affecting the overall learning experience.
- Common Sense: LLMs can make mistakes that seem silly or illogical. Their lack of common sense can hinder their ability to provide accurate and reliable information, especially in complex medical scenarios.
- Bias: LLMs are trained on extensive datasets that can contain biases present in the source material. As a result, they may unintentionally produce biased text, perpetuating existing biases and potentially influencing learners' understanding in a skewed manner.
- Inaccuracy: LLMs are still undergoing development and there are instances where they produce inaccurate text, particularly in tasks that demand a high level of precision, such as explaining intricate medical concepts. This inaccuracy can lead to misconceptions and misinterpretations.
- Lack of context: LLMs are trained on massive datasets of text, but they do not have the ability to understand the context of the information they are given. This can lead to them generating responses that are irrelevant or even harmful. For example, an LLM might be asked to provide information about a rare disease, but if it is not given enough context, it might generate a response that is inaccurate or misleading.
- Lack of expertise: LLMs are not experts in any particular field. They can provide information on a wide range of topics, but they do not have the same level of knowledge as a human expert. This means that they should not be used as a substitute for human expertise in medical education.
- Hallucinations are a type of inaccuracy that raises concerns about any reliance on LLMs for professional tasks. The LLM can insist that for instance a reference exists when it has made

it up. This means that users can be convinced that the LLM is right even when it is not.

These examples are not soluble with current technology. The student needs to understand the problem and learn how to stay safe. Sometimes bringing the LLM in house and running it on the university servers is the right solution. There are times when the university will need to ask students to include sensitive information.

- Cost: Developing and maintaining LLMs requires significant computing power and resources, making them expensive to implement in educational settings with limited budgets. This financial barrier can restrict their widespread adoption although there are some newer models that are small enough to be run on the university server.
- Control Challenges: LLMs are complex systems and ensuring control over their output can be difficult. There is a risk of generating offensive or harmful content, highlighting the importance of carefully monitoring and guiding their usage.
- Potential for Harmful Content: LLMs have the capacity to generate content that can be used for malicious purposes, such as hate speech or propaganda. This emphasises the need for responsible and ethical use of LLMs in medical education.
- Privacy concerns: LLMs are trained on massive datasets of text and code, which raises privacy concerns about the potential for the model to learn sensitive information about individuals. This may be important if doctors fail to anonymise their patients data before submitting it.
- Overfitting: LLMs can be prone to overfitting, which means that they may learn the training data too well and not be able to generalise to new data. This can lead to problems in medical education, where the model may not be able to provide accurate or reliable information on new or emerging topics.
- Lack of transparency: LLMs are complex models and it can be difficult to understand how they work or to explain their decisions. This can make it difficult to trust the model to teach students the correct information and way of thinking about the subject.

Students will continue to use commercial online LLMs but should be encouraged to use a safe university LLM for sensitive and personal questions. To encourage this the university should avoid excessive regulation and encourage freedom of speech. They should discuss with students who breach guidelines rather than punish them. The university LLM must be a safe space for students to learn and experiment.

Despite these limitations LLMs are a huge advance in the technology of medical education. The comprehensive nature of the data sets means that unlike other types EdTech the LLMs will not run out of material. Problems such as the vagueness of the models understanding are likely to disappear as the number of tokens that they are trained on increases.

Medical knowledge assessments.

As LLMs become better at passing various medical knowledge assessments there is concern from medical educators. They are worried that students will use the LLM to generate answers to questions and make those questions invalid as a measure of student performance.

The correct response for the educators is to encourage the use of LLMs and then alter the assessment methods, not to try to prevent the use of the LLMs. This will allow students to gain the advantages of better training and understanding but still face a fair test on their abilities.

This may mean developing new types of test or increasing the standards expected of the students to pass. There is evidence from teaching theory that the overall performance of students may improve. This will create an ethical dilemma as to whether to allow the proportion of students who pass to increase. Also whether we should allow students who would not have been accepted to medical school in the past to enter the courses.

A dissertation is a long, in-depth research paper that is written as a requirement for graduation from a doctoral program. It is usually the culmination of years of study and research and it is a major test of the student's knowledge and skills. LLMs can assist a student writing long pieces of written work and can shorten the time.

There is an argument that long written work could be extended to make it more challenging. This would mean that degree students may be asked to produce theses rather than essays or dissertations rather than theses.

- Dissertations are typically between 100 and 200 pages long and they require a significant amount of original research. Dissertations are typically written for PhD degrees.

- Theses are typically between 50 and 100 pages long and they require some original research. Theses are typically written for master's degrees.

- Essays are typically between 10 and 20 pages long and they do not require original research. Essays are typically written for college or university courses.

Unless universities decide to return to formal observed written examinations the educator will need to assess how well the student has collaborated with the LLM. How well the student has achieved adaptive learning with the LLM and range of data that the student has considered. These factors will ensure that the assessment is comprehensive and valid.

LLMs are increasingly adept at solving clinical problems and it is possible that students by working with LLMs will be able to master this approach to higher standard. MCQs are likely to remain valid although the standards expected may need to be increased.

Medical students may become more eloquent as they interact with LLMs and this in turn may also improve the quality of the answers they give. The educators can use AI to check whether the student has rote learned an answer or has really understood the subject they are discussing.

Explaining medical knowledge to a patient is a task that may improve with use of LLMs. In this case having standardised explanations that are adaptable to the individual patient is an advantage. Explanations should be effective in helping the patient understand and do not need to be comprehensive.

The ability to answer patient questions would then only be a challenge if they ask unusual questions that could not be pre-prepared. If the educator wishes to check whether the advice is personalised, they should ask the examinee to provide alternative ways of giving the information. This task would demonstrate flexibility in the post LLM world.

Conclusions.

Large language models (LLMs) have the potential to greatly impact medical education. They can be utilised in various ways, including personalised learning, adaptive assessment, clinical decision support and research. LLMs can provide tailored content and feedback, assist in making better clinical decisions and enable students to explore medical topics in innovative ways.

To effectively work with LLMs in medical education, certain steps should be followed. These include defining the goals of collaboration, using natural language when interacting with the models, breaking down goals into smaller tasks, training the LLMs with appropriate data, seeking feedback from others, iterating on the generated content, being patient throughout the process and evaluating the results.

Iteration is a critical skill for those using LLMs and is a key way that the learner engages with the LLM and improves the output.

Prompts play a crucial role in guiding LLMs' output. Various types of prompts, such as instructional, question-based, creative, data-driven, step-by-step, multi-step, argumentative, hypothetical, self-reflective, open-ended, challenging and personalised prompts, can be used depending on the desired outcome. Effective prompt engineering can significantly improve the performance of LLMs and enhance their ability to provide accurate and relevant responses.

Training an LLM involves selecting the appropriate model, cleaning and preparing data, performing feature engineering, tuning hyperparameters and applying regularisation techniques. While there are models available that can be trained by non-specialists, access to sufficient and relevant data remains important.

Incorporating LLMs into medical education requires support from institutions and educators to help learners effectively utilise the technology. Although learning to use LLMs can be complex and outside the comfort zone of many doctors, the potential benefits make it worth the effort. As LLMs continue to advance, educators and learners need to stay informed and adapt their approaches to make the most of this powerful technology.

In summary, LLMs have the potential to revolutionise medical education by providing personalised learning experiences, adaptive assessments, clinical decision support and research capabilities. By following the steps for working with LLMs, utilising effective prompts and training the models appropriately, medical educators can harness the power of LLMs to enhance teaching, learning and patient care in the field of medicine.

Top tips.

Define the Goal: Clearly define the student's objective when using an LLM in medical education. Determine whether the goal is to create an essay, learn about a subject, find answers to questions, or explore a specific area.

Prompt engineering. All students should be trained to use a variety of standard prompts and encouraged to develop their own approaches. Diagnosis of the reasons for poor results will determine the student's AI learning needs.

Collaboration with LLMs: Students should learn how to collaborate with LLMs and educators should develop new assessment methods and training to ensure that students attain maximum benefit from the interaction.

Chapter 23: GLOBAL HEALTH IN MEDICAL EDUCATION

Global health lacks the cohesive theory that many other areas of study involve. Apart from the idea that the study is global little else links the concepts. The key elements appear to be public health approaches such as epidemiology, health policy and ethics. The special issues of infectious disease, humanitarian crisis and poverty are too variable for a unified global perspective.

For the educator this creates a problem, do they teach the students each topic as a separate learning objective? Or do they try to find a common theme that will hold the teaching together and build to a coherent whole? The former has the advantage that the UK can used to compare with other countries. The latter has the advantage that it is more engaging as a subject.

Issues such as climate change and pollution and migration have given Global Health a new focus. These problems appear to require international cooperation rather than individual action. They are a best tangential to Global Health as a subject and arguably outside of public health.

The idea of studying about public health from a global perspective is attractive because it makes the findings more applicable to medicine. The cause of many illnesses is social and political rather than to do with locality. Risk factors for poor health includes poverty, lifestyle choices, inequality and lack of research into the causes of disease.

The advantages of looking at health from a global perspective are that individual governments may have little control over their population's health. Factors such as war, migration, infectious disease and industry are largely determined by geographical realities than by political decisions of the individual government.

Although there are global agencies such as the WHO, NATO, UN and World Bank these have little power to influence global policies. The power is within a few countries, large corporations and financial institutions who really make the rules.

Issues such as climate change, pollution, global companies, migration and epidemics of infectious disease have pushed global health up the agenda. The problems remain - whose responsibility is global health, where will the funding come to make the sorts of changes and will anyone listen to what the individuals want or need?

Global health as a subject is considered in three groups which look at the problems from individual to medicine from a global perspective and then to international action. What is not considered in sufficient detail is the political dimension, war, economic policy, climate change, resource exploitation and globalisation are likely to have greater influences than the way that a health system is organised.

Social and Political Determinants of Health

This group of topics focuses on the social and political factors that influence health. These factors include things like poverty, inequality, discrimination and access to healthcare. They ask the student to consider what world they would like to see and how it would change health issues around the world.

Students need to be able to imagine a different set of rules and then the world that would be created. This mental exercise is not easy and looking at different examples is often used instead. The key is to look at each example as group of different rules and then consider the extent that they predict the health outcomes.

- Social determinants of health: This area of study focuses on the social, economic and environmental factors that influence health. Global health professionals study social determinants of health work to understand how these factors contribute to health disparities and to develop interventions to address them.

- Health policy: This area of study focuses on the development and implementation of policies that affect health. Global health policy professionals work to improve health outcomes in populations around the world by advocating for policies that promote health, such as policies that improve access to healthcare, reduce poverty and protect the environment.

- Health ethics: This area of study focuses on the ethical issues that arise in the context of global health, such as the right to health, the allocation of resources and the use of human subjects in research.

- Cultural competence: This topic focuses on the importance of understanding and respecting different cultures when working in global health.

- Global health law: This area of study focuses on the laws that govern global health, such as the laws that regulate trade in health products, the laws that protect human rights and the laws that address infectious diseases.

- Global health and development: This area of study focuses on the relationship between global health and development, such as the ways in which economic development can improve health outcomes and the ways in which health interventions can promote development.

These six areas are interested in how changes of policy could improve health outcomes in the world. The study of the individuals' experience of global health raises more questions than it can provide answers to. There is a risk that these topics can sound like preaching because they ask what principles the countries should follow.

As most countries have major difficulties with their health care systems it seems unfair for a rich country to complain about a poor country's choices. One approach is to apply global health principles to the UK health system and ask how far we achieve the standards we set. Issues such as drug misuse, mental health, home instability and access to healthcare can be compared with the performance in different countries.

Global Medicine

This group of topics focuses on the practice of medicine in a global context. This includes things like the epidemiology of diseases, the delivery of healthcare and the challenges of working in resource-limited settings.

Students become frustrated that the solutions rarely focus on practical steps. The apparent need for western medicine and idea rather than local doctors treating patients has paternalistic overtones. The skills seem to be distant from the real needs of ill people in other countries.

- Clinical medicine: This part of the course looks at the diagnosis and treatment of diseases in a global context. Students learn about the different diseases that are prevalent in different parts of the world, as well as the different ways to treat them.

- Research methods: This part of the course focuses on the methods used to conduct research in global health. Students learn about how to design and conduct research studies, as well as how to analyse and interpret data.

- Health systems: This area of study focuses on the organisations and processes that deliver healthcare. Global health professionals who study health systems work to improve the performance of health systems to improve health outcomes in populations around the world.

- Humanitarian health: This topic looks at the health of people affected by disasters, conflict and other humanitarian emergencies.

- Epidemiology: This area of study focuses on the distribution and determinants of disease in populations. Global health epidemiologists use this information to identify and address health problems in populations around the world.

- Public health: This area of study focuses on the prevention and control of disease and other health problems. Global health public health professionals work to improve health outcomes in populations around the world by developing and implementing interventions such as vaccination programs, sanitation initiatives and health education campaigns.

There is a risk that students will see all countries in an area as having the same problems and requiring the same solutions. The educator should instead find a general problem such as low funding for the health service and then consider solutions that have worked around the world.

Many paths to the same goal can both respect the different approaches and learn the lessons. The UK does not have all the answers and struggles in areas that other countries have found solutions. The student can be encouraged to see global health as a toolkit where they can select the right tool.

The educator must also consider how far epidemiology, research and public health can help solve their country's problems. The importance of other factors such as economic development, political instability and war can be considered. A population's health depends upon more that an effective health system.

The role of individual health professionals can end this section with a positive. The book Where There Is No Doctor - A Village Health Care Handbook can help students see how people can improve community health. Covid immunisations in the UK was mainly delivered by GPs rather than private contractors.

International Development

This group of topics focuses on the process of developing countries. This includes things like economic growth, poverty reduction and social development. Students struggle with political decision making and can find this area difficult to engage with. The problems that are presented can appear to be intractable and progress can easily reverse.

- International development: This topic looks at the role of international development in improving health.

- Gender and health: This topic focuses on the ways in which gender can influence health outcomes.

- Environmental health: This topic focuses on the ways in which the environment such as climate change and hunger can impact health.

- Humanitarian aid: This part of the course focuses on the provision of health care to people in crisis situations. Students learn about the different types of humanitarian aid organisations, such as the Red Cross and Doctors Without Borders.

This topic is about big infrastructure and aid programmes which doctors will rarely be involved in. Using a PBL approach questions such how could a global government improve global health? and what is the most effective way of spending money to improve health? can be engaging. The role of director general of the WHO could provide a resource for learners to consider.

How to interest students.

There are several areas that can engage student's interest and help them take a deeper look at the issues. The problem is that when covering the content in a short time makes engaging students a lower priority.

- Globalisation of health. Diseases that spread across borders such as HIV and Covid can help students consider Ebola and malaria as whole world problems.

- Visit developing countries. Some schools also have partnerships with hospitals or clinics in developing countries, which allow students to gain experience working in a global health setting. This can influence the choice of elective.

- Individual case studies. Students are more motivated when considering how an individual obtains the correct treatment. For instance, a patient with HIV/AIDS in South Africa would help students to understand the challenges of treating HIV/AIDS in resource-limited settings.

- Discuss the root causes. Considering a local disease hotspot and the root causes can help identify how social, economic and political factors can influence health.

- National Health design. By providing materials on a specific country's health system and using PBL a group can create a list of health priorities. This would help them understand the difficulties facing countries designing health systems.

- Global Health as a career. Discussing how doctors can get involved with global health, what training they require and what sort of roles can remove the mystery of global health.

- Primary care. Discussing the effectiveness of primary care in improving healthcare can transform the student's beliefs. Every dollar spent in primary care saves 2 in secondary care. Primary care doctors save 4 times as many lives a year per doctor than hospital doctors.

Students need to believe that there are solutions to global health problems. They need to feel that they can make a difference to this massive issue. This means that the educator must choose those topics that can make the most difference.

These areas can help the educator engage the student and see global health as a real issue. There are other areas that whilst less engaging are arguably of greater importance. Primary care is a possible solution to many of the most pressing problems as it is highly effective, low cost and saves money.

Primary care.

Global health needs simple and effective solutions and primary care is a medical solution to many global health problems. Immunisation has largely removed the threat of infectious disease in the global north. Identifying disease in the window of opportunity is not easy. Stronger primary care would arguably improve health in both the global north and south.

The primary care doctor can travel to the patient and provide continuity of care in the long term. They are able understand the local needs of their population and engage with other professionals. They can deliver programs of health such as screening, immunisation and timely treatments.

Many doctors are unaware that every additional primary care doctor will both save more lives than their hospital colleagues and save money overall. Students may question whether this is true of the global north and the educator can help them see that they have unreasonable prejudices. GPs are more valuable than hospital consultants for overall health because they prevent disease.

There are many reasons why primary care doctors are undervalued compared to their hospital colleagues.

- Prevention is less visible than treatment. When a patient goes to the hospital, they are usually sick and need immediate care. This makes it easy to see the value of the hospital doctor who provides that care. However, when a patient goes to a primary care doctor for preventive care, such as a checkup or vaccination, the benefits of that care may not be as obvious. This can lead to the perception that primary care doctors are not as important as hospital doctors.

- Technology is less important for prevention. Hospital doctors often use expensive technology to diagnose and treat diseases. This can make it seem that they are more valuable than primary care doctors, who do not typically use as much technology. However, technology is not always necessary for prevention. In fact, many preventive measures, such as exercise and diet, do not require any technology at all.

- Primary care doctors are often paid less than hospital doctors. This is because the reimbursement rates for preventive care are lower than the reimbursement rates for treatment. This can lead to primary care doctors feeling undervalued and underpaid.

- Lack of understanding why primary care is effective. Primary care doctors use biopsychosocial progress to make small steps towards better health. This is rarely taught at medical school so most doctors (even GPs) may not be aware of why primary care is effective.

- Poor PR. Primary care doctors have less prestige. Hospitals are seen as the place where serious medical care is delivered. Primary care doctors work in offices, not hospitals. They are seen as doing the drudge work. This gives them less prestige and less visibility and their contribution to health is ignored.

- Mental health and other Cinderella areas. Primary care doctors are often working in areas that are less attractive such as helping those with mental health problems. 90% of mental health problems are managed in primary care and secondary care needs substantial resources to deliver for a small number of patients.

- Complexity and multimorbidity. Primary care doctors are experts in managing complexity where the outcomes are less good than single diseases. They are able to optimise the treatment in the elderly where it is more difficult to recognise good outcomes.

- Accessibility. Although being able to access the primary care doctor is highly valued this leads to unreasonable expectations. Primary care is seen as an infinite sink where workload can be increased without increasing resources or staffing.

Students may consider global health as being outside of their own areas of interest. They may feel that they never want to work in poor countries and have little interest in tropical diseases. They will accept that they will need to see patients who were born abroad but feel that they should treat them with the same modern treatments as other patients.

They may believe that they are going to specialise and become a consultant so do not need the wide variety of skills that a primary care doctor needs to be effective. They may struggle to understand what primary care doctors do and why they are important. An educator should try to at least help them understand that without the humble GP they would be overwhelmed with a several times increase in their workload.

War and conflict

War and conflict have a devastating impact on global health. They can lead to increased mortality, morbidity and disability. They can also disrupt healthcare systems and services, making it difficult for people to access the care they need.

Students have high engagement in this area because the problems are more immediate and necessary. The ethical issues of imposing western values are distant and the individuals' needs are clearly identified. The starkness of war makes other global health issues seem less important.

Violence particularly sexual violence is very common around the world. That does not mean that the UK does not also have problems with violent injuries. The long-term effects of conflict on our soldiers and childhood adversity on many adults mean that the subject is very real for many people.

Here are some of the ways that war and conflict impact global health:

- Increased mortality: War and conflict can lead to increased mortality through direct violence, such as injuries and death from landmines, shelling and gunfire. They can also lead to indirect violence, such as death from malnutrition, disease and exposure to hazardous materials.

- Disruption of healthcare systems: War and conflict can disrupt healthcare systems and services, making it difficult for people to access the care they need. This can be due to damage to hospitals and clinics, the displacement of healthcare workers and the lack of access to essential medicines and supplies.

- Decline in public health. War and conflict can lead to a decline in public health. This can be due to a number of factors, including the destruction of infrastructure, the displacement of people and the lack of access to clean water and sanitation.

- Increased morbidity: War and conflict can lead to increased morbidity through injuries, diseases and mental health problems. Injuries can be caused by direct violence, such as gunfire and landmines, or by indirect violence, such as falls from buildings or in vehicles. Diseases can be caused by poor sanitation, lack of access to clean water and malnutrition.

- Mental health problems: War and conflict can also lead to mental health problems, such as post-traumatic stress disorder (PTSD), anxiety and depression. These problems can have a significant impact on individuals, families and communities.

- Increased risk of infectious diseases: War and conflict can increase the risk of infectious diseases through a number of mechanisms, such as:

  o Destruction of infrastructure: War and conflict can destroy infrastructure, such as water and sanitation systems, which can increase the risk of waterborne and vector-borne diseases.

  o Mass displacement: War and conflict can lead to mass displacement, which can increase the risk of infectious diseases through crowding and poor hygiene.

  o Sexual violence: War and conflict can lead to sexual violence, which can increase the risk of HIV and other sexually transmitted infections.

Students can be asked to consider the effects of violence in their own country, stabbings, riots, protests, soldiers fighting abroad, terrorism. These examples can be used to explore how even mild levels of conflict can be highly disruptive to a society. This can open the discussion to the experience of those in war-torn areas of the world.

One engaging method of teaching about the healthcare problems related to war is a fictious journey. A child's journey through war and migration can be seen through the lens of their health problems. The students can research the common health risks in each of the steps to predict what the child will have. They can then discuss how they would address the child's needs when they attend a GP surgery in the UK.

Health inequities

Health inequities are systematic differences in health outcomes between different population groups. These differences can be due to a variety of factors, including social, economic and environmental conditions. Health inequities are a major problem in global health and they contribute to a significant amount of preventable death and disease.

There are many different ways to measure health inequities. One common approach is to use the concept of the health gap. The health gap is the difference in health outcomes between two population groups. For example, the health gap between rich and poor people can be measured by looking at the difference in life expectancy, infant mortality, or rates of chronic diseases.

Another way to measure health inequities is to use the concept of health disparities. Health disparities are differences in health outcomes that are unfair and avoidable.

Students often have mixed feelings with some believing that those who have poor health outcomes are responsible for those outcomes and others that unfairness leads to the poorer outcomes. Both ideas have some truth, many people with bad experiences have good health outcomes. Health can be irreversibly damaged by a bad experience.

There are a number of things that can be done to reduce health inequities. These include:

- Investing in social determinants of health. This includes things like improving education, providing affordable housing and creating jobs.

- Reducing discrimination. This includes things like addressing racism, sexism and other forms of discrimination.

- Promoting healthy lifestyles. This includes things like educating people about healthy eating and exercise.

- Providing access to healthcare. This includes making sure that everyone has health insurance and that healthcare is affordable.

It is important to recognise that whilst health inequities are complex and have many causes individuals affected may blame the society. The deprived groups are more likely to see themselves as victims and others as oppressors. This leads to reduced cohesion and less acceptance of social norms.

Health inequities whether real or perceived can lead to significant changes to the health of the population. There may be increased mortality and morbidity due to lifestyle changes adapting to poverty. The people involved can have reduced productivity and cause social unrest due to their sense of unfairness.

Health inequities are usually a sign of a deeper problem such as discrimination or a failing system. In a sense it is not important who is right about the causes if the inequity is present. In the short term this means that governments need to provide substantially larger resources and use multi-agency working to get the problems under control.

It is not sufficient to arrange equal access to healthcare and avoid discrimination. Societies must react to health inequities by promoting social justice and providing additional assistance to those with worse health outcomes. For example, young people with drug, alcohol and mental health problems need to see that the resources provided are increasing.

This is a counter intuitive response to unfairness as it means taking resources away from other needy people. The advantage to society of giving those suffering from health inequity greater resources is that it is more cost effective. Providing enough resources to solve the problems is cheaper than providing a sticking plaster.

Highly organised and targeted action is more likely to achieve a threshold of change. Any complex system will resist change, those people who are given the resources will argue that they are insufficient and undermine the effort. The extra funding will last long enough for there to be a change, what happens next is up to the community.

Conclusions.

Global health in medical education presents both challenges and opportunities for educators and students alike. One of the main challenges is the lack of a cohesive theory that links the various concepts within global health. However, the key elements of public health approaches such as epidemiology, health policy and ethics provide a foundation for understanding and addressing global health issues.

For educators, the question arises whether to treat each topic in global health as a separate learning objective or find a common theme to create a coherent whole. Both approaches have their advantages, with the former allowing for comparisons between different countries and the latter being more engaging for students.

Studying public health from a global perspective is attractive because it highlights the social and political determinants of health, which often play a significant role in disease causation. Factors such as poverty, lifestyle choices, inequality and lack of research into the causes of disease can have a profound impact on health outcomes and require a global perspective for effective solutions.

It is important to recognise that global health is influenced by factors beyond the control of individual governments. Issues such as war, migration, infectious disease and industry are largely determined by geographical realities rather than the political decisions of individual nations.

While global agencies like the World Health Organisation (WHO), NATO, the United Nations (UN) and the World Bank exist, they have limited power to influence global policies. The real power lies with a few countries, large corporations and financial institutions, raising questions about responsibility, funding and the inclusion of individuals' voices in global health decisions.

Global health in medical education can be organised into three groups: social and political determinants of health, global medicine and international development. These groups focus on understanding the factors that influence health, the practice of medicine in a global context and the process of development in countries. While these topics provide important insights into global health challenges, it is crucial to also consider the political dimension, including war, economic policy, climate change, resource exploitation and globalisation, as they can have a significant impact on health outcomes.

To engage students, various techniques can be employed, such as exploring the increasing globalisation of health, using case studies from developing countries, discussing the root causes of health disparities, examining national health systems, considering global health as a career and emphasising the importance of primary care. Primary care, in particular, offers simple and effective solutions to many global health problems and its value should be recognised and promoted.

War and conflict also play a significant role in global health, leading to increased mortality, disruption of healthcare systems, decline in public health, increased morbidity and mental health problems. It is important to address the impact of war and conflict on global health, as they have far-reaching consequences for individuals, communities and societies.

In conclusion, global health in medical education is a complex and multifaceted field that requires a holistic understanding of the social, political and economic factors that influence health. By integrating global health principles into medical education, students can develop the knowledge and skills needed to address the global health challenges of the present and future. It is essential for educators to engage students and help them recognise the importance of global health, including primary care, in achieving better health outcomes for individuals and communities worldwide.

Top tips.

Global includes the UK. Use the UK as an example when discussing global issues such as violence, drugs, infection, inequities and NCD. This reduces the risk that the students will see global health as third world problems.

Public Health: Focus on the social, economic and environmental factors that influence health. This includes studying social determinants of health, health policy, health ethics, cultural competence, global health law and global health and development.

Highlight the Role of Primary Care: Recognise the importance of primary care in addressing global health problems. Understand how primary care can provide simple and effective solutions to various health issues and improve health outcomes.

Chapter 24: THE CAUSES OF HEALTH DISPARITIES

Healthcare disparities are differences in the quality of healthcare that people receive based on their race, ethnicity, gender, sexual orientation, socioeconomic status, or other factors. These disparities can lead to worse health outcomes for people in marginalised groups.

There is an important difference between healthcare inequities and disparities. Whereas in the former the causes are mainly due to unfair decisions in the latter they have arisen out of other reasons as well. Whilst healthcare disparities includes inequities the solutions for the inequities will not work for disparities.

There is a risk when teaching about healthcare disparities that the educator takes a single viewpoint. Whilst increased funding and recognising structural racism is important there are other aspects. It is not possible to put right a lifetime of poor experiences, so some disparities are inevitable whatever changes are made.

The student should be able to recognise how to prioritise limited resources to maximise benefit. This cost benefit analysis may indicate that those with mental illness can benefit most from social changes such as affordable housing. Taking a primary care or public health view can enrich the student's experience of this topic.

Determinants of health care disparities.

Health disparities are differences in health status between different population groups. These disparities can be seen in a variety of areas, including life expectancy, infant mortality and rates of chronic diseases. Students should focus upon the ways in which the various determinants combine rather than each one individually.

There are many factors that contribute to health disparities, including:

- Poverty: Having less money means that fewer choices are available. They need to devote more time to managing their money. They find it more difficult to get a job because they do not have the right resources such as clothing or transport. Poverty can easily become a trap where being poor itself reduces access to employment, housing, safety and education.

- Social environment. People who live in neighbourhoods with high rates of crime and violence and have less access to healthy food and safe places to exercise must work harder to stay healthy.

- Environmental factors: People who live in areas with high levels of pollution or who are exposed to environmental toxins are more likely to experience health disparities. This is because these exposures can lead to a variety of health problems, including respiratory illnesses, cancer and birth defects.

- Family and community support. People with poor family or community have worse health because they have less access to opportunities and more exposure to risk factors.

- Behavioural factors: People who engage in unhealthy behaviours, such as smoking, drinking alcohol excessively and not exercising, are more likely to experience health disparities. This is because these behaviours can increase the risk of a variety of health problems, including heart disease, stroke and cancer.

- Access to healthcare: People who do not have access to healthcare are more likely to experience health disparities. This is because they are less likely to receive preventive care, such as vaccinations and cancer screenings and they are more likely to delay or forgo treatment for chronic diseases.

- Access to Education. Those people in society with a good education have increased choice as to where they live, the work that they can do as well as how to navigate the healthcare systems. They have a better understanding of their own health and can access healthcare more appropriately.

- Genetic factors: Some people are simply more at risk for certain diseases than others. Early death in family members leads to bereavement and less support.

- Historic discrimination. Minorities may have suffered discrimination in the past and the effects can remain present. This includes where a community lives, attitudes of the society in general, growing up in a less wealthy family and long-term effects in family members.

- Geography: People who live in rural areas are more likely to experience health disparities than people who live in urban areas. This is due to a number of factors, including access to healthcare, transportation and healthy food.

- Society health beliefs. Some societies have health beliefs that influence their uptake of care for instance a belief that older people's illnesses are just old age or drug misuse is their own choice. This can influence self help behaviour and the provision of resources by the society.

These determinants are not all fixable and it may be necessary to ignore some determinants to improve the overall effectiveness of the program. Equally failure to address key determinants may lead to the efforts being wasted. Fixing housing without mental health or vice versa is ineffective. Intersectionality refers to the phenomenon where multiple determinants intersect in the same person.

Students should be encouraged to consider combinations of the determinants but avoid believing that there is one recipe that solves all problems. Hunger is the main problem until hunger is solved, infections are the problem until we have antibiotics and so on. Solving the immediate crisis leads to problems in a different area so plans must be future proof.

This means that the students should predict the next problem when trying to solve the current problems. Ensuring access to the treatment for HIV led to marginalisation of primary care in many countries. The 'one disease' model was highly effective at achieving fair access to anti-retrovirals but missed the opportunity to improve all healthcare.

The key neutral causes of healthcare disparities are access to social support, exposure to risk factors, lack of trust in the resources available, lifestyle choices and access to healthcare. The rest of the chapter considers how to approach these areas in a way that encourages student engagement and deep understanding of the issues.

Lack of trust in the resources available.

Many people lack trust in their healthcare systems and this impacts on the quality of care that they receive. Trust is hard won and easily lost and on an individual level will always remain challenging. The greater problem is when the population as a whole starts to mistrust parts of their healthcare system.

The educator needs to help the students explore their own ideas on this topic. They should understand that trust impacts upon more than healthcare disparity. Lack of population trust means that the whole healthcare system will fail. No amount of money and resources can compensate for a population that does not trust medical advice.

Starting with individual allows the student to explore the difficulties when offering treatment to an individual. This allows them to learn that patient's background of trust in healthcare. They will then be able to identify how trust can influence disparities of health.

Looking at population trust then allows the student to consider the problem from a public health or political standpoint. Many of their solutions such as increasing funding and providing support will then be challenged. Finally looking at solutions to improving trust will help them see that trust is built with personal relationships not money.

Individual trust

There is a large overlap between the communication skills needed to work in primary care and to improve trust for individuals. There are other issues which can be addressed by a public health approach. Providing resources to remove barriers is the first step. The health care professional can only use their communication skills to improve the patient's trust if a patient attends for treatment.

There are a number of reasons why individuals may not trust the healthcare resources available to them. These reasons include:

- Past experiences with discrimination or mistreatment in the healthcare system. People who have had negative experiences in the healthcare system may be less likely to trust providers or institutions.

- Cultural differences. People from different cultures may have different expectations of the healthcare system. They may not be familiar with the system or they may not feel comfortable with the way it is structured.

- Unfairness. Even a false belief of unfairness can impact the person's health and trust in healthcare. Real unfairness will cause damage to even those who are not being adversely affected. The trust in healthcare depends upon fairness to be present and seen to be present.

- Systemic problems. There are many systemic problems that are recognised to cause healthcare disparities. When these persist and are not resolved those disadvantaged can believe that they are deliberately maintained.

- Language barriers. People who do not speak English as their first language may have difficulty communicating with providers. This can lead to misunderstandings and mistrust.

- Financial barriers. People who cannot afford healthcare may be less likely to seek care. This can lead to worse health outcomes.

Lack of trust in the resources available can have a number of negative consequences for people's health. These consequences include:

- Delayed or missed care. People who do not trust the healthcare system may delay or miss care altogether. This can lead to worse health outcomes.

- Increased use of emergency services. People who do not trust the healthcare system may only seek care when they are in an emergency. This can lead to higher costs for the healthcare system and worse health outcomes for individuals.

- Self-treating. People who do not trust the healthcare system may try to treat their own illnesses. This can be dangerous, especially if the illness is serious.

Lack of trust on an individual level will initially decrease the costs associated with their care. With time the individual will present with more advanced and more expensive problems and get less benefit from their treatment. This means that paradoxically decreasing trust initially appears to be beneficial.

A hostile practice will have lower healthcare costs, lower levels of illness and perhaps even higher approval for those that do attend. Only with time the failure to engage with the practice population will become apparent. The patients will learn to look for a quick fix, wait for the out of hours or accept their sickness rather than access effective care.

Population trust.

Where a population loses trust in their healthcare there are many of the same features as with individual loss of trust. Populations can also put pressure upon government, change to private or non-medical providers and cause breakdown of systems such as immunisation and social disorder.

An example is the failure to provide effective mental health services. This has led to increasing prevalence and severity of mental illness, increased drug and alcohol abuse and suicidal behaviour. The costs of this failure go beyond the direct costs of medical treatments into increased need for social care, prisons and increasing areas of deprivation.

- Increased pressure on the government: When people lose trust in the healthcare system, they may put pressure on the government to do something about it. This can lead to healthcare reorganisations which make it more difficult to deliver care.

- Increased use of private or non-medical providers: When people lose trust in the healthcare system, they may be more likely to undergo private investigations and treatments leaving the NHS to pick up the bill for follow up.

- Breakdown of systems such as immunisation: When people lose trust in the healthcare system, they may be less likely to follow public health recommendations, such as getting vaccinated. This can lead to outbreaks of preventable diseases.

- Social disorder: When people lose trust in the healthcare system, they may be more likely to engage in social disorder, such as violence or vandalism in healthcare buildings. This can lead to further barriers to healthcare.

It is difficult for politicians to maintain population trust as they largely depend upon ideas from healthcare. When creating solutions to healthcare disparities it is important to recognise that a failing healthcare system effects everyone. Even where a two-tier system exists those rich enough to pay can still be exposed to the risk of poor health due to social disorder.

Solutions.

The solutions to issues of trust are arguably at the heart of improving healthcare. As the quality of healthcare falls then the worst hit will be those at the bottom. Trust is the fuel that keeps healthcare floating but most solutions are based on other ideas. The cost effective approach to give priority to solutions which increase trust.

When governments try to improve healthcare, they typically address the most difficult and costly problems. This leads to greater healthcare disparities as a cheap but effective solution will not be attractive to the voters. The professionals who advise governments should therefore explain why steps such as GP access will help them trust healthcare in general.

There are a number of things that can be done to address the issue of lack of trust in the healthcare resources available. These things include:

- Improving the quality of care delivered: People need to be confident that they will receive high-quality care when they need it. This means improving the quality of care across the board but especially at the first points of contact.

- Providing culturally competent care. Providers should understand the cultural needs of their patients. Patients will only seek care when they trust the healthcare practitioners will be able to help them. Being able to recognise cultural cues can improve healthcare.

- Breaking down communication barriers. Communicating even with an interpreter is difficult and takes a long time. Providers and patients need a common language to ensure smooth access and mutual trust.

- Removing barriers to healthcare. People should be able to access healthcare without unnecessary barriers. This may be the indirect costs or choosing to pay for private care. Any barrier leads to lowered trust because they feel discriminated against.

- Making the healthcare system more transparent and accountable: People need to be able to trust that the healthcare system is working in their best interests. This means making sure that the system is transparent and accountable.

- Addressing the stigma of mental illness: There remains a large gap between the funding of mental illness both in primary and secondary care and physical illness. This gives the impression that mental illness cannot be treated effectively and people then lose trust that they can get help.

Surprisingly most of the solutions for improving healthcare and reducing disparities are cheap. They may even save money particularly if the general social costs are included. E.g. providing GPs with short term extra funding could increase mental health support and address local backlogs.

The solutions require access to practitioners who understand mental illness, communication and culture. The solutions need practitioners who can explain the reasons for the decision and help them access the right care. The solutions need people who are available, qualified and skilled rather than high-cost technological fixes.

GPs are excellent at innovating cost effective solutions so no increase in managers would be required. The advantages and disadvantages of blind faith in GPs rather than micromanaging GPs can be discussed. Students should debate whether the government trusting GPs might have positive outcomes.

Evaluation of Interventions is essential and the educator could ask the students for examples of how they would measure success. This will help them see that changes are slow and there are few hard outcome measures. Biopsychosocial progress is a measure that has promise in this area.

Access to healthcare

Healthcare cannot provide care effectively if the public does not self-care but those who are poor will need more advice to effectively self-care. This means that having good access to healthcare is essential to reduce health disparities. Those with more skills are more able to navigate complex systems and will receive more advice.

The key problem in many western healthcare systems is a lack of primary care doctors. This appears to be as much about overregulation as actual lack of personnel. There are hundreds of thousands of doctors in the UK so any shortage of staff appears to be related to the rules on who is allowed to work.

In deprived areas there are also other problems that are listed here and these will need to be addressed even if sufficient GPs can be found.

- Increasing the number of primary care providers. Primary care providers are the first point of contact for many patients. Increasing the number of primary care providers would help to improve access to care and reduce wait times.
- Healthcare literacy. Healthcare access is often based upon the communities views the right problems to see the GP about. Having better ways of describing symptoms and problems with each other can improve self-care and appropriateness of attendance.
- Improving the coordination of care. The coordination of care is the process of ensuring that patients receive the care they need from the right providers at the right time. Improving the coordination of care would help to improve patient outcomes and reduce costs.
- Reducing administrative barriers. Administrative barriers, such as paperwork, phoning for an appointment and long wait times, can make it difficult for people to access healthcare. Allowing patients to book online or email for advice can improve this.
- Community engagement. Communities can help support healthcare providers in many ways from volunteering to education. Grassroots initiatives can address social problems that the healthcare professionals cannot.
- Expanding access to other health care professionals. Dental and vision care are often not well served in many populations. Investing in community-based health care professionals can improve access generally.
- Reducing direct costs of healthcare. Reducing the cost of prescription drugs, dental treatment and private investigations would help to make healthcare more affordable for everyone.
- Providing transportation assistance to healthcare appointments. Transportation can be a barrier to accessing healthcare for many people. Providing transportation assistance would help to ensure that everyone has access to the care they need.

- Expanding access to telehealth. Telehealth is the use of technology to provide healthcare services remotely. Expanding access to telehealth would help to make healthcare more accessible for people who live in rural areas or who have difficulty getting to a doctor's surgery.
- Investing in preventive care. Preventive care is the care that is given to patients to prevent them from getting sick. Investing in preventive care would help to improve public health and reduce healthcare costs.

There are many problems that prevent good access to healthcare and solving some will improve general access, others are particularly useful for disadvantaged populations. When discussing how improving access with reduce healthcare disparities the educator should focus on simple low-cost solutions.

Students can be encouraged to look for win-win solutions which improve both healthcare disparities and overall healthcare. Zero sum game is initially attractive as it is appears fairer but in the long run the poor will lose out. A solution that offers benefits for the rich is more likely to be accepted than one that only offers an advantage to the poor.

Lifestyle choices.

Lifestyle choices can play a significant role in health disparities. For example, people who smoke, drink excessively, or eat unhealthy diets are more likely to develop chronic diseases such as heart disease, stroke and cancer.

These diseases are more common in people of lower socioeconomic status, who are more likely to live in areas with fewer healthy choices and more unhealthy choices. Addressing the inequities of living in a deprived area can help reduce unhealthy lifestyles.

There are a number of things that can be done to address health disparities but few are primary health issues. GPs can screen for poor lifestyles and offer additional services to those with mental health. They can open surgeries in poorer areas and develop additional services.

Many lifestyle choices can only be improved by increased flexibility in poorer areas. Allowing the area to impose restrictions on fast food, permitting targeted funding, short term resources when required, policing and social work, outreach work and addressing local needs.

The students can consider a case study of a person risk factors for heart disease tries to improve their health. The social barriers to accessing smoking cessation, better food and doing more exercise. The costs of reducing barriers to health can be compared with the costs of treating poor health.

- Improving access to healthy food in deprived areas: This can be done by expanding the availability of healthy food options in grocery stores and restaurants in these areas. It can also be done by providing subsidies to help people purchase healthy food.

- Targeting resources on those with the worst lifestyles: This can be done by providing targeted interventions, such as smoking cessation programs and weight loss programs, to people who are at high risk for chronic diseases.

- Stop smoking clinics in poorer areas: This can help to reduce smoking rates in these areas, which would lead to improved health outcomes.

- Improving mental health for those at risk: This can be done by increasing the availability of mental health services in deprived areas and by providing education and support to people who are at risk for mental health problems.

- Reducing discrimination in housing, employment and education: This can be done by passing laws that prohibit discrimination and by enforcing these laws. It can also be done by educating people about the importance of non-discrimination.

- Expanding access to healthcare in deprived areas: This can be done by increasing the number of healthcare providers in these areas and by making healthcare more affordable.

- Improving the quality of healthcare in deprived areas: This can be done by providing training and support to healthcare providers in these areas and by investing in new technologies and equipment.

- Involving poorer communities in improving their lifestyles: This can be done by working with community leaders and organisations to identify the needs of the community and to develop solutions that are tailored to the specific needs of the community.

- Identifying local resources for exercise: This can be done by creating maps of local parks, trails and gyms. It can also be done by providing information about local fitness classes and programs.

This focus on deprived areas is not altruistic or positive discrimination. These areas have the highest rates of disease so that the benefits from any intervention are greatest. The people with lifestyle problems are more likely to cost the health system money and least likely to contribute in taxes. They also have the highest birth rates and therefore the greatest contribution to the next generation.

The value of providing extra resources to this group is that it is the most cost-effective method. Targeting at those with greatest needs has the greatest benefit for the lowest costs. There is some evidence that improvements in lifestyle for the poorest can actually reduce the costs overall.

Social support.

Social support from the family, social group and wider community improves prognosis of many diseases. The reasons for this improvement are likely to be complex and multiple. A person who has social support will usually make better choices, has access to shared resources and protection from adverse events.

Being part of a group also appears to have psychological benefits, emotional stability, shared purpose and social conformity. Although poverty is a risk factor for poor social support loneliness is not restricted to those who are poor. The whole society will benefit from living in a community with stronger ties and more cohesion.

Friendships and families are key elements of social support and the quality of those elements is a large determinant of long term health. A child who grows up in a low-quality social environment will on average have worse education, access to healthcare, behaviour problems and poorer health beliefs whatever the income of their parents.

The educator may find this area challenging to teach as it is not clear what the healthcare professional can do to improve social support. The traditional approaches have limited effectiveness as single interventions however combinations can have excellent results.

- Community health workers: Community health workers are individuals who are trained to provide social support and health education in their communities. Providing direct social support in the home and teaching about self-management of healthcare conditions is effective but time-consuming.

- Groupwork program. The Sure Start program has many of the advantages of Community health workers but is provided in a group environment. This has led to increased cost effectiveness although it is not suitable for all clients.

- Support groups: Support groups are groups of people who meet regularly to discuss their experiences with a particular health condition. They can provide emotional support, education and practical advice.

- Carer support: Carers such as mothers or those caring for disabled people often require assistance. Focusing limited healthcare resources on these carers improve the health of the carer themselves but also those that they care for. The general benefits make this intervention particularly cost effective as well as reducing healthcare disparities.

- Telehealth: Telehealth services allow people to communicate with healthcare providers remotely. This can be especially helpful for people who live in rural areas or who have difficulty accessing healthcare. Often these services are used to provide social support to lonely people so a diverse team is useful.

- Family therapy: Although formal family therapy is costly and difficult to organise community workers often visit families at home. This gives the opportunity to speak with the members of the family and friends and understand their concerns.

- Supporting Self-help: Encouraging contacting the friends and family, getting involved the community with support can be helpful. Many people struggle to know how to make contact or manage their interactions so support from a health care professional can be useful. The professional's involvement can be relatively minor for the benefit attained.

- Social Media: Online relationships do not suit everyone and for some it makes them lonelier and feel cut off. Health care professionals should consider the suitability of this type of interaction and risk factors such as the risk of online stalking. Signposting to supportive online groups can help.

- Education: Whether taking a class or enrolling on a degree learning can give purpose to those who are struggling. The advantage of this type of help is that educational establishments have resources and skills is helping those with problems. Health care professionals can help by identifying any learning problems that need adjustments.

Improving social support is within the skillset of most health care professionals and should be seen as part of their role in reducing healthcare disparities. The benefit from these interventions is slow to appear but generally require modest resources.

The health care professional's key role is to provide psychological support and problem solve. Students can consider why they would find this type of work difficult. Some will find it emotionally challenging to talk to people who are struggling. Others will recognise that they too have socially empty lives and feel upset.

The concept of psychosocial progress can be useful to assess the effectiveness of social interventions. The small improvements in personal and social functioning will improve the overall health. Patients are more likely to comply with health checks and self care if their lives are improving even slightly.

Exposure to risk factors.

There is a large overlap between risk factors for health disparities and adverse childhood experiences (ACE). It is important to recognise that almost all people have some adverse childhood experiences. The students can be asked to discuss why people are reluctant to discuss their own adverse childhood experiences.

Some educators ask students to share their adverse childhood experiences however this is problematic. Apart from the risk of triggering psychological breakdown there are issues of confidentiality. Those who have shared may be concerned that they will be judged by their peers or the educator.

For this reason, students should be cautioned to avoid disclosing their adverse childhood experiences. They should be advised against discussing them with their peers. They should be signposted to student healthcare support and their personal tutor. This will help them understand why many people are correctly reluctant to discuss adverse childhood experiences.

This may appear paradoxical for the students, people should share their experiences particularly with their doctors. They will ask how doctors can help patients if they do not disclose what made them unwell in the first place. The students can then be asked what help they would provide for these patients.

The management of ACEs is complex and can be learned by doctors but is a special skill. This means that doctors need to work with social workers if they are going to help their patients. The educator can ask the students whether they intend to undertake the necessary training to be able to manage their patient's ACEs.

The idea of this exercise is to help students understand the difficulties of disclosing ACEs. This helps them develop strategies for approaching patients with ACEs. A key idea is that many people without overt mental illness struggle with ACEs. A simple approach that all doctors can learn is to explain the risk factors associated with ACEs.

- Stress response system. ACEs can affect the system responsible for regulating the body's reaction to stress. When the stress response system is damaged, it can lead to chronic inflammation, which can damage the body's tissues and organs.
- Brain development. The brain is particularly vulnerable to stress during childhood. When children experience stress, it can change the way that their brains develop. This can lead to problems with attention, memory and learning.
- Emotional regulation. Both abnormal stress responses and brain development can make emotional regulation more difficult. This can make it more difficult to make good decisions.
- Personality disorder. Those with a history of ACEs have an increased risk of developing a personality disorder. This appears to be a defence response to their emotional regulation problems and ongoing life stressors. They can find that their brain does not work the same as other people's.
- Poor education. Learning involves more than intelligence, the person must concentrate and practice the material. Brain changes and abnormal stress response can interfere with learning. Children can find that they bring their emotional responses from home into school.
- Reduced supportive relationships. Having ACEs makes it more difficult to have the strong social connections needed to buffer the effects of ACEs.
- Violence. People with a history of ACEs may use violence as a way of coping. They are at very much higher risk of being victims of violence because they have problems with recognising dangers and are less good at judging character.
- Unhealthy behaviours. People with ACEs are more likely to smoke, drink alcohol and use drugs to cope with stress. They are at increased risk of addiction likely due to brain changes. These unhealthy behaviours can also contribute to worse health.
- Infections and allergies. The immune system is impacted by stress. This can lead to lowered resistance to infections and risk of diseases such as fibromyalgia and chronic fatigue.
- Increased risk of mental health problems. A history of ACEs makes the person more susceptible to mental health problems. They may develop PTSD from the ACE itself but have a higher risk when dealing with later experiences. Often they struggle to enjoy good experiences.

Many students are reluctant to request support for these risk factors because they believe that social workers do a poor job. Whilst the newspapers are full of stories suggesting that social workers are incapable to protecting children the truth is somewhat different. The best way of addressing this misconception is by asking a social worker to participate in a teaching session.

The failure of medical health professionals and social workers to work together is a major cause of healthcare disparities. The social workers have techniques to address many of the risk factors. Doctors prefer to manage the risk factors without training or the necessary skills.

Breaking down the barriers between these two professions will take more than educational experiences but it is a start. Most social workers are natural problem solvers and most doctors have a lot in common with them. Social worker techniques involve many familiar to specialists in areas such as psychiatry but they also use the law.

Social workers having access to a stick may be uncomfortable to doctors but it means that new choices are available. Many mental health crises have been averted by the social worker and doctor playing bad cop – good cop. If the educator is unfamiliar with the role of a social worker then healthcare disparity is an excellent opportunity to learn.

Conclusions.

Health disparities are complex and multifaceted issues that stem from various causes. Poverty, social environment, environmental factors, lack of family and community support, behavioural factors, limited access to healthcare and education, genetic factors, historic discrimination, geography and societal health beliefs all contribute to health disparities. While increased funding and addressing structural problems are important, it is crucial to recognise that solving healthcare disparities requires a multifaceted approach that considers the interplay of these determinants.

Lack of trust in the healthcare resources available is a significant factor contributing to health disparities. Both individual and population trust are essential for a functioning healthcare system. Addressing this issue involves improving the quality of care, providing culturally competent care, breaking down communication barriers, removing financial barriers, making the healthcare system transparent and accountable and addressing the stigma of mental illness.

Access to healthcare is another key factor that affects health disparities. Increasing the number of primary care providers, improving care coordination, reducing administrative barriers, expanding access to other healthcare professionals, reducing direct costs, providing transportation assistance, expanding telehealth and investing in preventive care are all crucial steps to improve access to healthcare.

Lifestyle choices also play a role in health disparities. Unhealthy behaviours such as smoking, excessive alcohol consumption and poor diet contribute to the development of chronic diseases that disproportionately affect marginalised populations. Addressing these disparities requires promoting healthier lifestyles and providing education and resources to support individuals in making healthier choices.

In addressing health disparities, it is important to consider cost-effectiveness and prioritise solutions that benefit both disadvantaged populations and the overall healthcare system. By implementing comprehensive strategies that address the various determinants of health disparities, it is possible to make improvement even if equitable healthcare for all individuals is not possible.

Top tips.

New theories: The current theories of health disparities and associated social determinants have not led to solutions. There is a need to find a way of simplifying the complexity.

Adverse Childhood Experiences (ACEs): ACEs contribute to health disparities through long term impacts on the individual's health. Prevention and treatment of the effects of ACEs is a key priority in reducing inequities.

Collaborative working. The best results achieved is provided by different professional groups working together. Primary care doctors working with social workers is a collaboration which is more successful than standard care.

Chapter 25: PROFESSIONAL STANDARDS.

Professional standards are a set of expectations for the knowledge, skills and behaviours that doctors should demonstrate in order to be effective in their roles. These standards are designed to help doctors reflect on their practice, identify areas for improvement and develop a plan for professional learning.

Professional standards are important for a number of reasons. First, they help to ensure that doctors provide high-quality care to their patients. Second, they help to protect patients from harm. Third, they help to maintain the public's trust in the medical profession.

Teaching professional standards is challenging because much of the guidance is written in general way that is not easy to apply to practice. Situational judgement and ethics attempt to address this problem but do not indicate what professionalism is. The student can learn all the rules without understanding what they are intended to achieve.

The concept of professional standards is controversial and the educator needs to address this issue in their teaching. The key complaint is that statements on professional standards paradoxically worsen standards by devaluing individual contributions.

Students should learn that they need to develop their own professionalism and not to rely upon any one size fits all solution. They should expect to be challenged and be able to defend their approach to professionalism. Where approaches differ from standard guidelines they should be prepared to consider the situation. Their opinions upon professionalism should not be biased.

Key areas of practice model.

The first model for professional standards for doctors to consider is key areas of practice. All doctors need various skills to be effective and the model considers those skills. What the model does not explain is what professionalism is beyond being a good person.

The simple division of tasks in the model makes it clear that simply having knowledge and skills is not sufficient. A doctor who is dishonest, lacks integrity and respect will be a danger however good their knowledge and skills. Students can be asked whether they believe professionalism is essential.

- Knowledge of medical science: Doctors should have a comprehensive understanding of medical science, including anatomy, physiology, biochemistry, pharmacology and pathology.

- Clinical skills: Doctors should be able to perform a physical exam, order and interpret diagnostic tests and develop and implement treatment plans.

- Communication skills: Doctors should be able to communicate effectively with patients, their families and other healthcare professionals.

- Professionalism: Doctors should demonstrate professional behaviour, including honesty, integrity and respect for patients and their families.

This is a good opportunity to discuss what the student's own beliefs about professionalism are. This is an important foundation for the further discussion because some students will try to argue that professionalism does not exist outside of good medical practice.

Discussing why being a good person is an important part of being a doctor helps ground further teaching in this area. It is possible to ask the students to define what being a good person means to them. Often students will notice that there are many behaviours that are relevant to life in general but some are specific for being a doctor.

Ordinary Professionalism

Professionalism is a set of values and behaviours that are expected of people who are employed in a profession. It is characterised by a commitment to excellence, a high standard of conduct and a respect for others. Professionalism is important in the workplace because it helps to create a productive and respectful environment. It also helps to build trust and confidence between colleagues and clients.

The ordinary professionalism model grounds the standards within those behaviours that are expected of any good person. Few professionals would challenge the basic assumption that a doctor should be a good person. The assumption in the model that doctors should therefore be better than ordinary good people is largely unchallenged.

There are many different aspects of professionalism, but some of the most important include:

- Honesty and integrity: To be a good person honesty is an essential trait. A doctor might be expected to adhere to a higher standard of honesty and trustworthiness.

- Competence: Professionals should take responsibility to ensure that they are competent in their field. This appears to go beyond the normal standards as doctors must check that they have knowledge and skills necessary to do their job well.

- Respect: Professionals should respect the rights and dignity of others. They should be polite and courteous, even when they disagree with someone. Doctors are often asked to tolerate rudeness and abuse from patients or their relatives.

- Diligence: Professionals should be diligent in their work. They should be reliable and hardworking as would be expected from any worker. The standard expected from doctors is higher, they should not go home at the end of the shift if there are insufficient resources.

- Responsibility: Professionals are responsible for their actions. They take ownership of their work making records and addressing any mistakes. They also have a duty of candour which is a positive duty to confess when a mistake has occurred and draw attention to it.

- Appearance: Professionals dress and groom themselves appropriately for the workplace. They are clean and tidy and they avoid wearing anything that is too revealing or too casual. Doctors are expected to go beyond this and should also move and talk in way that is expected of them.

- Communication: Professionals communicate effectively. They are clear and concise in their speech and writing and they are always respectful of others' time. Doctors' communication is scrutinised regularly and any minor errors can be the subject of a complaint. The doctor may be responsible for how the patient sees their communication rather than just whether it was appropriate.

- Ethics: Professionals behave ethically. They follow the rules and regulations of their profession and they always act in the best interests of their clients. Doctors have higher ethical standards to follow with many rules and regulations that do not apply to normal people.

This model is useful to show creep in standards, the entirely reasonable statement that a doctor should be respectful becomes the more troubling statement that doctors should accept abuse. The reasonable requirement for diligence becomes an imperative to cover for management deficiencies.

The risk from these standards is that they provide an excuse for others to fail. The doctor does not require enough time to do their job or sufficient resources. They do not require support when making difficult decisions, they can be complained about and criticised for minor errors. They can be forced to work when ill or exhausted and still measured against impossible standards.

This model gives specific examples of professional behaviour and students should understand the difference between the general principles and the creep. The model finds the balance between common sense and idealism. There is however no sense of the professional being a human being or having a bad day or anyone but the doctor being responsible for what goes wrong.

The Seven Principles of Public Life (also known as the Nolan Principles)

Professionalism as a set of rules is taken further with the Nolan Principles which the educator can use as an example of how to get professionalism wrong. The Nolan Principles model has been seen as blaming the individual for systemic problems and as being systemically biased against minorities. The UK government has adopted the principles and I have quoted them verbatim. They appear superficially reasonable but have been widely criticised.

- *'Selflessness: Holders of public office should act solely in terms of the public interest.*
- *Integrity: Holders of public office must avoid placing themselves under any obligation to people or organisations that might try inappropriately to influence them in their work. They should not act or take decisions in order to gain financial or other material benefits for themselves, their family, or their friends. They must declare and resolve any interests and relationships.*
- *Objectivity: Holders of public office must act and take decisions impartially, fairly and on merit, using the best evidence and without discrimination or bias.*
- *Accountability: Holders of public office are accountable to the public for their decisions and actions and must submit themselves to the scrutiny necessary to ensure this.*
- *Openness: Holders of public office should act and take decisions in an open and transparent manner. Information should not be withheld from the public unless there are clear and lawful reasons for so doing.*
- *Honesty: Holders of public office should be truthful.*

- *Leadership: Holders of public office should exhibit these principles in their own behaviour. They should actively promote and robustly support the principles and be willing to challenge poor behaviour wherever it occurs.'*

The Seven Principles of Public Life are generally accepted as a good framework for ethical conduct in public office. However, there are some potential arguments against them.

- The principles are too vague. The principles are broad and open to interpretation, which can make it difficult to apply them in specific cases. For example, what does it mean to act "solely in terms of the public interest"? What does it mean to be "impartial"? These are questions that can be difficult to answer definitively.
- The principles are unrealistic. The principles assume that public office-holders are always able to act in a selfless and impartial manner. In reality, public office-holders may be motivated by a variety of factors, including personal ambition, financial gain, or the desire to help their friends and family.
- The principles are not enforced effectively. There is no single body that is responsible for enforcing the Seven Principles of Public Life. This means that it can be difficult to hold public office-holders accountable for their actions.
- The principles are too focused on the individual. The principles focus on the individual behaviour of public office-holders, rather than on the broader institutional and cultural factors that can contribute to corruption and unethical behaviour.
- The principles are not culturally sensitive. The principles are based on Western values, such as individualism and the rule of law. These values may not be shared by all cultures, which could make it difficult to apply the principles in some contexts.

Overall, the Seven Principles of Public Life are a necessary framework for ethical conduct in public office. They provide a set of general principles that can help public office-holders remain accountable to the public. They have substantial limitations and over-rigid application would make most political decisions impossible.

It can be argued that the Seven Principles of Public Life apply to doctors as medical practitioners are members of the establishment. The current trends in professional standards suggest that doctors are seen in this way. Students may be uncomfortable with the idea that they are entering public life. They may feel that a vocation should be protected from public scrutiny or even that they are just doing a job and have a right to privacy.

Benefits and problems with professional standards.

Doctors who fail to meet professional standards may face disciplinary action, such as suspension or revocation of their license to practice medicine. Doctors generally support the use of professional standards to maintain the reputation of their profession and prevent dangerous doctors from harming patients.

Doctors are concerned when professional standards are used to drive good doctors out of the profession, impose management decisions or obstruct good quality care. Educators can discuss with students what they can do to achieve the benefits and avoid the problems with professional standards.

Here are some of the benefits of professional standards for doctors:

- Improved patient care: Professional standards help to ensure that doctors provide high-quality care to their patients. This is because the standards set out the knowledge, skills and behaviours that doctors should demonstrate in order to be effective in their roles.

- Protection of patients: Professional standards help to protect patients from harm. This is because the standards set out clear expectations for how doctors should interact with patients. For example, the standards state that doctors should always act in the best interests of their patients and that they should never discriminate against patients based on their race, religion, gender, or any other factor.

- Maintenance of public trust: Professional standards help to maintain the public's trust in the medical profession. This is because the standards set out clear expectations for how doctors should behave. For example, the standards state that doctors should always be honest and trustworthy in their interactions with patients and colleagues.

These benefits are necessary and proportionate to the risks that medical practice presents to the public. Poor quality care, patients being harmed by doctors and erosion of the public trust can all lead to long term disability and death. These risks are substantial and push regulators towards restrictive standards.

Some of the problems that current models of professional standards can encounter are as follows.

- The rules are biased towards doctors who have had access to public school education and a stable childhood.

- The rules are often based on a white, Western, middle-class perspective, which can exclude the experiences and perspectives of doctors from other backgrounds.

- The rules can be used to reinforce social hierarchies and power imbalances.

- The rules are open to interpretation and can be used to exclude specific types of behaviour, such as wearing odd clothing or explaining something with humour.

- Much of what is considered professionalism is based on the patient's perspective, which can be subjective and biased.

- There is no appeal process or way to challenge a decision about professionalism.

- Doctors who are disabled are forced to comply with the rules, even if that disadvantages them.

- Decisions about professionalism are made by a committee who may not share their reasoning with the doctor.

- The public discourse about professionalism is limited.

- The rules are often outdated and do not reflect the realities of modern practice.

- The rules are not always clear, which can lead to confusion and uncertainty.

- The rules are often too rigid and do not allow for individual expression or creativity.

- The rules are often enforced inconsistently, which can lead to unfairness.

- The rules are often used to punish doctors for minor infractions, which can have a chilling effect on free speech and whistleblowing.

- The rules are often used to protect the interests of the profession, rather than the interests of patients.

- The rules can be used to silence dissent or to punish doctors who speak out about important issues.

- The rules can create a culture of fear and intimidation, making it difficult for doctors to report concerns about patient safety or unethical behaviour.

Professionalism may be a series of rules to constrain the doctor's autonomy, a list of instructions to being a good doctor or ways to punish doctors who get out of line. For many students they will appear to be a way of excluding disabled and minorities without having to say so.

The rules do appear to be highly biased to the 'right sort' of doctor who has had access to public school education and a stable childhood. Many of the rules can be interpreted to exclude specific types of behaviour. Does wearing odd clothing make you a bad doctor? Does explaining something with humour or in an unconventional way prevent you from giving good care?

The problem appears to be that much of what is considered as professionalism is from the point of view of the patient. A patient who feels that the doctor was not competent, respectful, diligent can raise a complaint. Their opinions might be based upon the colour or sex of the doctor but they are not challenged as long as they limit their complaint to these factors.

There is no appeal or way of challenging the issue of professionalism. A doctor who is disabled must comply with the rules even if that disadvantages them. Any decision about professionalism is taken by a committee who may not share their reasoning even to the doctor. Public discourse about professionalism appears limited and the educator may find that the students are less than happy with the present situation.

Research into professional standards.

The type of data that would be useful to inform debate about professional standards is not always collected. Any system should be monitored for adverse effects and professional standards have great potential for harm. Educators can help students understand their role in professional standards by discussing what data would be useful.

The following topics could be discussed with the students to help them understand what they could do to improve professionalism. By discussing what the results might show and what actions might be taken as a result the students will gain a deeper understanding of the subject.

- The role of professional standards in maintaining public trust in the healthcare system. How do professional standards help to ensure that the public has confidence in the healthcare system? What are the challenges of maintaining public trust in an increasingly complex and fragmented healthcare system?
- The impact of professional standards on patient outcomes. Do professional standards lead to better patient outcomes, reduced cost and improved safety? Or do they simply create a more bureaucratic and paperwork-intensive environment that makes it more difficult to provide high-quality care and make errors more likely?

- The role of professional standards in promoting equity and justice in healthcare. How do professional standards help to ensure that all patients receive the same level of care, regardless of their race, ethnicity, gender, or socioeconomic status?
- The relationship between professional standards and innovation in healthcare. Do professional standards stifle innovation by making it difficult for new treatments and technologies to be adopted? Or do they help to ensure that patients receive up to date care?
- The role of professional standards in promoting diversity and inclusion in the medical profession. Do professional standards help to ensure that the medical profession is representative of the population that it serves? Or do they create a culture of conformity that makes it difficult for doctors from minority groups to succeed?
- The impact of professional standards on the quality of life of healthcare professionals. Professional standards can have a significant impact on the quality of life of healthcare professionals. For example, professional standards can lead to increased stress and burnout, or they can make it difficult for professionals to balance their work and personal lives.
- How do professional standards differ across different countries? The current models on professional standards may be missing key approaches that should be incorporated. They may have solutions to our problems and be able to tailor the standards more appropriately.

These topics for research are complex and engaging and the educator can bring the ideas together by making the issue more personal. Each student needs to find their own solution to professionalism. Changing the focus from asking what professionalism is, to what it means to the individual, can help resolve the confusion in this subject.

The reason is that one-size-fits all solutions to issues such as human behaviour are always limited. The students need to understand that by imposing rules upon each other they are denying their humanity. This causes bias and stress with worsened team cohesion and communication. The correct approach is recognise diversity and value different members of the team.

How can doctors develop their own professionalism?

Developing a sense of professionalism is partly about understanding what a good person is and partly about teamwork. Teamwork involves understanding the roles that the individual and their colleagues take within groups. Each doctor must approach their work focusing on their strengths.

Professionalism is understanding how to be a good person using the tools that they have access to. It is not trying to change the doctor's personality so that it fits a standard model. It is recognising that the doctor's personality will define the type of professional they will become.

- Reflect on their values and beliefs. What is important to them in their personal and professional lives? What are their core values? Once they have a good understanding of their own values, they can start to align their behaviour with those values.

- Identify conflicts with ethical codes. These codes outline the standards of conduct that are expected of doctors. By recognising when there may be conflict between their beliefs and the ethical codes they can learn how both to stay true to their beliefs and follow the code.

- Use a respectful manner. There are many approaches that a doctor can use when dealing with patients, colleagues and other healthcare professionals. Using a respectful approach first is more likely to get a good response. The person's response to the respectful approach is a good guide as to what approach should be taken next.

- Have a reputation for honest and trustworthy. Doctors who have a good reputation particularly for honesty are more likely to trusted. Being aware of one's reputation and working to build a good reputation can be a useful investment.

- Show an interest providing high-quality care. Doctors and other professionals often are aware of how good their colleagues are clinically. Showing an interest in providing high-quality care can help colleagues feel confident in the doctor. Colleagues are more likely to step in and help a doctor who is struggling if they indicate that they want to provide high quality care.

- Model positive role models. Find doctors who you admire for their professionalism and integrity and watch how they interact with others. Colleagues will recognise the steps you take as they know what you are trying to achieve. You can also learn a lot from observing how they handle difficult situations.

- Be a team player. Doctors work in a variety of settings and they often need to collaborate with other healthcare professionals to provide the best possible care for their patients. This means listening to others' perspectives, understanding why they disagree and be willing to compromise.

- Lifelong learning. Staying interested in patients, their illness and medicine in general can make it easier to align professional standards and the doctor's own professionalism. It makes conflicts less likely to occur because the doctor will understand why they need to change their approach in a specific circumstance and be flexible.

- Other roles. One way of developing professionalism is taking on roles such as mentoring, education, management or leadership. Where the doctor's values align with these roles they can be useful in helping the doctor develop. Role conflicts can occur which paradoxically can make the doctor's values appear aligned when they are not.

- Reflection and feedback. Where a situation has occurred the student can learn from that situation through reflection and feedback. This ensures that in future the behaviours are better aligned to the doctor's professionalism.

Some students will question the focus on appearing to comply with the rules. They will ask whether it is good for a doctor to pretend as this will lead to stress. They will be concerned that some of these approaches appear to be manipulative or trying to persuade others. The educator can help the students see that professionalism is about how others see doctors.

A doctor who is caring, compassionate and honest but is seen by others to be uncaring and dishonest has not succeeded. These techniques are based upon the fact that students are human beings with their own views. Human beings will not always be able to perfectly align with professional standards and ethics.

All doctors need to take care of their reputation and find workarounds for where they do not fit with perfection. Choosing role models, trying to work as a team and starting with a respectful approach may not make you a better doctor but it reduces resistance from colleagues to your approach. Showing an interest in things like lifelong learning, high standards and reflection can make fitting in easier.

The educator's role in teaching about professional standards is not to try to indoctrinate the students in a particular model. The educator should try to help students consider their own approach to professionalism. Students should recognise that authenticity is far more effective than a jobsworth following of rules.

Resist the creep of professionalism:

The definition of professionalism is constantly evolving depending upon political factors. The concept of professionalism can be used to justify unethical or discriminatory practices.

The concept of professionalism is often used to put pressure on doctors to comply with an idealised view of what a doctor should be. This can lead to unrealistic expectations, burnout and a loss of autonomy.

Doctors need to be aware of the ways in which the concept of professionalism can be used to manipulate or control them. Doctors should not be afraid to challenge the status quo and to speak up for what they believe in.

Challenge unrealistic expectations. When you are asked to do something that is not in the best interests of your patients or your own well-being, speak up. Explain why the request is unreasonable and offer alternative solutions.

Doctors need to work together to resist the creep of professionalism. This means complaining about managers who are imposing unrealistic expectations.

Create a culture of support. Talk to your colleagues about the challenges of maintaining professional standards in today's healthcare environment. Share tips and strategies for coping with stress and burnout.

Involve medical leaders. Encourage medical leaders to work to promote physician wellness and professional autonomy. These leaders can provide you with support when challenging professional creep.

By working together, doctors can resist the creep of professionalism and create a healthcare environment that is supportive, respectful and conducive to providing high-quality care.

Conclusions.

Professional standards play a crucial role in guiding the knowledge, skills and behaviours expected of doctors. They help ensure high-quality patient care, protect patients from harm and maintain public trust in the medical profession. However, teaching professional standards can be challenging due to the general nature of the guidance and the lack of clarity on what professionalism truly entails.

Different models of professional standards are available such as Key areas of practice, Ordinary professionalism and Principles of public life. These models emphasise the importance of knowledge, clinical skills, communication, professionalism, honesty, integrity, respect, diligence, responsibility, appearance, ethics and leadership.

While professional standards have benefits such as improved patient care, patient protection and maintenance of public trust, they also face several problems. These include biases, cultural insensitivity, reinforcement of power imbalances, subjective interpretations, lack of clarity, rigidity, inconsistent enforcement, punishment for minor infractions, silencing dissent and a culture of fear.

It is important for educators to engage students in discussions about their beliefs and understanding of professionalism, as well as the potential problems and biases within professional standards. Encouraging students to develop their own professionalism and critically evaluate the standards is vital. Students should be prepared to challenge and defend their approach to professionalism, reflecting on individual situations and the broader context.

Further research into professional standards and their impact is necessary. Collecting data and monitoring the effects of professional standards can inform the ongoing debate and help identify areas for improvement. Students can contribute to this research by exploring what data would be useful and considering the actions that could be taken based on the findings.

In conclusion, professional standards are essential in promoting excellence, accountability and ethical conduct in the medical profession. However, it is important to recognise their limitations and address the problems they can present. By fostering critical thinking and open discussions, educators can empower future doctors to navigate professional standards and contribute to their continuing improvement.

Top tips.

Developing your own Professionalism: Doctors can develop their professionalism by recognising that it comes from their personal skills and values. Professionalism comes from within rather than an imposed set of rules.

Identifying conflicts with ethical codes. The doctor can find solutions to apparent conflicts between their beliefs and ethics. It is possible to align authenticity and professionalism and no doctor should feel that they have to live a lie.

Resist creep: Professionalism can become idealised concept which sets unreasonable standards. Work with colleagues to defend you and your team's professional standards and challenge unrealistic expectations.

Chapter 26: PATIENT SAFETY

Teaching patient safety has challenges as it is difficult to get the balance between specific advice to avoid a mistake and general comments. Using specific examples can help illustrate general mistakes but students will often fix upon the specifics. Safety theories can help make broader points but they are dry and it is difficult to achieve engagement.

The educator should help the students recognise the complexity of patient safety. They should recognise that there is no one-size-fits-all approach. The responsibility for patient safety is shared by all staff. Health and safety is not an add on, for instance if staff are unwell the patient safety implications cannot be fixed by resilience training.

What does patient safety mean in practice?

The students can be asked to brainstorm as many examples as possible of patient safety issues. This approach will increase the types of problem they see as safety issues. The educator can then ask whether they consider other items below as patient safety issues.

Rather than challenge student's perception of what is patient safety it is worth making a note of what they say. There are many fallacies in patient safety which need careful unpicking. A common resistance to patient safety is that Health and Safety can obstruct care and is an unnecessary burden.

It is worth addressing this fallacy when it arises by agreeing that Health and Safety cannot be imposed upon a system. Patient safety must be supported and professionals trusted that they are motivated to keep patients safe. Any improvements in patient safety must come from increased knowledge and skills.

- Delayed diagnosis: This can happen when a patient's symptoms are not taken seriously or when they are not given the correct tests. This can lead to the disease progressing and becoming more difficult to treat.
- Incorrect treatment: This is when a patient is given the wrong treatment or the wrong dose of medication. It can also be the right treatment at the wrong time. This can also lead to serious complications or even death.
- Complications of surgery: These can include bleeding, infection and organ damage. Post-op infections can occur after any surgery, but they are more common after certain types of surgery, such as bowel

surgery or surgery on the spine. Post-op infections can be serious and can lead to sepsis, which is a life-threatening condition.

- Drug side effects: These are the unwanted effects of medications. Drug side effects can range from mild to severe. Some drug side effects can be life-threatening.
- Patient falls: Falls are a common risk in hospitals and other healthcare settings. They can be caused by a variety of factors, such as poor lighting, slippery floors and inadequate staffing. Falls can lead to serious injuries, such as fractures and head injuries.
- Violence and abuse: This is any act of physical, sexual or verbal aggression that is directed towards a patient or healthcare provider. Violence in healthcare settings can be caused by a variety of factors, including stress, frustration and mental illness. Violence in healthcare settings can lead to serious injuries, including physical assault and even death.
- Psychological harm: This is any emotional or psychological injury that is caused by the healthcare system. Psychological harm in healthcare settings can be caused by a variety of factors, including misdiagnosis, incorrect treatment and lack of communication. Psychological harm in healthcare settings can lead to long-term emotional problems, such as anxiety, depression and post-traumatic stress disorder.
- Healthcare-associated infections. Healthcare-associated infections (HAIs) are infections that patients acquire while receiving care in a healthcare setting. HAIs can be caused by bacteria, viruses, fungi and parasites.
- Patient neglect: This is when a patient's basic needs are not met, such as food, water, or medication. Patient neglect can lead to serious complications, such as dehydration, malnutrition and pressure sores.
- Complications of treatment: Even when healthcare providers provide the best possible care, there is always a risk of complications. Complications can be caused by the underlying disease, the treatment itself, or the patient's individual circumstances.
- Unsafe environment: This can include factors such as poor staffing, inadequate equipment and unsanitary conditions. Unsafe environments can increase the risk of harm to patients.
- Rationing. There are many types of reduced access from drug shortages, high costs of private treatment, waiting lists, poor access to GPs or specialists, disparities in care such as less funding for mental illness.

- Laboratory errors: These can include mislabelling samples, misreading results, or failing to report results with unnecessary investigations and treatment.
- Unnecessary tests and procedures: These are tests and procedures that are not necessary for the patient's care but are performed to reach targets.
- Inadequate communication between healthcare providers. This can lead to repeated questioning and patient dissatisfaction but also errors in diagnosis and treatment causing injury.
- Inadequate informed consent. This is when patients are not given enough information about their treatment options so that they can make informed decisions. This can lead to patients feeling pressured into accepting treatment that they do not want or need.
- Dysfunctional departments. Failure by management to address dysfunctional departments can lead to multiple poor outcomes for instance maternity departments or mental health services.
- Inadequate research: There is not enough research on some important medical conditions. This can make it difficult to diagnose and treat these conditions.
- Misinformation: Patients may be exposed to misinformation about medical conditions and treatments, which can lead to them making poor decisions about their care.

The aim of this section is to help broaden the students' ideas of what patient safety is and how they can be part of the solution. The educator can use positive reinforcement saying things like 'that sounds as if it is something you already do to keep patients safe' or 'you seem to know a lot about patient safety'.

Students may choose to share their own experiences of patient safety and want to discuss what went wrong. Looking at specific examples may not assist understanding so encourage the quieter members of the group to offer their opinions or feedback with risk factors below.

Risk factors for patient safety.

To bring some order to the brainstormed list the educator needs to characterise the patient safety problems. This can be difficult because it is not always easy to see the connections between risk factors and safety problems. It may be easier to provide the list of risk factors and ask the students to characterise them.

The more perceptive students may note that the risk factors are present in most of the examples above. The educator should provide encouragement for engagement rather than clever answers. Maintaining group cohesion is the key task.

- Communication: Clear and concise communication between patients, providers and other members of the healthcare team is essential for preventing errors. This means that everyone involved in the patient's care needs to be able to understand each other's instructions and information. It also means that everyone needs to be able to speak up if they have any concerns.

- Training: Providers and staff need to be properly trained in the procedures they are performing. This includes knowing the correct dosages of medications, the proper way to use medical equipment and the signs and symptoms of potential complications.

- Human factors. These include factors such as fatigue, stress and distractions that can lead to errors. Fatigue can impair judgment and decision-making, while stress can lead to carelessness. Distractions can also lead to errors, such as when a provider is interrupted while giving medication or when a patient is not paying attention to their care instructions.

- Technology: The use of technology can help to prevent errors, such as barcoded medication administration and electronic health records. Barcoded medication administration helps to ensure that the correct medication is given to the correct patient at the correct dose. Electronic health records can help to improve communication between providers and track a patient's care over time.

- Environment: The physical environment of the healthcare setting can also contribute to patient safety. For example, well-lit and organised workspaces can help to prevent mistakes. This requires appropriate use of the available resources.

Some students will find these risk factors to dry and vague to engage with. It is worth encouraging students to share experiences of when these factors caused problems. This can improve engagement and help all the students understand why these factors are important.

Useful questions are 'to what extent can you control these risk factors?' and 'who controls them?' The learning point is that individuals can influence some of these risk factors. The group can make a large difference to the risk factors but often it is managers that create the problems.

Health care professionals often try to ignore management considering that it is irrelevant. By identifying the risk factors associated with patient safety as management issues this changes the dynamic. The students should be encouraged to express their stresses when dealing with managers.

Often students fixate upon the need to increase resources. The educator should ask the student to explain how increasing resources would make the patient safer. For instance, would increased nurses on the shift translate to better care if they are all used to increase data input?

Encouraging a broader range of solutions can move the discussion from blame of other to personal responsibility. The educator can then introduce the theories that managers use to solve problems of safety. Expressing the theories as an insight into management thinking rather than something that the studnets must do themselves can help retain engagement.

Theories of system failure.

There are many serious criticisms of the theoretical framework behind patient safety. The theories can be complex to understand and implement, it is difficult to monitor progress. They can be too narrow or simplistic and effective interventions need further work.

The educator is likely to have limited time to discuss these theories and may wish to pick one or two to study in more detail. Having a full session on management theories can help students really understand the tools that are available. When discussing safety with managers they can show knowledge and insight.

The models fail to address the breadth and complexity of patient safety or the risk factors above. The students should be able to recognise that a manager's perspective will always be solving the patient safety problem. They may recognise that patient safety needs to be incorporated into the healthcare structure.

- Human error theory by James Reason: This Swiss Cheese Model suggests that errors are caused by a combination of factors, including individual factors (such as fatigue, stress, or lack of knowledge), organisational factors (such as poor communication or inadequate training) and system factors (such as design flaws or equipment failures).

- Reliability theory by Dekker: This theory focuses on the design of systems to prevent errors from occurring. It suggests that systems should be designed to be as reliable as possible and that they should be able to recover from errors that do occur.

- Resilience engineering by Hollnagel: This theory focuses on the ability of systems to adapt to and recover from unexpected events.

It suggests that systems should be designed to be flexible and adaptable and that they should be able to learn from errors so that they can be prevented in the future.

- Organisational safety culture by Westrum: This theory suggests that the culture of an organisation can have a significant impact on patient safety. Organisations with a strong safety culture are more likely to have a focus on preventing errors and they are more likely to learn from errors that do occur.

- Design of Everyday Things by Norman. This theory suggests that many errors in healthcare are caused by poorly designed systems or devices. For example, a medication label that is difficult to read or a piece of equipment that is difficult to operate can increase the risk of errors.

- Social cognitive theory by Bandura. This theory argues that behaviour is influenced by a combination of personal factors (such as knowledge and skills), environmental factors (such as the culture of the organisation) and social factors (such as the behaviour of others).

The educator should encourage the students to consider how difficult it is for a manager to make improvements to patient safety. The students may suggest that the theories are not fit for purpose or that they do not apply to a complex system like healthcare. They may suggest that management should work in healthcare environments rather than offices to improve their insight.

Understanding why management theories fail will encourage some of the students to recognise the need for doctors and managers to collaborate. This insight indicates that the students have recognised that if they do not get involved then the outcomes will be worse. An educator can reinforce this insight by observing that it is individual action that keeps people safe.

At this stage of the teaching experience the group energy should be assessed. If the group energy is very low then working with the following list individually would be appropriate. Ask them to rate the following tips on a scale from one to 10. If it is high then choosing 2 or three of the practical tips for small group work will increase deep learning.

Practical tips to improve patient safety.

The practical tips section of the training experience is potentially the most useful part of the training. The students can recognise why specific situations cause a risk to patients' safety. They can identify the risks of that situation and understand why management theory cannot provide a solution.

Translating their knowledge into practice is more challenging, there is practical resistance such as established systems. There is also emotional resistance to taking on the responsibility for patient safety. Patient safety is a new concept for many students and there is usually cognitive dissonance. Students may feel that patient safety is someone else's job not theirs.

Organisational:

- Learn from other organisations. Clinical negligence lawyers and experts have great experience in the sorts of problems that go wrong in healthcare. They are usually delighted to share their experiences.

- Emotion reports. Having a regular report on the emotional health of the team can identify when dysfunction is occurring. The reports should provide the manager with an understanding of how the issues are impacting the staff and offer steps that could improve their emotional health.

- Staff morale. Where staff feel empowered, rested and are working as a team they are less likely to make mistakes and more likely to recognise and raise errors that do occur. Fatigue is a common symptom of poor staff morale.

- Promoting a team atmosphere. This can help to create a culture of safety where everyone is aware of the risks and is working to prevent them.

- Work environment. The work environment should be designed to minimise the risk of errors, this means improving the quality of life issues such as quiet and rest time.

- Safety research. Where a problem occurs repeatedly it may be necessary to commission research to find a solution. It may not be easy to find a solution without further understanding of the cause of the problem.

- Root cause analysis. A formal root cause analysis is beneficial for problems that have high importance but appear intractable. A violent patient or medical care disaster are examples of problems that need to be further analysed to learn lessons.

Patient centred.

- Comprehensive assessment. The more comprehensive the doctor's initial assessment of the patient the more likely that all the patient's problems will be identified. This allows doctors to put the issues together and recognise complex patterns of illness.

- Medical Summary. A summary of previous problems makes it easier to orientate when seeing the patient again. This reduces the chance of an error or misunderstanding.

- Management plans. Having a written management plan can make it easier on subsequent assessments to work out what is happening and what needs to be done next. This can reduce the risk of an issue not being addressed on follow up.

- Special plans. Some problems are both common and specialised such as fall prevention, infection control and pressure area care. Having specialised protocols can ensure that patients get high quality care despite being on an ordinary ward.

- Electronic follow up. By including electronic alerts in the health record the patient can be automatically followed up for ongoing health care problems.

Systematic.

- Fail safe. Many systems can be made fail safe so if the patient fails to return for follow-up then they are not forgotten. Considering whether a system is fail safe or fail dangerous can avoid errors.

- Making Complaints. Where a management decision causes problems for the team it can be difficult to address its consequences directly. Making complaints that identify the specific consequences of that decision directed at the manager involved can be effective for bringing it to the attention of the management team.

- Looking for patterns. Many errors appear unrelated but have a common cause. Reviewing problems that have not be properly resolved can lead to unexpected insights. Systems can often be failing for a while before anyone recognises that they are causing harm.

- Error reporting. Errors should be reported and analysed so that lessons can be learned and improvements can be made. Feedback to the staff on the findings of the reports can help them offer solutions.

- Using monitoring technology. This can help to identify and prevent problems early on. Medical devices should be designed and used safely.

- Information technology. Checklists, electronic health records, AI diagnostic tools should all be used appropriately when they have a role in patient safety.

Human factors:

- Training. Healthcare providers need to be trained in patient safety principles and how to prevent errors.

- Following proper handwashing procedures. This is one of the most important things that can be done to prevent the spread of infection.

- Verifying all medical procedures. This helps to ensure that the correct procedure is being performed on the correct patient.

- Making sure patients understand their treatment. This can help to reduce the risk of medication errors and other mistakes and make them more likely to ask relevant questions.

To cover all the areas above would take longer than is available in most curricula. The educator should cover about 2 areas so that the students can see how they could change patient safety. A useful approach is to ask the students what they think is the advantage and disadvantage of the tip.

They may spontaneously identify that other people are involved in the implementation of the patient safety tip. This can lead to the recognition that a plan will be required to make this happen. For many students planning is a skill that they are unfamiliar with. Asking them to consider how they could assist a manager who is trying to plan improvements in patient safety can be a better approach.

Planning improvements in patient safety:

Students may have experience of planning care and this experience can be used to normalise the processes that a manager uses. The manager should treat any risk factors and diagnose the problem. They should monitor the problem and act when the problem moves outside of the safe limits. They should work with their team to get the best results.

This can feel very similar to managing for instance cardiovascular risk. Checking the person's cholesterol and sugar and making a diagnosis of hypertension or diabetes are important. The effects of treatment should be monitored and the treatment changed if it is not working. If the patient has a heart attack then steps should be made to put the problem right and prevent it from happening again.

1. Identify and assess risks: The first step is to identify and assess the risks that patients face in the healthcare setting. This can be done by conducting root cause analyses of adverse events, reviewing incident reports and conducting surveys of patients and staff.

2. Implement preventive measures: Once the risks have been identified, preventive measures can be implemented to reduce the likelihood of errors. These measures may include changes to procedures, training, or technology.

3. Monitor and evaluate the effectiveness of preventive measures: It is important to monitor and evaluate the effectiveness of preventive measures to ensure that they are working as intended. This can be done by collecting data on adverse events and comparing it to historical data.

4. Learn from errors: When errors do occur, it is important to learn from them so that they can be prevented from happening again. This can be done by conducting root cause analyses and sharing the findings with staff.

5. Create a culture of safety: A culture of safety is one where everyone is committed to preventing errors and where individuals feel comfortable reporting them when they do occur. This can be created by providing training on patient safety, rewarding reporting and holding people accountable for their actions.

6. Continuously improve. Patient safety is an ongoing process. You need to continuously review your risk assessment and make changes as needed. You should also regularly review your reporting system to see if there are any trends or patterns that need to be addressed.

The educator may have students who are fully engaged and wish to be part of the patient safety systems. They should not expect this of the students as the purpose of this training is to remove resistance to patient safety interventions. Students should be encouraged to consider whether the proposed intervention is appropriate.

Often a manager needs to be helped to recognise that the proposed intervention will not be effective. There may be another better intervention that would be more effective. Learning the language of management can help students see their role in patient safety.

Conclusions.

Teaching patient safety poses challenges in finding the right balance between specific advice and general concepts. It is important for educators to help students recognise the complexity of patient safety and understand that there is no one-size-fits-all approach. Patient safety is a shared responsibility among all healthcare staff and it should not be seen as an add-on or something that can be fixed solely through resilience training.

To expand students' understanding of patient safety, educators can encourage brainstorming and discussion of various examples of patient safety issues. It is essential to address fallacies and misconceptions surrounding patient safety, such as the belief that health and safety measures obstruct care. Instead, it should be acknowledged that patient safety requires support, trust in healthcare professionals' commitment to safety and continuous improvement through increased knowledge and skills.

The chapter also highlights a range of patient safety issues, including delayed diagnosis, incorrect treatment, surgical complications, drug side effects, patient falls, violence, psychological harm, healthcare-associated infections, patient neglect, abuse, complications of treatment, unsafe environments, laboratory errors, unnecessary tests and procedures, inadequate communication, rationing, inadequate informed consent, dysfunctional departments, inadequate research and misinformation. By discussing these examples, students can broaden their understanding of patient safety and their role in ensuring it.

Identifying risk factors for patient safety is another crucial aspect of the chapter. Factors such as communication, training, human factors, technology and the environment can significantly influence patient safety outcomes. Educators should encourage students to reflect on these risk factors and consider their impact on patient safety. Understanding that individuals can influence some of these factors and that management plays a role in creating a safe environment can empower students to actively contribute to patient safety improvement.

The chapter also introduces various theories of system failure, including human error theory, reliability theory, resilience engineering, organisational safety culture, design of everyday things and social cognitive theory. While these theories may face criticism and implementation challenges, they offer insights into management thinking and provide a framework for understanding patient safety from a systemic perspective.

Lastly, the chapter provides practical tips to improve patient safety. These tips encompass organisational, patient-centered and systematic approaches to enhance safety, such as learning from other organisations, monitoring staff morale, promoting a team atmosphere, conducting comprehensive assessments, implementing fail-safe systems, utilising technology and encouraging error reporting and analysis. By translating knowledge into practical solutions, students can better grasp the importance of patient safety and their role in its implementation.

Overall, teaching patient safety requires educators to navigate challenges, broaden students' perspectives and provide practical tools for improvement. By fostering engagement, understanding risk factors and exploring theories and practical tips, students can become active participants in promoting and ensuring patient safety in healthcare settings.

Top tips.

Help students recognise the complexity of patient safety and understand that there is no one-size-fits-all approach. They should recognise the importance of simple steps such as staff morale and having the right equipment.

Address fallacies and misconceptions surrounding patient safety, such as the belief that health and safety measures obstruct care. Learning how to align patient safety with good medical care will integrate safety into clinical practice.

Identify risk factors for patient safety, including communication, training, human factors, technology and the environment. The students can then recognise when dysfunctional behaviour is compromising patient safety.

Chapter 27: QUALITY IMPROVEMENT IN HEALTHCARE.

Teaching QI is difficult because it has a poor reputation amongst clinical staff and managers find this difficult to understand. They are surprised that clinical staff should resist change when medicine is continuously developing. One suggestion is that clinical staff do not understand the various QI methods.

The importance of stakeholder engagement to any change means that issues such as trust must be addressed. There is general concern about constant reformations of the health service both nationally and locally. Deteriorating services despite increased resources makes people think that waste must be increasing. Trust that taxes will be well spent is dwindling and there is increasing reluctance to spend more.

Quality improvement (QI) in healthcare is the process of identifying and addressing problems in the delivery of healthcare to improve patient outcomes. QI is a systematic approach to problem-solving that uses data and evidence to identify areas for improvement, develop and implement interventions and evaluate the impact of those interventions.

Quality improvement (QI) should be a systematic and continuous effort to improve the quality of care and outcomes for patients. QI involves a variety of stakeholders, including patients, healthcare providers, administrators and policymakers. It is often patchy and intermittent and causes undesirable side effects.

Different QI methods

The educator may find that students are resistant to a discussion of the methodology. It may be necessary to explore their resistance and to give examples of systemic problems that need QI to solve. There are some overlaps between general principles of analysis and the QI techniques.

Clinical staff who learn and understand the different QI methods are generally supportive of the approaches. They are logical and effective and they should lead to improvements in healthcare. The evidence is however patchy and it can be difficult to understand why methods fail.

Suggestions for the lack of success are that the necessary additional resources for change may not be available. Clinical staff may sabotage the changes, undermine the process or fail to engage with the training. It is possible that the methods were not followed correctly.

There are many different QI methods and tools that can be used to improve healthcare. Some common methods include:

- Root cause analysis: This method is used to identify the underlying causes of a problem.

- Data collection and analysis: This involves collecting data on patient care, such as outcomes, processes and resources. The data is then analysed to identify areas for improvement.

- Benchmarking: This involves comparing the performance of one organisation to another. Benchmarking can help to identify best practices and areas where improvement is needed.

- Plan-do-study-act (PDSA) cycles: This is a cyclical approach to QI that involves planning, implementing, studying and acting on changes. PDSA cycles are often used to test small changes to care processes.

- Lean methodology: This is a set of principles and tools that can be used to improve efficiency and reduce waste in healthcare.

- Six Sigma: This is a methodology that uses statistical techniques and reducing variation and risk of defects to improve quality.

- Process mapping: This involves mapping out the steps involved in a particular care process, to identify potential areas for improvement.

- Intervention design: This involves developing and implementing interventions to challenge accepted practice.

The theories often seem to be esoteric and distant from the experiences of professionals. There is often substantial resistance to the conclusions as the plans rarely seem relevant to the real world. The additional resources dedicated to these approaches are often disproportionate to the problems. Often they would solve the problem if just spent directly on the problem.

The management often appears to rely upon inconsistent and unreliable data when making decisions. They use targets but do not recognise the risk of gaming or distortion of the healthcare delivery system. Many processes increase problems such as dysfunctional relationships and fail to create improvement.

Plans can be implemented without proper testing leading to failed experiments that compete for resources with standard care. All change is disruptive and many staff learn to resist all change when plans repeatedly fail. The staff start to believe that the real motivation is to cut costs rather than improve quality.

The strongest criticism is that QI is basically flawed because the theory of continuous change is not appropriate. Medicine is continually developing so most areas of healthcare must remain stable to provide a solid base. Change must be limited to that which is necessary to improve care and should not be systematic.

Possible benefits of QI.

When discussing benefits of QI the educator should differentiate between what the managers wish to achieve and the real world results. One question that can help this process is 'is it possible that data collection could identify a patient safety issue?' The students can then see the difference between the potential and what happens and develop ideas why this occurs.

Managers argue that QI is an important part of healthcare because it can help to improve patient outcomes, reduce costs and improve the quality of care. QI can be used to improve a wide variety of healthcare processes, including:

- Patient safety: QI can be used to identify and address risks to patient safety.

- Clinical care: QI can be used to improve the quality of clinical care, such as the accuracy of diagnoses and the effectiveness of treatments.

- Patient experience: QI can be used to improve the patient experience, such as by reducing wait times and increasing patient satisfaction.

- Organisational efficiency: QI can be used to improve the efficiency of healthcare organisations, such as by reducing waste and improving communication.

- Improved staff satisfaction: QI can also lead to improved staff satisfaction, as it can give staff a sense of ownership and empowerment in the improvement process.

The problem is that these benefits do not appear to materialise in practice. The staff satisfaction in the NHS is notoriously poor, the organisational efficiency is so poor that some care standard in 1990 is no longer available, patient experience is at its lowest level and medical errors is a major cause of death.

Not all these problems are due to the failure of QI but failing healthcare systems in many countries is not good for QI's reputation. The inconsistency between QI's apparent solid logical basis and its complete failure in healthcare remains a mystery to those involved.

QI theories are sophisticated and versatile tools that have great potential to help healthcare teams provide exceptional care. They are not easy to use and have substantial risks associated with them. The key problem in the use of QI theories is the alignment problem.

The Alignment Problem.

The educator may improve engagement by asking the group why there is a difference between the real-world results and the theory. The group may be able to identify much of the alignment problem without being told. The educator may only need to facilitate occasionally to keep the group performing well.

A basic theory of QI is that the manager's analysis is correct and the clinicians should align to the management view. There is talk about a culture of quality improvement where all parties are aligned but little progress has been made. The clinicians often complain about management not being aligned to good clinical practice.

The correct approach is to work with all parties to achieve alignment then decide what to do. This may sound logical, but in QI it is the other way around. The more that one side considers that they are right and the other side is not, the less alignment there will be. Alignment is one part of teamwork and failing to work as a team will always be damaging, whatever the skills of the participants.

The depth of the problems with alignment can be seen by inconsistencies within QI theory. For instance, one theory focuses upon human errors and another on systematic errors. Neither theory has all the answers however they are both used as if they are the only correct answer.

This is compounded when the theories are applied to real world problems. The specific situation that is causing problems is often more complex than can be captured by QI theories, even if used in combination. This means that the solutions and priorities proposed will not work in practice.

To solve the alignment problem so that QI can be effective in healthcare there are several steps that are required.

- Common understanding: Stakeholders in quality improvement (QI) often have different perspectives on the problems that need to be addressed. This can make it difficult to reach a common understanding of the problem and to develop effective solutions. To address this, it is essential that all stakeholders have a shared understanding of the root causes of the problem, as well as the potential solutions.

- Multiple theories. When trying to solve a problem, it is important to consider multiple theories or perspectives. This will help to identify the root causes of the problem and to develop solutions that are likely to be effective. The process of solving problems must be flexible and adaptable, willing to change course if necessary and to be open to new ideas.
- Trust and respect: There may be a lack of trust and respect between stakeholders, which can make it difficult to have any engagement with the QI process. To build trust they should be transparent and honest, consistent and fair.
- Power imbalances: Power imbalances can create barriers to effective QI, which can make it difficult for all voices to be heard. For example, managers may have more power than clinicians and can force through poor quality decisions.
- Leadership. Leaders play a key role in creating a culture of alignment in patient safety. They must be able to set a clear vision for patient safety, to build trust and respect among stakeholders and to create an environment where everyone feels comfortable speaking up.
- Wasted resources: It is inevitable that there will be mistakes and wasted resources when trying something new. The stakeholders should agree that the resource allocation is necessary and proportionate before QI is tried. For instance, a simple solution that has been forgotten could save the need for the QI process.
- Collaboration: Some stakeholders will have diametrically opposed views which need to be incorporated into the final decisions. These stakeholders are important because they are more likely to understand why the decisions will fail.
- Common agreed goal: No agreement is likely if there are no common goals, all sides must agree an overall goal rather than simply focus upon short term goals. For example, managers may be more focused on reducing costs, while clinicians may be more focused on improving patient care.

The alignment problem is arguably an existential challenge facing healthcare. Until and unless managers and healthcare professionals align their views the situation will worsen. Few healthcare professionals understand the managers point of view. The managers are trying to make things better but cannot understand the resistance that they face.

Educators can use the alignment problem as way of helping students understand why the problem continues. The phrase 'the beatings will continue until the morale improves' may be used by the group. This should be challenged, medical practice is difficult and managers have a useful role to play.

Teamwork requires all participants to be prepared to listen to and collaborate with the others. If doctors fail to explain why the managers are making mistakes it is not right to blame managers for this failure. Improved communication and understanding by both doctors and managers may lead to a culture of trust and respect.

Conclusions.

Quality improvement (QI) in healthcare is a crucial process for identifying and addressing problems in the delivery of healthcare in order to improve patient outcomes. However, teaching QI can be challenging due to the poor reputation it holds among clinical staff and the lack of understanding of QI methods. There is a need for increased stakeholder engagement and trust-building to address resistance to change and reform in the healthcare system.

While there are various QI methods and tools available, their implementation is often patchy and intermittent, due to undesirable side effects. Theories and approaches may seem distant from the real-world experiences of healthcare professionals, causing scepticism and resistance. Insufficient resources, staff sabotage and poor implementation of QI methods can contribute to their failure.

Despite the potential benefits of QI, such as improving patient outcomes, reducing costs and enhancing the quality of care, these benefits often do not materialise in practice. Issues such as low staff satisfaction, organisational inefficiency, poor patient experience and medical errors persist. The reputation of QI is further affected by the worsening performance of healthcare systems in many countries.

The alignment problem between managers and clinicians is a significant challenge in QI. There is a need for a common understanding, multiple perspectives, trust, respect and effective leadership to address this problem. Power imbalances and wasted resources also hinder the success of QI initiatives. Collaboration among stakeholders with differing views and the establishment of common goals are essential to overcome these challenges.

The alignment problem represents an existential challenge for healthcare. It is crucial for managers and healthcare professionals to align their views and foster improved communication and understanding. Blaming one side or the other does not lead to effective solutions. Instead, creating a culture of trust and respect through improved teamwork can pave the way for successful QI initiatives.

In summary, QI has the potential to significantly improve healthcare outcomes, but its implementation faces challenges related to stakeholder engagement, resource allocation and the alignment of perspectives. By addressing these challenges and promoting collaboration, transparency and effective leadership, healthcare systems can harness the power of QI to deliver better care and outcomes for patients.

Top tips.

Real world QI results. Encourage students to critically analyse the gap between QI theory and real-world results. Explore the reasons behind this discrepancy and identify ways to improve the effectiveness of QI in practice.

Explore alignment: Help students understand the alignment problem between managers and clinicians, where different perspectives hinder effective QI. Promote common understanding by frank discussions about the proposed QI methods.

Discuss resource allocation: Highlight the importance of appropriately allocating resources for QI initiatives. Avoid wasting resources on ineffective approaches and ensure that resource allocation is proportionate to the problem being addressed.

Chapter 28: EVIDENCE BASED MEDICINE.

Evidence-based medicine (EBM) is a process of making clinical decisions by integrating the best available research evidence with clinical expertise and patient values. EBM is based on the idea that the best way to provide high-quality care is to use the best available evidence to guide decision-making.

EBM is a valuable tool for healthcare professionals. It can help to ensure that patients receive the best possible care based on the best available evidence. However, it is important to remember that EBM is not a substitute for clinical judgment. The clinician must always use their own judgment and experience when making decisions about patient care.

NICE- 'It is not mandatory to apply the recommendations and the guideline does not override the responsibility to make decisions appropriate to the circumstances of the individual, in consultation.'

In one sense all medicine should be evidence based but EBM has been developed as a way of developing consensus. It has been successful in finding agreement on many difficult issues. It has been less successful in resolving the tension between finding the optimal treatment for the individual and a standardised treatment that works best for a society.

The risk of EBM is that it removes reasonable treatments from the patient. Where there is uncertainty as to the best treatment then patients should have the ultimate decision. Guidelines make it difficult to give the right treatment for an individual. A patient can be denied a reasonable treatment which has accepted effectiveness.

Patients have a role in determining what treatment they have. The Montgomery case made it clear that patients should be provided with all the information that a reasonable person requires and all the information that they as an individual require. This means that patient must be able to choose to vary from EBM guidance against their doctor's advice.

Teaching evidence-based medicine as a technique is not complex. AI such as Med Palm 2 has the potential to make EBM much easier. The students may argue that they already use the technique, so they do not need to be taught. This belief can be difficult to overcome and lead to lack of engagement.

Proponents of EBM have been unfairly cast as interested in one-size-fits-all approaches when in reality they are aware of the need to individualise care. Process has a key role in EBM - what are the correct steps to get to good outcome? Many clinical errors are due to failure to follow the correct process rather than flaws in guidelines.

EBM questions.

There are several questions that can be used to improve engagement by challenging student's assumptions. These assumptions cause resistance to EBM and can be overcome by good questions. In teaching the educator will become aware of further assumptions. Educators can share these assumptions and questions with their colleagues.

- How much time does it take to do a literature review on a subject and really understand the choices?
- How would you approach a complex case where the evidence is not available and you have to balance conflicting aims?
- What is the theoretical maximum percentage that a guideline will provide the correct answer to a clinical condition?
- Do you follow the guidelines or do you use your own clinical judgment to find the correct treatment for a patient?
- If a patient wants a treatment and there is equipoise should they be able to have the treatment that they want?

These questions are designed to help the student understand that EBM is at the heart of clinical practice. That guidelines are helpful to remind the professional of what is expected. Students need to be aware of EBM as there are many tools that depend upon the technique and they need to use them correctly.

The five steps of EBM.

Although much of the EBM knowledge base is already in guidelines the student should know the steps. This is because they will come up against problems that are not covered by guidelines. The steps are also useful to critically appraise available guidelines.

1. Ask a clear question. The first step is to identify a clinical question about a patient's clinical area. This question can be about the best treatment for a particular condition, the best way to prevent a disease, or the best way to manage a patient's care. This question should be specific, answerable and relevant to the patient's care.

2. Best evidence. Find the best available evidence to answer it. This evidence can be found in medical journals, systematic reviews and clinical practice guidelines. Basic science can be a good source of insight.

3. Appraise. Critically appraise the evidence to determine its quality and relevance. This involves assessing the study design, the methods used and the results of the study.

4. Integrate. Integrate the evidence with clinical expertise considering the patient's individual circumstances and preferences when making a decision.

5. Evaluate. Evaluate the outcome of the decision by tracking the patient's progress and adjusting the plan as needed.

Many guidelines fail to ask a clear question, the management of hypertension assumes that it is a single disease. There are subtypes which require different approaches. The best evidence may not be in the medical literature and medicine can be an echo chamber. Guidelines that do not recognise that some individuals will not benefit from the standard treatment and offer alternatives have limited utility.

Asking the students to provide an EBM answer on a subject that is controversial can help them understand the process. They may come to different conclusions but should have found the same evidence. The educator can then add further details that shift the decision to one side or the other showing how the evidence strengthens and weakens.

Benefits of EBM:

The benefits of EBM are largely unproven because it is difficult to do a trial with randomisation. The development of the NICE guidelines has had some issues but generally they are exceptionally useful. Their focus upon the process of delivering care has meant that they can inform practice better than a list of treatments.

- Improved quality of care: EBM can help to improve the quality of care by ensuring that patients receive the best available evidence-based treatments. This can lead to better outcomes for patients, such as shorter hospital stays, fewer complications and improved quality of life.
- Improved patient satisfaction: EBM can also help to improve patient satisfaction by ensuring that patients receive care that is based on their individual needs and preferences. This can lead to patients feeling more confident in their care and more likely to adhere to treatment plans.
- Reduced medical errors: EBM can help to reduce medical errors by providing clinicians with the information they need to make safe

and informed decisions. This can lead to fewer mistakes being made in the diagnosis and treatment of patients.

- Increased efficiency: EBM can also help to increase efficiency by ensuring that healthcare resources are used in the most effective way possible. This can lead to lower costs for healthcare providers and better outcomes for patients.

- Improved communication: EBM can also help to improve communication between clinicians, patients and other healthcare providers. This can lead to better understanding of the patient's condition and treatment options and more informed decision-making.

Codifying clinical practice has had a profound impact on clinical practice in the UK. Many of the clinical decisions are taken by reference to guidelines rather than clinical judgment. This has led to increased consistency and overall is likely to have improved outcomes. The reduction in unwarranted variation has led to improvements in poor care.

Challenges of EBM:

Most of the challenges of EBM relate to inappropriate use of the technique. The use of guidelines means that it rare that an individual clinician needs to search for the right answer. Guidelines are kept up to date and generally unbiased and are unambiguously simple. They should be used in conjunction with clinical judgement and are not a substitute for individual care.

The educator should help the students recognise the appropriate use of EBM. EBM provides guidance as to the correct process and treatment options to offer. It does not say what the doctor must do for their patient although this is not always clearly worded in the guidance. The student should recognise that they must keep good records especially when their patient does not fit with the normal pattern.

- Time. It can be time-consuming and challenging to find and appraise the best available evidence.

- Inconsistent. The evidence may not always be clear or consistent, which can make it difficult to make decisions.

- Reluctance. Clinicians may not always be willing or able to use EBM in their practice.

- Applicability. The evidence may not be applicable to the individual patient. The best available evidence may be based on studies of a population of patients, but the individual patient may have different characteristics that make the evidence less applicable.

- Outdated. The best available evidence is constantly evolving, so it is important to make sure that the evidence you are using is up-to-date. However, it can be difficult to keep up with the latest evidence, especially if you are a busy clinician.

- Biased. The evidence may be biased if the researchers who conducted the study had a vested interest in the outcome of the study. For example, a study that was funded by a pharmaceutical company may be more likely to find that the company's drug is effective.

- Interpretation. The evidence may be complex and difficult to understand, especially if you are not familiar with research methods. This can make it difficult to decide whether the evidence is strong enough to support a particular decision.

- Lack of resources: EBM requires access to high-quality research evidence, which can be expensive and time-consuming to obtain.

- Lack of training: Clinicians may not have the training or skills necessary to critically appraise research evidence and apply it to their practice.

- Resistance to change: Some clinicians may be resistant to change and may not be willing to adopt new evidence-based practices.

- Cultural barriers: Cultural factors can also pose challenges to the adoption of EBM. For example, in some cultures, there is a strong emphasis on traditional medicine and practices, which may make it difficult to implement evidence-based practices.

- Political barriers: Political factors can also pose challenges to the adoption of EBM. For example, in some countries, there may be a lack of political will to support the implementation of evidence-based practices.

A major resistance to the use of EBM is that some people argue that guidelines must be followed. These people may be in positions of power but they should be challenged. The educator can discuss issues such as professionalism, ethics and teamwork in this context.

Managers may use EBM to create targets and it is not ethical to use EBM to bully colleagues. Professionals take pride in doing the right thing and will stand up for their practice. Where EBM is being used to create targets then the team should work together to resist this.

Conclusions.

Evidence-based medicine (EBM) is a valuable approach to clinical decision-making that integrates the best available research evidence with clinical expertise and patient values. EBM helps ensure that patients receive high-quality care based on the best evidence, although it should not replace clinical judgment.

While EBM has been successful in finding consensus on many difficult issues, it faces challenges in balancing individualised care with standardised treatments that work best for society. Patients have the right to make informed decisions that may vary from EBM guidance, as highlighted by the Montgomery case.

Teaching EBM is essential to equip healthcare professionals with the necessary skills to critically appraise evidence, understand the EBM process and effectively use tools like guidelines. Engaging students with thought-provoking questions can help them appreciate the importance of EBM in clinical practice.

The benefits of EBM include improved quality of care, increased patient satisfaction, reduced medical errors, increased efficiency and improved communication among healthcare providers. Codifying clinical practice through guidelines has led to greater consistency and reduced unwarranted variation, potentially improving outcomes.

Challenges of EBM include the time and effort required to find and appraise evidence, unclear or inconsistent evidence, resistance to its use, applicability to individual patients, outdated or biased evidence, difficulty in interpretation, lack of resources and training, resistance to change, cultural and political barriers and the risk of using guidelines as rigid rules instead of guidance.

It is important to recognise appropriate use of EBM, as it provides guidance while allowing for individualised care based on patient needs. EBM should not be used to replace clinical judgment but to inform and support decision-making. Resistance to the use of EBM should be understood and ethical considerations, professionalism and teamwork should be emphasised in its implementation.

Overall, EBM is a valuable tool that, when used appropriately, can improve patient care, outcomes and satisfaction. Continued education and critical appraisal of evidence are essential for healthcare professionals to effectively incorporate EBM into their practice and adapt to the evolving landscape of medical research.

Top tips.

Learn the five steps of EBM: asking a clear question, finding the best evidence, critically appraising the evidence, integrating it with clinical expertise and evaluating the decision. Use the technique to analyse guidelines in your area of practice.

Recognise the role of clinical judgment: While EBM and guidelines are crucial in guiding decisions, they should not replace clinical judgment. Always consider the individual patient's circumstances and preferences when making treatment choices.

Respect patient autonomy: Include patients in decision-making when there are multiple reasonable management approaches. This may involve using EBM to investigate the patient's preferences and consider whether their wishes are reasonable.

Chapter 29: PROFESSIONAL DEVELOPMENT FOR MEDICAL EDUCATORS

Professional development for medical educators is essential to ensuring that they have the knowledge and skills necessary to provide high-quality education to medical students and other healthcare professionals. As medical educators cover a vast area of knowledge this can appear impossible to achieve.

The key areas that medical educators should focus on in their professional development are the process of learning and how to teach. The educator does not need to have an active knowledge of all the theories but must be able to teach them. This can appear paradoxical as how can an educator teach something that they do not remember?

The answer is that it is not necessary to know something to understand it. The educator must understand the content of their teaching but does not need to memorise it. The learning materials will contain the information necessary to master the subject, the educator just needs to guide the students through the subject.

For this reason professional development for medical educators focuses upon the methods rather than learning information. Educators should however be aware of topics that they have difficulty understanding. Many of the most challenging topics have been discussed in this book. There are however aspects of clinical medicine which also cause problems.

Professional development is targeted at the essential elements (see below), the gaps in their understanding and unfamiliar topics. This can substantially reduce the amount of training that they require. There are other tricks that educators can use to manage their learning load such as preparing learning materials.

- Teaching methods and techniques: Medical educators should be familiar with a variety of teaching methods and techniques, so that they can choose the most effective approach for their learners. They should also be able to adapt their teaching methods to the needs of different learners.

- Knowledge: They should be able to demonstrate that they are up to date with their knowledge base for instance by sitting the same examinations as their students.

- Learning theories: Medical educators should have a basic understanding of learning theories, so that they can design and deliver educational experiences that are effective for their learners.

- Assessment: Medical educators should be able to design and use effective assessment tools to measure the learning outcomes of their learners.

- Curriculum development: Medical educators should be able to develop and implement effective curricula that meet the needs of their learners.

- Educational technology: Medical educators need to be familiar with the use of educational technology in teaching and learning. This includes tools such as LLMs, e-learning platforms, simulation software and video conferencing.

- Patient respect: Medical educators should be familiar with the principles of patient respect and other ethics how to incorporate them into their teaching sessions.

- Communication: Medical educators should be effective communicators, both verbally and in writing. They should be able to communicate complex concepts in a clear and concise way.

- Professionalism: Medical educators need to be role models for professionalism in teaching and learning. This includes demonstrating respect for learners, colleagues and patients.

- Other areas: Educators should add to this list to reflect their personal learning needs, for instance an educator who struggles with teamwork should identify learning needs in this category.

During appraisal or review of the continuing professional development the educator should consider whether they are addressing all the areas of their career. They may wish to reflect on their study over a 5 year cycle or continuously update a chart. I recommend reviewing each area at least once every 3 years to plan further learning.

In general, a red flag for a particular area is a reluctance to consider if there are any problems with that area. If the educator has regular appraisals they could be asked to describe their response to new changes in their field. 'How are you managing LLMs?' or 'how do you know what to include when teaching about headaches?'.

Extended roles for medical educators.

Not every educator will take on extended roles, some may be full time clinicians but having extended roles means further areas to keep up to date with. Planning for appropriate development goals in multiple areas is more complex. The key is to ask yourself what knowledge and skills is required and how to keep these up to date.

For many roles there will be overlap for part of the role for instance leaders need to use education techniques to influence their colleagues. There are parts of any role which are unique to that role and will need to individual focus. Teaching materials for each of the roles can help guide development planning.

The following are aspects of each role that the educator will need make specific plans to achieve. A common approach is to argue that although the educator takes on that role they are not involved in that aspect of the role. This is an error, if an educator takes on a role they must be proficient in all aspects of that role.

- Leadership: Compare the educator's skills with leadership skills and identify areas of weakness. How does a leader affect professionalism?

- Advocacy: Critically appraise the presentation of a problem that faces medical students and trainees. How effective was this presentation in reducing resistance to providing an effective solution.

- Quality improvement: Consider alignment issues in QI, what skills are required to create good alignment and what needs to be learned.

- Mentoring: Assess a mentoring interaction, how approachable, what did the student require, able to help?

- Technology: Medical educators should be familiar with the latest educational technologies and how to use them effectively.

- Interprofessional education: How uncomfortable does the educator feel when approaching other professionals and do other professionals respond to the approach?

- Research: Medical educators may want to consider developing their research skills so that they can contribute to the body of knowledge in medical education in areas such as educational scholarship or faculty development.

All professionals see additional roles as minor additions to their main role. This is mistaken as each role has its own professional knowledge and skills that need to be maintained. Where a professional takes on multiple additional roles there is a risk that they may not be able to do any well.

Whilst it is not possible to learn the whole of areas such as management or research or AI the educator must learn enough to be safe. This means that they should undergo basic training and allocate enough resources to keep learning. As a rule of thumb this translates to about 500 hours total for a hobby and 2000 hours if the role is paid.

Doctors have additional responsibilities for keeping up to date with an area than professionals in that area. A hospital manager does not need to pass any examinations or do any study. A doctor in the same role will fall foul of their professional regulator if they do the same.

Processes for professional development.

Educators can be as unstructured in their approach to education as any other professional. It is therefore important to have a systematic approach to learning to ensure that no gaps occur. The educator should use the following or a similar approach formally so that they can demonstrate that they have undertaken a thorough review.

Using a list of common areas and writing reflections against each item is a good start. This can help the educator identify significant problems that are obvious. They may wish to undergo further assessment to determine their needs. This may mean accessing specialist assessments.

1. Review all the areas of professional practice. This is the foundation of PDP and includes identifying your current knowledge, skills and attitudes in relation to your profession. You can do this by reflecting on your own practice, seeking feedback from others, or completing a self-assessment.

2. Identify gaps in knowledge, skills and attitudes. Once you have a clear understanding of your current level of practice, you can identify the areas where you need to improve. This could include areas such as knowledge of new research, skills in using new technologies, or attitudes towards working with different types of people.

3. Plan steps to address each gap. Once you have identified the gaps in your knowledge, skills and attitudes, you can start to plan how you will address them. This could involve attending training courses, reading books or articles, or shadowing other professionals. Set clear goals and be realistic about timescales.

4. Implement training to address each gap. Once you have a plan in place, you can start to implement the training that you need to address the gaps in your knowledge, skills and attitudes. This could involve taking a course, reading a book, or shadowing another professional.

5. Network with colleagues. Your colleagues will have strengths in your areas of weakness. Working with colleagues as mentors or in groups will allow you to learn more quickly, identify gaps and find suitable resources more quickly.

6. Assess the effectiveness of the training. Once you have completed the training, you need to assess how effective it has been. This could involve reflecting on your own practice, seeking feedback from others, or completing a self-assessment.

Complaints and feedback are often opportunities to reflect on possible gaps and consider further learning. Curriculum design is a commonly cited area that causes stress and should be considered regularly. Undergoing specialist training can address these areas of low confidence.

The number of areas that the educator needs to be up to date on may be large but there are ways of making the learning more efficient. It is important to ensure that the educator has a system for monitoring their current performance. This may include sitting regular examinations or having regular feedback from observed teaching. It is recommended that the educator develops a comprehensive system of assessment for all the areas above.

Produce Teaching Materials

Educators have a trick that can simplify their learning - produce teaching materials on each of the topics that they cover. This makes more sense as it is a normal part of the educator's work, reflects workload and shows that they are up to date. There does need to be some element of reflection to ensure that it is not a tick box exercise.

Assessment is a key part of the educator's role so they have easy access to opportunities to self-assess. This may be part of the field testing of the assessments or can be after the assessment has occurred. There are advantages of this approach as it is formative and has high accuracy.

There are some areas that cannot be assessed easily and alternative methods such as preparing teaching materials may be used. As an educator's strength is in communication and helping others to learn this has an advantage. The educator can write an article about for instance learning theories and share it with their colleagues. They then help their colleagues keep up to date with the area and get feedback.

Some educators will be able to find evidence of their competence in areas such as communication and respect from other roles. Many will need to undergo other forms of assessment and 360 degree assessment is popular. The problem is that patient feedback and colleague feedback is largely based on the quality of the relationship rather than skills.

It is therefore better to arrange a formal assessment if possible or attend a course on clinical skills if not. There are restrictions on doctors sitting examinations such as those held by the Royal Colleges but there are informal providers. Another approach is to enlist the help of a colleague whose role includes assessment of professionalism or communication skills.

For new and emerging areas such as LLMs the educator may struggle to keep up to date with all the advances. They may not be able to write good teaching materials and may not have colleagues who can either. In this case it is better to head hunt those with the correct knowledge and network with them.

Asking an expert in the use of LLMs in medical education to come and give a talk could ensure that they and their colleagues are updated. Educators often have access to opportunities to invite speakers and many experts are happy to give a talk for little or no payment.

Conclusions.

Professional development for medical educators is a multifaceted and ongoing process that plays a crucial role in ensuring high-quality medical education. The chapter highlights the key areas that medical educators should focus on, including teaching methods and techniques, knowledge, learning theories, assessment, curriculum development, educational technology, patient respect and ethics, communication, professionalism and other areas based on personal learning needs.

Extended roles for medical educators, such as leadership, advocacy, technology, interprofessional education and research, are also discussed as important areas to consider for professional development.

The chapter outlines a systematic approach to professional development, including steps such as reviewing current practice, identifying gaps, planning steps to address those gaps, implementing training, networking with colleagues and assessing the effectiveness of the training.

The production of teaching materials is highlighted as an alternative approach that aligns with the educator's workload and demonstrates their up-to-date knowledge. Assessment methods are emphasised, including formal assessments, attending courses, seeking feedback from colleagues and utilising opportunities for self-assessment.

Overall, the chapter emphasises that professional development for medical educators is an ongoing process that requires continuous learning and growth. Medical educators should actively seek out opportunities to enhance their knowledge and skills to provide the best possible education to their learners.

Top tips.

Systematic learning. Develop a systematic approach to professional development by reviewing all areas of your practice, identifying gaps, planning steps to address them and implementing training accordingly.

Be realistic: Use available methods such as sitting the same examinations or formal assessments as your students. Allocate sufficient time and resources to maintain reasonable progress in all areas of your practice.

Teaching materials. Producing teaching materials involves understanding the material, reflecting the topic and choosing material that helps other to learn. They can also be produced for areas that the educator does not currently teach.

Chapter 30: SCHOLARSHIP AND RESEARCH IN MEDICAL EDUCATION

Scholarship and research in medical education is important to educators as it is a way of progressing in their career and developing their roles. There are three types of research available, self-funded role based, Masters courses or scholarship depending upon skills. An experienced educator should be able to conduct self-funded research to the point when they need to apply for funding to complete the research.

If the educator lacks the necessary research skills or had difficulty with graduate level long essays then a supervised Masters is better. Depending upon the educator's job role the appropriate type of research should be obvious. Most educators will be creating new educational resources or assessing how well students are learning.

If the educator is not involved with any of these areas then they should consider what research they may have access to. A literature review is possible but is not an easy choice as it is study heavy. The results are often difficult to get published and it may be better to write articles instead.

Scholarship and research in medical education is a broad field that encompasses a wide range of activities, including:

- Theoretical research that seeks to understand the underlying principles of medical education.

- Empirical research that investigates the effectiveness of different educational interventions.

- Evaluation research that assesses the impact of educational programs on student learning and patient outcomes.

- Developmental research that creates new educational materials and resources.

- Dissemination research that shares the findings of educational research with the wider community.

- Professional development that supports the learning and growth of medical educators.

- Scholarship of teaching and learning that documents and reflects on the practice of teaching and learning in medicine.

Having research published can open the chance to do further research and build an academic career. The educator's role would then include lecturing and supervising other researchers. This is demanding work and more varied than clinical or preclinical teaching. Each student will choose a different area of study keeping the educator on their toes.

Some educators will want to become researchers themselves and the steps described can help with this decision. The workload is heavy, research is competitive and challenging as it requires new skills and the costs can be high. Many academically gifted people have significant impairments when it comes to writing so an educator should be prepared to coach writing skills.

How to become a researcher.

The opportunities of scholarship and research in UK medical education include a wide range of areas. The application processes are similar to other areas of research with scholarships available but the funding is limited. It is important to consider what options are available before committing to a particular area of research.

When choosing an area of study the researcher should consider which journal they wish to publish in and its impact factor. Different journals have different scopes and the desired journal may not publish in an area of interest. It is worth looking at the submission guidelines early in the research as they may change the way that the research is undertaken.

The necessary research skills will vary with different research projects although it is possible to collaborate with other researchers to gain new skills. Attending research method courses and helping other researchers can be helpful. Networking is important to all researchers to give opportunities to collaborate and learn about the area.

Getting published opens doors so it is important to prioritise any chance to get your work in print. Even if it is a news and views article or a letter it may catch the attention of a colleague who can help support your career and research. It often takes many attempts to get published, so it is important to be persistent.

Self-funded research has advantages over paying fees for a course or applying for a scholarship. Scholarship funding is very competitive and the paperwork is often extensive. It can be easier to fill in the paperwork if the researcher already has some results.

As much of medical education research has low costs and there are lower ethical barriers it makes sense to iterate before applying. Developing a good research project often takes a number of iterations. Starting with an observation or an essay can allow the researcher to explore the area superficially before tackling the deeper aspects.

It is better to have several areas of interest and developing them all rather than trying to focus on one area too soon. The more areas that the researcher explores the more likely that one will become a passion. Publishing a few short pieces is better than depending on one piece. Having several articles can help work out which area generates the most interest.

It can be difficult to develop a clear research question and many researchers make the mistake of trying to force the process. It is better to delay the application and spend more time exploring the literature than to apply too early. Even when a possible topic seems compelling it is better to do so initial work to see if the results are as expected.

At this stage the researcher will have published an initial article in the area, have an important question to address and be confident that no one else has studied this area. They will have initial results that are promising and should then be able to write the perfect research study. This is to ensure that they understand how this topic should be researched properly.

The decision to proceed with the research by completing the application form for funding or self-funding should be based upon this 'perfect study'. If the study requires substantial funding then they will need a scholarship. The researcher may decide to cut expenses and aim lower for their research publication or try to get the full funding.

Masters courses.

First-time researchers often need a lot support from a supervisor and will find that they get stuck at an early stage. They will struggle with the early research and writing an article or planning how to explore their ideas. A Masters course can be a great option in these cases.

Masters courses offer formal teaching on how to conduct literature reviews, design research projects, collect and analyse data and write research papers. Supervisors help identify weak areas and provide guidance on improving research skills. Networking with other researchers can provide feedback on your work and find collaborators for future research projects.

On a Masters course the researcher should expect to have teaching in all the necessary research skills. They should expect that their supervisor asks interesting questions about their proposed research. This is to help them self-reflect and identify areas of weakness.

The student will need plan and complete their research project. Universities break this down into steps starting with the idea for the research project. As the project is short and has a low likelihood of being published it is not essential that it is an important question.

The next step is to conduct a literature review and identify the relevant research. This is useful later because it provides a list of references that can be copied into the dissertation. It is usually best to summarise the main points of each article in the reference so that the correct reference can be identified.

Start to firm up the plan to include specific details on how the research will be conducted and a timeline. This is useful for the supervisor because they can check if the researcher is falling behind. If the supervisor has not asked relevant questions then the researcher should ask for a further review by a senior supervisor.

It can be difficult to work out what is missing from a research project particularly the first time around. The supervisor needs to understand what the researcher is trying to achieve. The supervisor should be aware of the subject to enough depth to have an idea about the likely results that will be obtained.

It is important to check whether the researcher has the correct research skills to perform the research and the supervisor may need to arrange further training. If the researcher is struggling with writing clearly and concisely they will require assistance. Although LLMs can help researchers become more eloquent there is a high risk of plagiarism and writing training is a better option.

Here are some tips on how to improve your writing skills:

1. Identify the main points you want to make. What are you trying to say in your writing? What are the key messages you want your audience to take away? Once you know what you want to say, you can start to organise your thoughts and ideas.

2. Arrange the points in a logical order. The order of your points is important. You want your writing to flow smoothly and make sense to your reader. Consider the most logical way to present your points and then arrange them in that order.

3. Use headings for the points. Headings can help to break up your writing and make it easier for your reader to follow. They can also help to emphasise the key points of your writing.

4. Write each point as a single sentence. This will help to keep your writing clear and concise. It will also make it easier for your reader to follow your argument.

5. Use clear and concise language. Avoid using jargon or technical terms that your reader may not understand. Instead, use simple language that is easy to understand.

6. Proofread your writing carefully before you submit it. This will help to catch any errors in grammar, spelling, or punctuation. It will also help to ensure that your writing is clear and concise.

Benefits of scholarship and research in medical education:

There are few other ways to improve career prospects and reputation in education that are as effective as research. Research can have direct health benefits as many medical accidents are caused by poor training. Learning to improve medical education to address these known gaps can reduce the risk from the doctors in the future.

There are many new technologies in medical education but it is not clear whether they are improving outcomes. Researchers are the front line of these developments and can be highly influential in the decision making of what to teach future doctors. This in turn have major implications on the health of the population.

- Improved student learning: Scholarship and research in medical education can help to identify the most effective teaching methods and learning strategies, which can lead to improved student learning.
- Increased patient safety: Scholarship and research in medical education can help to identify and address factors that contribute to medical errors, which can lead to increased patient safety.
- Improved quality of care: Scholarship and research in medical education can help to improve the quality of care that patients receive by ensuring that medical students are well-trained and prepared to practice medicine.
- Advancement of the field: Scholarship and research in medical education can help to advance the field of medicine by identifying new knowledge and best practices.

Scholarship and research in medical education is an important part of the field of medical education. It helps us to improve the quality of medical education and to ensure that our students are getting the best possible education. If you are interested in getting involved in scholarship and research in medical education, there are many opportunities available to you.

Conclusions.

Scholarship and research in medical education play a crucial role in advancing the field and improving the quality of medical education. By conducting research, educators can identify effective teaching methods, enhance student learning, increase patient safety and improve the overall quality of care.

There are various types of research available, including self-funded role-based research, pursuing a Masters degree, or seeking scholarships depending on the individual's skills and interests. Each educator should carefully consider their job role and the areas they are involved in to determine the most suitable type of research.

Becoming a researcher in medical education requires developing research skills, collaborating with other researchers, attending research method courses and networking to find opportunities for collaboration and learning. Publishing research findings is crucial for building an academic career and gaining recognition in the field.

Masters courses can provide valuable support and formal teaching on research skills, allowing first-time researchers to receive guidance from supervisors, improve their research abilities and network with fellow researchers.

Improving writing skills is essential for effective communication of research findings. Identifying key points, organising them logically, using headings, writing concisely and proofreading carefully are all important aspects of improving writing skills.

Scholarship and research in medical education offer numerous benefits, including improved student learning, increased patient safety, improved quality of care and the advancement of the field. It provides opportunities to address gaps in medical training, influence the adoption of new technologies and shape the future of healthcare.

Overall, scholarship and research in medical education are integral to the continuous improvement and development of medical education practices. Engaging in research not only enhances educators' careers but also contributes to the betterment of medical training, ultimately benefiting students, patients and the healthcare system as a whole.

Top tips.

Start with the question: Asking questions and finding the answers to those questions will prepare you for research. Finding an important question which does not have an answer provides motivation and focus.

Developing the research. Create a clear and focused research question based upon the type of research that suits your skills, goals and job role. Plan what steps will be required to achieve the research including training.

Prioritise Publication: Getting research published opens doors for further research opportunities and enhances your academic profile. Consider the scope and impact factor of the journal you wish to submit to

Chapter 31: REFLECTING IN MEDICAL EDUCATION

Reflection is a process of thinking about and evaluating an experience to gain a deeper understanding. It is an essential part of medical education, as it helps students to develop their clinical skills and judgment.

The process of reflection has not been fully understood and there are significant risks. Those who have low reflection find the process of reflection unpleasant and confusing. There is a risk of psychological breakdown if a person was forced to reflect without psychological support.

Reflection has overlap with psychological counselling as both require an interest in understanding behaviour and feelings, having insight and engaging in self-reflection activities. These activities can cause a disruption to the person's sense of self which can create an identity crisis.

Educators should ensure that they are fully trained in reflection and psychological first aid if any student becomes overwhelmed. Those who have psychological skills should avoid trying to counsel the student. The focus when teaching reflection is the student's safety and maintaining consent. Having a safe word, explaining the risks and allowing students to not participate are all important.

The educator should encourage the group to monitor each other alter them if any students are looking unwell. The process should be paused if any student has problems. They should be reassured that many excellent doctors struggle with reflection.

Reflection methods.

There are many different ways to reflect in medical education. Some common methods include:

- Writing a reflective journal: This is a great way to document your thoughts and feelings about your experiences. You can write about anything that you find interesting or challenging and you can use your journal to explore your own learning and development.

- Writing reflective essays: This is a traditional method of reflection in which students write about a specific experience they have had. The essay should explore the student's thoughts, feelings and emotions about the experience, as well as what they learned from it.

- Critical incident reporting: This involves writing about a specific event that occurred during a clinical rotation.

- Guided reflection: This involves discussing a particular experience with a facilitator or mentor. This can help identify key learning points and develop strategies for improvement.

- Reflective practice groups: This involves meeting with a group of peers to discuss their experiences and reflections.

- Talking to a mentor or supervisor: This can be a helpful way to get feedback on your practice and to discuss your experiences. Your mentor or supervisor can help you to identify areas where you need to improve and they can offer guidance on how to develop your skills.

- Using a reflective framework: There are a number of different reflective frameworks that you can use to guide your reflections. These frameworks can help you to structure your thinking and to identify the key learning points from your experiences.

All these methods are time consuming and unnecessary unless the issue is important. It can be argued that reflection only works if professionals actually engage in it. There are no benefits from suggesting forms of reflection which do not actually get used.

Some students are naturally reflective and will often spontaneously offer reflections. Many students will resist requests to reflect and provide superficial reflections that lack insight. It is unclear whether these students can be taught to reflect and they are just resistant.

Individual teaching may be used to help those with the greatest difficulty with reflection. The risk of this approach can be mitigated by ensuring that the student fully consents to the process. This unfortunately means that some students will not give consent and will not be able to achieve the goal.

Reflection sentences

Reflection sentences are a short and concise way to capture the essence of an experience. They can be used as an alternative to formal reflection, which can be more time-consuming and complex.

There are several advantages to using reflection sentences. First, they are quick to write, so students can generate more of them in a shorter amount of time. This can help students to reflect more frequently on their experiences, which can lead to deeper insights.

Second, reflection sentences are often more authentic than longer pieces of writing. This is because they capture the student's initial thoughts and feelings about an experience, which are often more genuine than the thoughts and feelings that they may have later on.

Third, reflection sentences can be used to track progress over time. By comparing reflection sentences from different points in time, students can see how their thinking and understanding have evolved.

There are also some potential disadvantages to using reflection sentences. One concern is that they may not be as deep as longer pieces of writing. However, the evidence suggests that this is not always the case. In fact, reflection sentences can often be just as insightful as longer pieces of writing, if not more so.

Another concern is that reflection sentences may not be as helpful for students who are struggling to articulate their thoughts and feelings. However, this can be overcome by providing students with prompts or questions to help them get started.

Reflection sentences may further advantages because they are more flexible, can be used to capture a greater range of experiences and can help the student select an experience for deeper reflection.

Overall, reflection sentences are a valuable tool for reflection. They are quick to write, authentic and can be used to track progress over time. While they may not be as deep as longer pieces of writing, they can be just as insightful.

Practical steps to reflect.

Reflection is an important part of medical education, but it can be difficult to know where to start. If you are new to reflection, there are a few things that you can do to get started:

- Set aside some time for reflection: Reflection takes time, so it is important to set aside some time for it each week. Even 15 minutes a day can make a difference.

- Start by choosing a specific experience to reflect on: When you are first starting out, it can be helpful to choose a specific experience to reflect on. This could be a patient encounter, a clinical rotation, or even a lecture.

- Be honest with yourself: When you are reflecting, it is important to be honest with yourself about your thoughts and feelings. This can be difficult, but it is essential for learning and growth.

Reflection is a valuable skill that can help you to become a better doctor. By taking the time to reflect on your experiences, you can learn from them and improve your practice.

What does reflection achieve?

The process of reflection is associated with higher performance, increased learning, improved decision making, enhanced creativity and increased self-awareness. These benefits make the attainment of reflection a key learning goal for educators. It is clear that many professionals do not reflect on a daily basis. This may represent a missed opportunity for improved performance.

- Identify their strengths and weaknesses: By reflecting on their experiences, students can identify areas where they need to improve their knowledge, skills, or attitudes.
- Develop critical thinking skills: Reflection can help students to develop their critical thinking skills by challenging their assumptions and biases.
- Improve their communication skills: Reflection can help students to improve their communication skills by learning how to express their thoughts and feelings clearly and concisely.
- Increase their self-awareness: Reflection can help students to increase their self-awareness by becoming more aware of their own thoughts, feelings and behaviours.

The key question that has not been properly addressed is whether training can improve reflection and if so what type of training is appropriate. Measuring ability to reflect is at an early stage and has some limitations.

Measuring reflection.

The Self-Reflection (SRIS-SR) scale is a tool that can be used to measure reflective abilities. The scale asks questions such as interest in understanding behaviour and feelings, having insight and engaging in self-reflection activities.

The SRIS-SR can be used to identify people who need help with reflection. For example, if a student scores low on the scale, it may be an indication that they need help learning how to reflect. Educators can use the SRIS-SR to provide specific assistance to these students.

In addition to identifying people who need help, the SRIS-SR can also be used to track progress in reflection. If a student scores low on the scale at the beginning of a semester, but then scores higher at the end of the semester, it is an indication that the student has made progress in their reflective abilities.

Measuring reflective abilities can also be used to assess the effectiveness of reflection training exercises. There is a risk of bias with self-report of reflection behaviours particularly when the educator acts upon the results.

Training reflection.

There are a number of proposed methods for helping educators to teach students how to reflect. Their effectiveness is not proven but could be tried with consent with those who struggle with reflection. There are potential risks of using unproven techniques to achieve reflection and educators should make careful records.

- Questioning: One of the best ways to help people reflect is to ask them questions. These questions can be open-ended, such as "What did you learn from that experience?" or "What could you have done differently?", or they can be more specific, such as "What were your thoughts and feelings during that situation?" or "What were the factors that contributed to your decision?".

- Journaling: Journaling is another great way to help people reflect. This involves writing down their thoughts and feelings about a particular experience. Journaling can be done in a free-form way, or it can be more structured, with prompts to help people focus on specific aspects of their experience.

- Reflective listening: Reflective listening is a technique where the listener repeats back what the speaker has said, in their own words. This helps the speaker to hear themselves think and to clarify their thoughts.

- Role-playing: Role-playing can be a helpful way to help people reflect on their behaviour. This involves acting out a particular situation, with the person taking on different roles. This can help them to see the situation from different perspectives and to understand how their behaviour might be perceived by others.

- Feedback: Feedback from others can be a valuable source of information for people who are trying to reflect on their behaviour.

This feedback can be positive, negative, or neutral. It can be given in a formal setting, such as a performance review, or it can be given informally, such as in a conversation with a colleague.

- Critical thinking: Critical thinking is a skill that involves analysing information and making judgments. It can be used to help people reflect on their experiences and to identify patterns and themes.

If a student becomes unwell during the process of reflection then allow them to do what they need to in order to recover. This may be getting angry and shouting or sitting quietly on their own or rocking. In general the effects will wear off over the next 15 minutes without needing to obtain psychological assistance.

Conclusions.

Reflection is a crucial aspect of medical education that helps students develop their clinical skills, judgment and self-awareness. It is associated with various benefits, including higher performance, increased learning, improved decision making, enhanced creativity and increased self-awareness.

However, the process of reflection is not fully understood and there are risks involved, particularly for individuals with low reflection abilities. Reflection can be unpleasant and confusing for them, potentially leading to psychological breakdowns if not supported properly. It is important to provide psychological assistance when necessary and not force reflection upon individuals who are resistant or unprepared.

There are several methods of reflection in medical education, such as writing reflective journals or essays, engaging in critical incident reporting, participating in guided reflection sessions or reflective practice groups and seeking feedback from mentors or supervisors. Reflective frameworks can also be used to structure thinking and identify key learning points. However, it is crucial to ensure that these methods are meaningful, relevant and actually utilised by professionals, as there are no benefits to suggesting forms of reflection that are not actively engaged in.

Reflection sentences are a concise and authentic alternative to formal reflection methods. They allow for quick capturing of thoughts and feelings, enabling students to reflect more frequently and gain deeper insights. Reflection sentences can also track progress over time and be just as insightful as longer pieces of writing.

To facilitate reflection, individuals can set aside dedicated time for reflection, choose specific experiences to reflect on and be honest with themselves about their thoughts and feelings. Reflective abilities can be measured using tools like the Self-Reflection (SRIS-SR) scale, which can help identify individuals who may require assistance and track their progress. However, self-reporting of reflection behaviours should be interpreted with caution, as biases may exist.

Teaching reflection to students can be approached through various methods, such as questioning, journaling, reflective listening, role-playing, feedback and fostering critical thinking skills. It is important for educators to be cautious and maintain careful records when using these techniques as they are unproven.

In summary, reflection is a valuable skill in medical education that should be nurtured and supported. By engaging in reflection, students can identify their strengths and weaknesses, develop critical thinking and communication skills and increase their self-awareness. It is essential to provide appropriate training, ensure the effectiveness of reflection methods and offer psychological first aid when needed.

Top tips.

Assess reflective abilities: Use tools like the Self-Reflection (SRIS-SR) scale to measure reflective abilities. This can help identify students who need special support to progress in reflection.

Consider reflection sentences: Try using reflection sentences as a quick and concise way to capture the essence of an experience. They can be just as insightful as longer pieces of writing and help track progress over time.

Reduce resistance: Break refection down into steps and help the student practice each step. Describe the situation in detail, explore their feelings and thoughts about the experience identify what they learned and how to apply that learning in the future.

Chapter 32: TEACHING LEADERSHIP SKILLS

Teaching leadership skills varies in difficulty from the straightforward e.g. problem solving and teamwork to the challenging e.g. vision and motivation. Each of these leadership skills can help a person taking on a leadership role be more effective. Whether a professional will then become a full-time leader depends on the individual's motivation and abilities.

As with any team role people vary in how suited they are to leadership. Those who are natural leaders will have higher motivation and ability to lead. They still require training to ensure that they have the skills necessary to be successful. There are different ways to leadership and a single leadership style will not suit everyone.

An educator should help the students recognise their own team roles and any strengths and weaknesses that they have in leadership. Most professionals will undertake some leadership roles during their careers so will need to learn how to lead. Encourage students to see leadership skills as necessary for their future career.

Leadership is essential for a political career and explaining the difference between this and other leadership roles can be helpful. Political leadership requires natural qualities that not everyone has. Political figures also need substantial training to become good at their role which is not required for other leadership roles.

Seeing leadership as a team role implies that the professional will have support from other team members. It is important to recognise that even the best leaders will not have all the necessary skills and will rely upon others. Leading is a collaborative task and students should be able to identify those who have skills that they are missing.

Introduction to leadership.

An educator should introduce a session on leadership by using a formal structure. This allows the students to see that there is nothing different about this topic than other topics they have learned. Reinforcing that this is not different can reduce the mystery of leadership as a topic.

- Start with the basics. Before you can teach learners how to be leaders, you need to make sure they understand the basics of leadership. This includes understanding the different types of leadership, the skills and qualities of a good leader and the different leadership styles.

- Be clear about your expectations. What do you want learners to be able to do by the end of the program? Make sure you are clear about your expectations so that learners know what they are working towards.
- Use a variety of teaching methods. There is no one-size-fits-all approach to teaching leadership skills. Use a variety of teaching methods to keep learners engaged and to help them learn in different ways.
- Provide opportunities for practice. The best way to learn leadership skills is by practicing them. Provide learners with opportunities to practice their skills in a safe and supportive environment.
- Give feedback. Feedback is essential for any leadership development program. Provide learners with specific and constructive feedback so that they can learn from their experiences and grow as leaders.

Normalising the topic of leadership is essential to improve engagement. If the students are thinking about leaders they are likely to disengage. They need to see that all professionals undertake leadership roles even if they are not leaders. Being a leader and leading are different tasks.

Key skills for leadership.

There is an overlap between the skills required as a professional and those that are needed for to lead. Communication, decision making and problem solving are unlikely to pose problems for most professionals. The other skills of motivation, vision and teamwork may not be included in usual training.

- Communication: Leaders need to be able to communicate effectively with their team members, stakeholders and other leaders. This includes being able to listen effectively, give clear instructions, create rapport and motivate others.
- Decision-making: Leaders need to be able to make decisions quickly and effectively. This includes being able to gather information, weigh the pros and cons of different options, identify the best course of action and make a decision.
- Problem-solving: Leaders need to be able to solve problems effectively. This includes being able to identify the problem, gather information, develop solutions and implement solutions.
- Motivation: Leaders need to be able to motivate their team members to achieve their goals. This includes being able to set clear

expectations, provide positive reinforcement and deal with difficult situations.

- Vision: Leaders need to have a vision for the future of their team or organisation. This includes being able to articulate the vision, inspire others to share the vision and develop a plan to achieve the vision.
- Teamwork: Leaders need to be able to work effectively with others. This includes being able to build trust, delegate tasks and resolve conflicts.

Although these skills are desirable the students may have resistance to learning them. They may feel that they are complex to learn, outside of their comfort zone and unnecessary. The educator can discuss with their students whether they feel those skills will be useful to them as a doctor.

Reassuring the students that they can learn these skills, that they can be used with patients and the training is not difficult can help remove these resistances. Giving the students the illusion of choice by asking them which skill they want to learn first can also be effective.

How to teach leadership skills.

There are many different ways to teach leadership skills and the educator will need to choose the best way to teach each skill. The choice will depend on the skills in the group, the material to be covered and the resources available. Repeated short learning experiences are likely to better than prolonged tasks.

- Role-playing: This involves giving participants the opportunity to practice leadership skills in a safe and controlled environment. For example, you could have them role-play a meeting where they have to give a presentation or delegate tasks.
- Simulations: This involves using a computer program or other simulation to create a realistic leadership experience. For example, you could have participants take part in a simulated service development or a simulated health crisis.
- Case studies: This involves presenting participants with a real-world leadership challenge and asking them to develop a solution. For example, you could give them a case study about a hospital that is facing financial difficulties and ask them to come up with a plan to turn things around.
- Coaching: This involves providing individual feedback and guidance to participants on their leadership skills. For example,

you could meet with them regularly to discuss their strengths and weaknesses and to help them develop a plan for improvement.

• Workshops: This involves providing participants with a structured learning experience on leadership skills. For example, you could run a workshop on topics such as communication, decision-making, or conflict resolution.

Leadership skills can be taught during a teaching session for another topic. Students are often encouraged to use leadership skills to help them achieve other tasks. This should be avoided because trying to do two things at once reduces the performance of both. It is better to have the leader concentrate just on a leadership skill.

Teaching motivation as a skill.

There are two skills that will need formal teaching as the student will not be familiar with them. The first is motivation and the second is vision. The educator will be familiar with this skill as they use it to help engage students in their tasks. Students are often reluctant to speak to colleagues because they are not sure what to say. The educator needs to address this reluctance by discussing with the students why they feel that way.

Set clear expectations.

• Work with the group to identify common goals and objectives.
• Break large goals down into smaller manageable steps.
• Create clear instructions on how to achieve the step.
• Provide the resources needed to achieve them.

Provide positive reinforcement.

• Speak to the different team members and find out how they are doing.
• Give feedback on their performance in a positive way.
• Praise, encouragement, when people meet or exceed expectations.
• Asking those who are struggling what they need to achieve their tasks.
• Find something positive to say such as 'you are working hard'.

<u>Deal with difficult situations.</u>

- Engage with those who are having setbacks or challenges.
- Listen to the person's ideas.
- Work out why they are having difficulties.
- Work with the person to develop a plan to overcome it.
- Help them manage emotions such as boredom or frustration.

Students will often disbelieve that motivation is as simple as is suggested by the steps above. They may require several demonstrations to be convinced that these steps are effective. Giving them the check list and asking them to perform the steps will help them see how it works. A leader's job is to remove barriers and this is enough to motivate people.

Teaching vision as a skill.

Many leadership roles come with a specific aim or objective but if this is not present it can be difficult to focus the efforts without a vision. A vision is basically a self-imposed objective that the leader creates to help them structure their activities.

Visions have the advantages of increasing clarity and focus on goals, helping make better decisions, increasing motivation as others can see what needs doing. When teaching the skill is important to differentiate between the choice of vision which is a creative process and implementing a vision.

- Consider options for a vision. A vision should be aligned with the aims of the team and the organisation, should be achievable but challenging and ideally engaging. A clear and compelling picture of the future that you want to create.
- Articulate the vision. This means helping them to clearly define what they want to achieve and why it is important to them. It also means helping them to break down their vision into smaller, more achievable goals.
- Inspire others to share the vision This means helping them to communicate their vision in a way that is clear, compelling and inspiring. It also means helping them to create a sense of shared ownership of the vision so that others are motivated to help achieve it.
- Develop a plan to achieve the vision. This means helping them to identify the resources they need, the steps they need to take and the timeline they need to follow. It also means helping them to overcome obstacles and setbacks along the way.

There are a number of techniques that can be used to help students create visions. The educator should focus on whether a vision is required for a particular leadership role, if the group can help with the vision and how to achieve the vision.

- The vision board: This is a classic exercise that helps people to visualise their goals. Have people create a vision board by cutting out images and words that represent their vision for the future.
- The future story: This exercise helps people to develop their imagination and to see the possibilities for the future. Have people write a story about the future that they would like to see.

The students should also learn one essential skill that is generally useful. The ability to make their point concisely and in an engaging way. The elevator pitch is one exercise that can help students learn this skill. Crafting the words into a pitch is challenging because each word must do some of the work.

- The elevator pitch: This exercise helps people to develop their communication skills. Have people practice giving a short pitch about their vision to a group of people.

The students should start with a strong hook to grab attention and then make the message clearly and concisely. They should use imagery such as metaphors or analogies and be passionate. Careful preparation before the group meets means that the student will be have all the resources needed to create a vision.

Educators will need to cover the other skills of communication, decision making, problem solving and teamwork. These skills will already have been covered in other topics but a reminder of the principles can help. There are various leadership theories which can help the students understand where these skills fit into the leadership role.

Trait theory

Trait theory is a leadership theory that focuses on the innate qualities of leaders. It is interesting for students to consider because it helps discriminate between leaders and leadership roles. A student may feel that they do not have the traits to be a great leader and should be encouraged to see what team role they are best at.

Trait theory is one of the oldest and most widely studied leadership theories. It has been responsible for much of the mystery associated with leadership. Trait theory helps identify those who have the potential to be great leaders.

It does not predict whether they will actually be effective, as other factors are also important.

- Intelligence: Effective leaders are typically intelligent and have a good understanding of the world around them. They can think critically and solve problems effectively and create compelling visions.

- Charisma: Effective leaders are typically charismatic and able to inspire and motivate others with their communication skills. They can build relationships and create a sense of excitement and enthusiasm.

- Decisiveness: Effective leaders are typically decisive and able to make quick decisions. They are not afraid to take risks and are able to adapt to changing circumstances.

- Self-confidence: Effective leaders are typically self-confident and believe in themselves and their abilities. They are not afraid to take charge and are able to inspire confidence in others. They can bounce back from setbacks and are able to learn from their mistakes.

Educators can ask students whether these traits have any negative aspects. This can help them understand why having these traits does not necessarily predict success. Learning to control these traits is as important as having them.

Behavioural theory

The behavioural theory model focuses on the behaviours that make a good leader. These behaviours can include things like delegation, communication and problem-solving. Leaders can range from autocratic through participative, democratic to laissez faire in their style and still get good results.

The behavioural theory of leadership identifies two main types of leadership behaviours:

- Task-oriented behaviours: These behaviours focus on getting the job done. Task-oriented leaders are typically good at setting goals, delegating tasks and motivating their team members.
- People-oriented behaviours: These behaviours focus on building relationships and creating a positive work environment. People-oriented leaders are typically good at listening to their team members, providing feedback and resolving conflicts.

Educators can use this model to explain why it is not always necessary to use all the leadership skills. If a leader is good at interacting with their team the members will be empowered by the positive environment to be more task oriented. If the leader is good at setting goals then the team will create a more positive work environment.

Contingency theory.

Contingency theory suggests that there is no one-size-fits-all approach to leadership. The best leadership style depends on the situation. It is a useful way of analysing the complexity of the leadership challenges.

- Leader-member relations: This refers to the quality of the relationship between the leader and the followers.
- Task structure: This refers to the degree to which the task is well-defined and structured.
- Position power: This refers to the amount of power and authority that the leader has.

The stronger the leader's position the less that they will need to use autocratic approaches and be free to use other styles. The model also explains why as the situation worsens the leader's range of options decreases.

Power and influence theory

Power and influence theory focuses on the way that leaders use power and influence to achieve their goals. Power comes from coercion, reward, charisma, expertise and the role itself. A leader can improve their position by how they use these sources of power.

- Rational persuasion: This is the use of logic and reason to convince others to follow a leader's lead.
- Personal appeals: This is the use of emotional appeals to convince others to follow a leader's lead.
- Legitimate power: This is the use of a leader's position or title to convince others to follow a leader's lead.
- Exchange: This is the use of rewards or benefits to convince others to follow a leader's lead.
- Coercive power: This is the use of threats or punishment to convince others to follow a leader's lead.
- Normative influence: This is the use of shared values and beliefs to persuade others to follow a leader's lead.

In practice, the leader will consider these options when trying to exert power to achieve their goals. They can then adapt their approach to suit a specific situation by using a variety of approaches. A common mistake for new leaders is to use excessive power to achieve their aims. This leads to them being seen as manipulative or coercive and can lead to conflict and resistance.

Authentic leadership

Authentic leadership focuses on being true to oneself and one's values. Authentic leaders are transparent and genuine and they are able to build trust and rapport with their followers. They achieve their reputation by aligning their actions with their beliefs. It is challenging to achieve this as there will usually be areas that are difficult to align.

- Self-awareness: Authentic leaders are aware of their own strengths and weaknesses and they are comfortable with who they are.

- Integrity: Authentic leaders act in accordance with their values, even when it is difficult.

- Transparency: Authentic leaders are open and honest with their followers and they are willing to share their mistakes.

- Humility: Authentic leaders are not afraid to admit when they are wrong and they are always willing to learn from others.

- Empathy: Authentic leaders are able to understand and connect with the needs of their followers.

- Courage: Authentic leaders are not afraid to stand up for what they believe in, even when it is unpopular.

Professionalism relies upon this type of leadership style as it is difficult to behave in a way that is inconsistent with one's beliefs. Educators can use the example of professionalism to explore why this approach is effective. Issues such as being too idealistic and oversharing can be problematic.

Transformational leadership

Transformational leadership focuses on inspiring and motivating followers to achieve more than they thought possible. Transformational leaders are typically charismatic and visionary and they are able to create a sense of excitement and purpose in their followers.

- Idealised influence: Transformational leaders are role models for their followers. They are seen as credible and trustworthy and they inspire their followers to emulate their behaviour.

- Inspirational motivation: Transformational leaders articulate a clear and compelling vision for the future. They are able to motivate their followers to share this vision and to work towards achieving it.

- Intellectual stimulation: Transformational leaders challenge their followers to think creatively and to solve problems in new ways. They encourage their followers to question the status quo and to come up with innovative solutions.

- Individualised consideration: Transformational leaders treat their followers as individuals. They are aware of each follower's strengths and weaknesses and they provide them with the support and coaching they need to succeed.

The educator can use this model to discuss both the dangers of the trait of charisma and that few leaders will actually use this approach.

Transactional leadership.

Transactional leadership focuses on the exchange of rewards and punishments to motivate followers. Transactional leaders set clear expectations and provide feedback and they reward followers for meeting those expectations.

Here are some of the advantages of transactional leadership:

- Clear expectations: Transactional leaders set clear expectations for their followers, which can help to reduce confusion and ambiguity.

- Regular feedback: Transactional leaders provide regular feedback to their followers, which can help to keep them motivated and on track.

- Rewards and punishments: Rewards and punishments can be effective motivators and they can help to ensure that followers meet their goals.

Here are some of the disadvantages of transactional leadership:

- Short-term focus: Transactional leaders focus on the short-term, which can lead to followers feeling disengaged and unmotivated in the long run.

- Autocratic: Transactional leaders can be seen as autocratic and controlling, which can lead to followers feeling resentful and disengaged.

- Not always effective: Transactional leadership is not always effective and it can be counterproductive in situations where followers need to be inspired and motivated to achieve more than they thought possible.

Many leaders will revert to this style as they appear to be doing their job competently. The problem is that this style is not very effective at building teamwork and motivation. The educator can use this style as an example where a leader can fail to do enough to be effective.

Servant leadership

Servant leadership focuses on the needs of followers rather than the needs of the leader. Servant leaders are humble and selfless and they are always willing to put the needs of their followers first. These leaders are seen as charismatic and build stronger relationships with their colleagues.

- Humility: Servant leaders are humble and put the needs of others before their own. They are not afraid to admit when they are wrong and they are always willing to learn from others.

- Empathy: Servant leaders are empathetic and understand the needs of their colleagues. They are able to see things from their colleagues perspective and they are always willing to help them.

- Listening: Servant leaders are good listeners and they are always open to feedback. They are willing to hear what their colleagues have to say and they are always willing to change their minds if they are wrong.

- Development: Servant leaders are always looking for ways to develop their colleagues. They provide them with opportunities to learn and grow and they are always willing to help them achieve their goals.

- Trust: Servant leaders are trustworthy and they build trust with their colleagues. They are honest and reliable and they are always willing to keep their promises.

The problems with servant leader style are that the leader may find making decisions difficult if they conflict with their team. They may find delegation difficult as it risks losing power and control. They spend a lot of time tending their colleagues which makes it difficult to get things done.

Charismatic leadership

Charismatic leadership focuses on the leader's personal qualities, such as charisma, vision and communication skills. Charismatic leaders are able to inspire and motivate followers and they often have a strong following.

Charismatic leaders are often eloquent speakers, have a compelling vision and excellent communication skills. They are motivating and can put forward creative and innovative solutions. They can inspire colleagues to make changes and overcome challenges by making them feel involved in something special.

They can lead to emotional dependency in their colleagues who want to the leader to tell them what to do. Charismatic leaders are often given more freedom than other leaders leading to abuse of power and overconfidence. They can overpromise and behave in ways that are manipulative and abusive.

Leadership as a journey

Leadership is a journey, not a destination. It is a process of continuous learning and growth, as leaders constantly adapt to new challenges and opportunities. There is no one right way to lead and what works for one leader may not work for another. However, there are some common principles that all great leaders share.

- Self-awareness. Leaders need to be aware of their own strengths and weaknesses, as well as their own values and beliefs. This self-awareness allows leaders to make better decisions and to build stronger relationships with their followers.
- Communicate effectively. Leaders need to be able to clearly articulate their vision and to motivate their followers to achieve that vision. They also need to be able to listen to feedback and to adapt their leadership style accordingly.
- Building relationships. Leaders need to be able to build trust and rapport with their colleagues, as well as with other stakeholders. This allows leaders to create a sense of shared purpose and to build a strong team.
- Continuous learning and development. Leaders need to be open to new ideas and to feedback. They also need to be willing to take risks and to learn from their mistakes.

Students may walk around the foothills of leadership or climb to the top of the leadership mountain. The leadership skills will help them with whatever tasks they face. They will give them skills that will make them more effective in many professional tasks outside of leadership roles.

Conclusion.

Teaching leadership skills is important for professionals who may take on leadership roles in their careers. Leadership skills vary in difficulty and include problem-solving, teamwork, communication, decision-making, motivation, vision and teamwork. While some individuals may have natural leadership abilities, training is still necessary to develop and enhance these skills.

To effectively teach leadership skills, educators should introduce the topic using a formal structure and clarify expectations. It is crucial to use a variety of teaching methods to engage learners and provide them with opportunities to practice and receive feedback. Normalising the topic of leadership helps students understand that leadership is a team role and that even the best leaders rely on the skills and support of others.

Motivation and vision are two important skills that need formal teaching. Motivation can be taught by setting clear expectations, providing positive reinforcement and addressing difficult situations. Vision as a skill involves considering options for a vision, articulating the vision, inspiring others to share the vision and developing a plan to achieve it. Techniques such as vision boards, future stories and elevator pitches can be used to help students develop their vision.

Trait theory, behavioural theory, contingency theory and power and influence theory are leadership theories that can help students understand different aspects of leadership. Trait theory focuses on innate qualities of leaders, while behavioural theory examines task-oriented and people-oriented behaviours. Contingency theory suggests that the best leadership style depends on the situation and power and influence theory explores how leaders use power and influence to achieve their goals.

Overall, teaching leadership skills requires a comprehensive approach that addresses different skills, theories and techniques. By providing students with the necessary knowledge and opportunities to practice, educators can help develop effective leaders who can positively impact their teams and organisations.

Top tips.

Key Leadership Skills: Discuss the 6 essential leadership skills - communication, decision-making, problem-solving, motivation, vision and teamwork. Explain that they will need training on motivation and vision.

Using leadership skills. Offer learners opportunities to practice leadership skills in a safe and supportive environment. This can normalise the concept of professional leadership and recognise the skills that they already have.

Self-Awareness: Feedback improves self-awareness which is the ability to understand one's own strengths, weaknesses, values and beliefs. It is a crucial skill for effective leadership, as it allows leaders to understand their own impact on others and make better decisions.

Chapter 33: MEDICAL HUMANITIES

Medical humanities is an interdisciplinary field that brings together the humanities, social sciences and arts to explore the human dimension of health and healthcare. It is a relatively new field, but it is growing rapidly in popularity as healthcare professionals and educators recognise the value of incorporating the humanities into medical education and practice.

Students can find the difference between science and humanities challenging. They may look for the take-away point, the key message and they find it lacking. The educator needs to explain that it is the journey to understanding and the experience of the art that will give them insight.

The educator's role is to help students understand that the humanities are not about finding answers, but about asking questions. They need to help students see the value in exploring the human dimension of health and healthcare and in using the humanities to gain insights into the patient experience.

One way to help students understand the importance of process in medical humanities is to have them engage with different art forms, such as literature, film and music. These art forms can provide students with a way to connect with the human experience in a way that traditional textbooks cannot. They can also help students to develop their own critical thinking skills and to see the world from different perspectives.

The importance of process and transformation in medical humanities makes this area difficult to teach. The educator may find that they try to find a quick fix to keep the interest of the students. They also need to go through the process themselves, reading the book, watching the film and then reflecting on their own experiences so that they can help their students.

There are many different ways to define medical humanities, but some of the key concepts include:

- The patient as a whole person: Medical humanities recognises that patients are not just their diseases. They are individuals with unique histories, cultures and experiences.

- The importance of communication: Medical humanities emphasises the importance of communication between healthcare professionals and patients. This includes verbal communication, as well as nonverbal communication such as body language and touch.

- The role of emotions: Medical humanities acknowledges the role of emotions in healthcare. Patients experience a wide range of emotions, from fear and anxiety to hope and joy. Healthcare professionals need to be able to understand and respond to these emotions in a way that is helpful and supportive.

- The importance of ethics: Medical humanities explores the ethical issues that arise in healthcare. These issues include informed consent, confidentiality and end-of-life care.

Medical humanities provide a type of experiential learning which is different from traditional methods. The learning requires active participation, the learner experiences the emotions and needs to reflect on the experience. The learning is more meaningful and can cause cognitive dissonance and change to the learner.

In the context of medical humanities, cognitive dissonance can occur when a learner experiences the emotions that are associated with illness, disability and death, but they do not yet have the knowledge or skills to understand or cope with those emotions. This can lead to a change in the learner's beliefs or attitudes about illness, disability and death.

When the learner experiences the world from the patient's perspective, they are better able to understand the patient's experiences and emotions. This can lead to more compassionate and effective care.

Literature:

Literature can be used to help doctors understand their patients experiences and the meaning they find in their illness. For example, reading about how a patient was told about their diagnosis in a book can help the doctor find a different way of sharing information. The patient can see this as caring and connecting with their sadness.

The following are examples of literature that the students may wish to experience themselves. They mainly explore the key concepts through a story and are well written and compelling. The educator can discuss with the students who have already read what they gained from the experience and encourage those that have not to consider whether they might benefit from the experience.

- Cancer Ward by Alexander Solzhenitsyn: This novel describes the experiences of patients in a Soviet cancer ward. It provides a vivid and unflinching look at the physical and emotional toll of cancer, as well as the challenges of providing care in a difficult and often dehumanising environment.
- The Idiot by Fyodor Dostoevsky: This novel tells the story of Prince Myshkin, a young man with a rare neurological disorder that leaves

him socially awkward and naive. The novel explores the themes of compassion, love and redemption and it offers a unique perspective on the experience of living with a disability.

- Cancer: The Gift of Imperfections by Angelina Jolie: This memoir tells the story of Jolie's decision to have a preventive double mastectomy after learning that she carries the BRCA1 gene mutation, which puts her at high risk for breast and ovarian cancer. The memoir is both personal and inspirational and it offers a powerful message of hope and resilience.
- Invictus by William Ernest Henley: This poem is a celebration of the human spirit in the face of adversity. It is often read at funerals and other memorial services and it offers a message of hope and strength to those who are struggling with illness or loss.
- Illness as a Metaphor by Susan Sontag: This book explores the ways in which illness is often used as a metaphor for other things, such as social or political ills. Sontag argues that this can be harmful, as it can lead to misunderstanding and stigma. The book offers a powerful critique of the way that illness is often portrayed in the media and in popular culture.
- A Room of One's Own by Virginia Woolf: This essay explores the ways in which women's writing has been shaped by the experience of illness and disability. Woolf argues that women's writing is often characterised by a sense of isolation and alienation and that this is due in part to the fact that women have historically been denied the same opportunities as men to receive an education and to develop their talents.
- The Yellow Wallpaper by Charlotte Perkins Gilman: This short story tells the story of a woman who is confined to her room by her husband, who believes that she is suffering from a nervous disorder. The story is a powerful exploration of the ways in which women's voices have been silenced and marginalised and it offers a critique of the medical establishment's treatment of women's mental health.
- The Bell Jar by Sylvia Plath: This novel tells the story of Esther Greenwood, a young woman who experiences a mental breakdown while working as a magazine intern in New York City. The novel is a harrowing but honest account of the experience of mental illness and it offers a powerful indictment of the ways in which society often fails to understand and support those who are struggling with mental health problems.
- My Own Country by Abraham Verghese: This memoir tells the story of Verghese's experiences as a doctor working in a small town in India. The memoir is a moving and insightful account of the

challenges of providing medical care in a resource-poor setting and it offers a unique perspective on the experience of illness and disability in a developing country.

- The Diving Bell and the Butterfly by Jean-Dominique Bauby: This memoir tells the story of Bauby, a French journalist who was left completely paralysed by a stroke. The memoir is written in the form of a series of eye blinks and it offers a powerful and inspiring account of the human spirit's capacity to overcome adversity.

- Night by Elie Wiesel: This memoir tells the story of Wiesel's experience in the Auschwitz concentration camp during the Holocaust. The memoir is a harrowing account of the physical and emotional toll of the Holocaust and it offers a powerful testimony to the human capacity for evil and resilience.

- When Breath Becomes Air by Paul Kalanithi is a beautifully written and moving memoir about the experience of facing death. Kalanithi, a neurosurgeon, was diagnosed with terminal cancer at the age of 36. The memoir chronicles his journey through diagnosis, treatment and ultimately death. Kalanithi writes with honesty and clarity about his thoughts, feelings and experiences. He also offers insights into the meaning of life and the importance of living in the present moment.

- Being Mortal by Atul Gawande is a thoughtful and compassionate book about the challenges of aging and dying. Gawande, a surgeon, writes about his own experiences with death and dying, as well as the experiences of his patients. He also explores the different ways in which people approach death and dying. Gawande's book is a valuable resource for anyone who is interested in learning more about end-of-life care.

- The Illness Narratives by Arthur Frank is a scholarly book that explores the different ways in which people tell stories about their illnesses. Frank argues that illness narratives can be a powerful way to understand the patient's perspective. He also offers a framework for understanding the different types of illness narratives.

Educators will have their own list of literature that they may feel is better suited than the list above. They will be able to talk from their own experiences of reading and how it changed their approach. It is not possible to predict which will be most effective; some books will have a major impact and others will have none on an individual.

There are no right or wrong experiences, each will have an impact on the doctor's understanding. The best way to find effective literature is to read and experience. Often the most unexpected book will cause emotional responses. The student can then reflect on why that writing had an emotional effect on them.

Art.

Art can be used to help patients express their emotions and to communicate with healthcare professionals. For example, a patient who is feeling anxious might draw a picture of their feelings. This can help the patient to understand their anxiety and to communicate it to their healthcare professional.

Art therapy is a recognised profession, it uses art as the medium for communication and expression to conduct psychological treatment. The patient draws or paints what they are feeling making the method particularly useful for those with language difficulties and difficult emotions.

- The Garden of Earthly Delights by Hieronymus Bosch (1503–1515) This painting is a complex and allegorical work that depicts the Garden of Eden, the Fall of Man and the afterlife. The painting is full of symbolism and imagery and it offers a rich and multi-layered meditation on the human condition.
- Guernica by Pablo Picasso (1937) This painting depicts the bombing of the Basque town of Guernica by German and Italian bombers during the Spanish Civil War. The painting is a powerful and moving anti-war statement and it offers a stark reminder of the horrors of war.
- Scream by Edvard Munch (1893) This painting depicts a figure with an agonised expression, against a blood-red sky. The painting is a powerful and disturbing image of anxiety and existential dread and it offers a meditation on the human condition.
- The Sick Child (1896) by Edvard Munch is a painting that depicts a young girl, presumably the artist's sister, who is dying of tuberculosis. The painting is characterised by its dark and sombre colours and its distorted perspective. The girl's face is pale and her eyes are closed and she is surrounded by a group of mourners. The painting is a powerful expression of the artist's grief and despair and it is considered to be one of the most iconic images of death in Western art.
- The Raft of the Medusa (1819) by Théodore Géricault is an oil painting that depicts the survivors of a shipwreck. The painting is set on a raft, which is overcrowded with people who are dying of thirst and starvation. The scene is chaotic and desperate and the painting is a powerful expression of the horrors of human suffering.

The painting was inspired by a real-life event and it was a major influence on the development of Romanticism.

- The Death of Marat by Jacques-Louis David (1793) This painting depicts the death of Jean-Paul Marat, a French revolutionary leader who was assassinated in his bathtub. The painting is a powerful and moving image of violence and death and it offers a meditation on the cost of revolution.
- The Pietà by Michelangelo (1499) This sculpture depicts the Virgin Mary holding the body of her son, Jesus Christ, after he was crucified. The sculpture is a moving and iconic image of grief and loss and it offers a meditation on the meaning of death.
- The Third of May 1808 by Francisco Goya (1814) This painting depicts the execution of Spanish civilians by French soldiers during the Peninsular War. The painting is a powerful and disturbing image of violence and death and it offers a meditation on the horrors of war.
- The Morgue by Honoré Daumier (1850) This painting depicts a morgue and it is a powerful and disturbing image of death and decay. The painting can be seen as a metaphor for the fragility of life and it offers a reminder of the importance of living each day to the fullest.
- The Cripples by Francisco Goya (1786–1788) This painting depicts a group of disabled people and it is a powerful and disturbing image of exclusion and marginalisation. The painting can be seen as a metaphor for the challenges faced by people with disabilities and it offers a reminder of the importance of equality and inclusion.
- The Third of May 1808 by Francisco Goya (1814) This painting depicts the execution of Spanish civilians by French soldiers during the Napoleonic Wars. The painting is a powerful and disturbing image of war and it offers a stark reminder of the horrors of violence.

Learning to respond to the emotions in pictures takes time and practice and there are many visually appealing artworks that can be used to practice. The student should be encouraged to also create their own artworks and reflect on their creations. This can take time and give rise to unexpected emotions.

Art galleries are powerful environments for contemplation of artworks. There is often a range of subjects and the student can spend time responding to a particular art piece. Educators should advise the student to look around the gallery and pick on one picture that speaks to them to spend time with.

Looking at the picture and being aware of the emotions that the person feels can reveal much about both. Often a person will feel angry or irritated, that they have 'done' the picture and should move on. They may feel embarrassed about spending time with the picture as they cannot hide their observing.

Film

Film can be used to help doctors understand what their patient's illness is like to live with. Watching film is more compelling than other forms of experience because of the actors' portrayal. The actor can connect with the observer and draw them into the experience.

Many students feel more comfortable watching a film than looking at art. This can lead to deeper involvement and feeling less self-conscious about observing. Film is a multimodal experience which can make reflection more difficult. It may be necessary to watch the film more than once to recognise where emotional responses come from.

- The Elephant Man (1980): This film tells the story of John Merrick, a man with severe deformities who is forced to live in a sideshow. The film is a powerful exploration of the social stigma of disability and the power of compassion.
- Philadelphia (1993): This film tells the story of Andrew Beckett, a lawyer who is fired from his job after revealing that he is HIV-positive. The film is a landmark portrayal of the AIDS crisis and the fight for gay rights.
- Terms of Endearment (1983): This film tells the story of Aurora Greenway, a widow who is diagnosed with terminal cancer. The film is a moving and often humorous exploration of love, loss and the meaning of life.
- The Curious Case of Benjamin Button (2008): This film tells the story of Benjamin Button, a man who is born with the physical appearance of an old man and ages in reverse. The film is a visually stunning and thought-provoking exploration of the nature of time and mortality.
- The Theory of Everything (2014): This film tells the story of Stephen Hawking, a theoretical physicist who was diagnosed with ALS at the age of 21. The film is a moving and inspiring portrait of a man who overcame incredible odds to achieve greatness.
- One Flew Over the Cuckoo's Nest (1975). This film tells the story of Randle Patrick McMurphy, a man who is committed to a mental institution. The film is a darkly humorous satire of the mental health system and the challenges of mental illness.
- Rain Man (1988) is a drama film that tells the story of a young man who discovers that he has an autistic older brother. The film

explores the relationship between the two brothers and it won four Academy Awards, including Best Picture.

- My Left Foot (1989) is a biographical drama film that tells the story of Christy Brown, an Irish painter and writer who was born with cerebral palsy. The film was directed by Jim Sheridan and stars Daniel Day-Lewis in the lead role.
- Dallas Buyers Club (2013) is a biographical drama film that tells the story of Ron Woodroof, a man who was diagnosed with AIDS in the 1980s. The film stars Matthew McConaughey and Jared Leto in the lead roles and it was directed by Jean-Marc Vallée.
- Awakenings (1990): This film tells the story of Dr. Malcolm Sayer, a neurologist who discovers a drug that can temporarily awaken patients with encephalitis lethargica, a rare neurological disorder that causes long-term coma. The film stars Robin Williams and Robert De Niro in the lead roles and it was directed by Penny Marshall.

This list is a starting point and gives the educator and group examples that they might already be aware of. It is important to focus on the emotional responses rather than a discussion of the story. Did the student learn anything or did they feel uncomfortable and why? Asking whether the student would watch the film again can give deeper explanations than asking if they enjoyed it.

Philosophy.

Philosophy can be used by doctor help patients think about their values and to make decisions about their care. For example, a patient who is considering end-of-life care may find and understanding of the meaning of illness can help them approach their death.

It is important to explain to students that they must immerse themselves in the philosophy to be able to give useful advice. The unpinning ideas are not 'philosophy' any more than looking at art will make you a better doctor. The student must reflect on the feelings that result from reading the philosophy materials.

Following are examples of areas of philosophy that could be of interest to a doctor who wants to help a patient make sense of their life. It is important to read widely on an area of philosophy to properly understand what it has to offer. The arguments are journey that a student must travel for enlightenment.

- Stoicism: Stoicism is a philosophy that teaches that we should accept the things that we cannot control and focus on the things that we can control. This can be a helpful philosophy for patients with chronic illnesses, as it can help them to accept their illness and to focus on living a meaningful life despite their illness.

- Existentialism: Existentialism is a philosophy that teaches that we are free to create our own meaning in life. This can be a helpful philosophy for patients with terminal illnesses, as it can help them to find meaning in their lives even in the face of death.
- Buddhism: Buddhism is a philosophy that teaches that suffering is a natural part of life and that we can overcome suffering through meditation and mindfulness. This can be a helpful philosophy for patients with any type of illness, as it can help them to cope with the emotional challenges of illness and to find peace in the midst of suffering.
- Virtue ethics: This philosophy focuses on the development of good character traits, such as courage, compassion and honesty. This can be helpful for patients who are struggling to cope with the challenges of illness, as it can provide them with a framework for making decisions and behaving in a way that is consistent with their values.
- Palliative care: This philosophy focuses on providing comfort and support to patients who are facing a terminal illness. This can be helpful for patients who are struggling with the emotional and spiritual challenges of dying, as it can help them to find peace and meaning in their final days.
- Bioethics: This philosophy explores the ethical dimensions of healthcare, such as the right to life, the right to die and the use of medical technology. This can be helpful for healthcare providers who are faced with difficult ethical decisions, as it can provide them with a framework for thinking about these issues.
- Utilitarianism: This philosophy judges the morality of an action based on its consequences. This can be helpful for patients who are trying to decide whether to undergo a risky treatment, as it can help them to weigh the potential benefits and risks of the treatment.
- Kantian ethics: This philosophy judges the morality of an action based on whether it follows the categorical imperative, which is a rule that states that we should always act in a way that we would want everyone to act. This can be helpful for patients who are trying to decide whether to break the law in order to get the care they need, as it can help them to weigh the moral implications of their decision.

The best way to use philosophy in healthcare is to tailor it to the individual patient and their specific needs. Philosophy is not a one-size-fits-all approach to healthcare. By understanding the patient's values and beliefs, doctors can better support them through difficult times and help them to make informed decisions about their care.

The best way for a doctor to learn philosophy is to immerse themselves in the philosophy and to reflect on the feelings that come from reading the philosophy materials. This will help them to understand the philosophy in a deep way and to be able to apply it to their patients' care in a meaningful way.

History

Studying the history of medicine can help students and healthcare professionals understand the social, cultural and ethical forces that have shaped healthcare. By studying how different cultures and societies have understood and treated illness over time, we can gain insights into the nature of disease and the challenges of providing care.

The educator may not have read all the books on this list but choosing one to read can help the student broaden their understanding. The list is not provided as a reading list but as a choice. The best book is one that gets read and any of these books will give the student a way of looking at medicine that they have not had before.

- The Anatomy of an Epidemic: A History of the Black Death, the Plague of Athens and Modern Medicine by Johnathan Hutchinson (2014) tells the story of the Black Death, one of the most devastating pandemics in human history. Hutchinson covers a wide range of topics, from the medical aspects of the Black Death to the social and economic impact of the plague. 8/10.
- The Birth of the Clinic: An Essay in the History of Medical Perception by Michel Foucault (1975) is a classic work of medical history that explores the development of modern medical practices. Foucault argues that the rise of the clinic in the 18th century led to a new way of understanding disease, one that emphasised the patient's body as a site of medical knowledge. 7/10.
- The Doctor's Dilemma: Essays on Ethics and Medicine by Arthur Caplan (2008) is a collection of essays on ethical issues in medicine. Caplan covers a wide range of topics, from the ethics of informed consent to the ethics of physician-assisted suicide. 8/10.
- The Emperor of All Maladies: A Biography of Cancer by Siddhartha Mukherjee (2010) is a Pulitzer Prize-winning history of cancer that explores the disease from its earliest origins to the present day. Mukherjee covers a wide range of topics, from the biology of cancer to the social and cultural history of the disease. 9/10.

- The Knife Man: The Extraordinary Life And Times Of John Hunter, Father Of Modern Surgery by Wendy Moore (2005) is a biography of John Hunter, one of the most important figures in the history of surgery. Moore covers a wide range of topics, from Hunter's early life and education to his groundbreaking work on surgery and anatomy. 8/10.
- The Gene: An Intimate History by Siddhartha Mukherjee (2016) is a book about the history of genetics and its impact on medicine. Mukherjee covers a wide range of topics, from the discovery of DNA to the development of genetic testing and gene therapy. 9/10.
- The Great Influenza: The Story of the Deadliest Pandemic in History by John M. Barry (2004) tells the story of the 1918 influenza pandemic, which killed an estimated 50 million people worldwide. Barry covers a wide range of topics, from the medical aspects of the pandemic to the social and economic impact of the flu. 9/10.
- The Great Mortality: An Intimate History of the Black Death by John Kelly (2005) is a history of the Black Death, the plague that killed an estimated 30-50% of Europe's population in the 14th century. Kelly tells the story of the plague through the eyes of its victims, survivors and the medical professionals who tried to treat it. 8/10.
- The History of the Present Illness: Medicine and the Problem of Medical Knowledge by Michel Foucault (1973) is a philosophical essay that examines the relationship between medicine and power. Foucault argues that medicine is not simply a science of healing, but also a way of controlling and disciplining the body. 7/10.
- The Immortal Life of Henrietta Lacks by Rebecca Skloot (2010) tells the story of Henrietta Lacks, a black woman whose cells were used to create the HeLa cell line, one of the most important cell lines in medical research. Skloot's book explores the ethical implications of using Lacks' cells without her consent and it also tells the story of Lacks' life and her family's struggle to cope with her death. 9/10.
- Pain: The Science of Suffering by Siddhartha Mukherjee (2017) is a look at the history of pain and how we understand it today. Mukherjee covers a wide range of topics, from the physical and psychological aspects of pain to the cultural and social meaning of pain. 9/10.
- The Poisoner's Handbook: Murder and the Birth of Forensic Medicine by Deborah Blum (2006) tells the story of the development of forensic toxicology in the early 20th century and the scientists who pioneered new methods for identifying poisons. 8/10.

- The Secret Life of Germs by Wendy Orent (2007) tells the story of the discovery of germs and how they have shaped our understanding of disease. Orent's book is a well-written and accessible introduction to the science of microbiology. 7/10.
- A Short History of Medicine by Roy Porter (1997) is a comprehensive and well-written overview of the history of medicine from ancient times to the present day. Porter covers a wide range of topics, from the development of medical theories and practices to the social and cultural history of medicine. 9/10.
- In Sickness and in Health: A History of Hospitals by Lindsay Prior (1998) is a fascinating look at the history of hospitals from their origins in ancient times to the present day. Prior covers a wide range of topics, from the physical design of hospitals to the social and cultural role of hospitals in society. 8/10.
- The Story of the Human Body: From Guts to Germs, the Weird and Wonderful Science of Our Anatomy by Bill Bryson (2019) is a fascinating and accessible look at the human body and how it works. Bryson's book is full of interesting facts and anecdotes. 9/10.
- The Story of Medicine by Howard Markel (2015) is a sweeping history of medicine from ancient times to the present day. Markel's book tells the stories of some of the most important medical discoveries and the people who made them. 8/10.
- The Story of Pain: From Prayer to Painkillers by Harold Merskey (2000) is a history of pain and its treatment. Merskey's book explores the different ways that pain has been understood and treated throughout history, from ancient practices like bloodletting to modern treatments like surgery and medication. 8/10.
- Under the Knife: A History of Surgery in 28 Remarkable Operations by Arnold van de Laar (2018) is a book about the history of surgery. Van de Laar's book tells the stories of 28 of the most important operations in history, from the first trepanation to the first heart transplant. 9/10.

These books explore a wide range of subjects but there many books that deal with specific subjects that are not covered here. This type of book is less humanity and more human story so does not have the same emotionality as the other areas. The history of medicine is a better fit to those who struggle with being challenged.

Conclusions.

Medical humanities is a dynamic and evolving field that bridges the gap between the sciences and the humanities, bringing a holistic and humanistic perspective to healthcare. By incorporating the humanities, social sciences and arts into medical education and practice, medical humanities allows healthcare professionals to better understand and connect with patients as whole individuals, beyond their diseases.

The journey of exploring medical humanities can be challenging for students, as they may seek concrete answers and find the experience lacking. However, educators play a vital role in helping students recognise that the value lies in the process of inquiry and the experience of the art itself, which can provide insights and transformative experiences. Engaging with different art forms such as literature, film and visual art can help students develop critical thinking skills, foster empathy and gain diverse perspectives on the human experience.

Key concepts in medical humanities include recognising the patient as a whole person, emphasising the importance of effective communication, acknowledging the role of emotions in healthcare and exploring the ethical issues that arise in healthcare settings. These concepts shape the understanding of healthcare professionals and contribute to more compassionate and patient-centered care.

Literature, art and film offer powerful mediums through which students and healthcare professionals can engage with the human dimension of health and illness. Literature provides stories that allow readers to explore diverse experiences and gain insights into the patient's perspective. Art, including paintings and sculptures, can evoke emotions, facilitate expression and foster communication. Films, with their multimodal nature and compelling narratives, offer a unique opportunity to understand what it is like to live with various medical conditions.

Experiential learning through medical humanities encourages active participation, reflection and empathy development. It can create cognitive dissonance, challenging learners' beliefs and attitudes about illness, disability and death. By experiencing the world from the patient's perspective, healthcare professionals can provide more compassionate and effective care.

Ultimately, medical humanities enriches the practice of medicine by fostering a deeper understanding of the human experience, promoting empathy and encouraging healthcare professionals to reflect on their own biases and assumptions. By integrating the humanities into medical education and practice, we can create a more humanistic and patient-centered approach to healthcare, ultimately improving the well-being and outcomes of patients.

Top tips.

Emphasise the Journey of Understanding: Medical humanities is not about finding definitive answers but rather about asking questions and exploring the human experience. Encourage students to engage in the process of inquiry and reflection to gain insights and transformative experiences.

Engage with Literature, Art and Film: Use different art forms to connect with the human experience in a way that traditional textbooks cannot. Literature, art and films provide powerful mediums for understanding patients' experiences and gaining diverse perspectives.

Acknowledge the Role of Emotions: Emotions play a significant role in healthcare, both for patients and healthcare professionals. Understanding and responding to patients' emotions in a supportive manner are essential for providing compassionate care.

Chapter 34: USING MODELS FROM SOCIOLOGY, PSYCHOLOGY AND ANTHROPOLOGY

Models are used in many areas of science and they can give insights that go beyond their area. Sociology, Psychology and Anthropology are three areas where understanding of medicine has come from another discipline. The educator can help students see the advantages of considering these models and being open to new ideas.

The models from sociology have elements that are interesting but need development to make them more relevant. The word 'sick role' is old fashioned and no longer acceptable and the inequality model has been overtaken by the inverse care rule. The models from psychology have made substantial changes to primary care such as the biopsychosocial model and CBT.

Educators can use these examples to teach students about the importance of the patient-centered approach. Complex problems are those that have multiple causes and are difficult to solve. They can show that there are techniques for managing complex problems and complexity as problem.

Models from anthropology have raised questions about the ways that doctors organise healthcare. Educators can use the insights in these models to question whether the culture/illness narrative, cultural meanings for medical issues and the role of healers could assist doctors in their roles.

Models from sociology.

Sociology insights have not been as effective as they first seemed. Concerns have been raised about the way that some models appear to stigmatise certain behaviours. Sociology potentially could help medicine understand the link between poverty and health.

Educators can use the models as discussion points to help students understand the limitations of these models. The ideas have some truth but critical assessment indicates that there are weaknesses. There is an inherent bias in some models which should be challenged.

- The 'sick role': This model describes the social expectations of how people should behave when they are sick. According to the 'sick role', people who are sick are expected to seek help from a healthcare provider, to follow the provider's instructions and to rest and recover.

This remains a useful model of illness behaviours and reflects social beliefs about needing to rest. The model does not explain phenomenon such the perception of 'worsening'. Even where the patient has clearly improved they will insist that their condition is worse than it was the year before.

A key prediction is that if the patient was told by their healthcare provider that they should return to work they would follow these instructions. This has not been fully studied and the hypothesis remains untested. Although any effect may be small it is recognised that doctors rarely challenge their patient's assumptions.

- The social construction of illness: This theory argues that illness is not simply a biological phenomenon but is also a social construct. This means that the way we define and understand illness is influenced by our culture and society.

This concept was convincingly applied to disability as environment influences disability. The anti-psychiatrists have argued that mental illness is a normal reaction to an abnormal situation. Work on poverty had early promise but experiments such as minimum wage has had limited success. The lack of evidence to support changes to the environment on mental health has reduced support for this model.

- The inequality model: This model argues that inequality can lead to poorer health. This is because people who are poor are more likely to be exposed to environmental hazards, have less access to healthcare and live in more stressful environments.

A further criticism is that the social construction of illness is it is too simplistic and appears to deny that the biological effects are substantial. The interaction between social and biological causes is a key element that has not been addressed.

The idea of inequality has been attractive as an explanation for differing health outcomes. Inequity has largely replaced inequality as the preferred concept. There is increasing interest in discrimination as a cause of inequity.

This model has not been as successful as the social determinants of health model. It is argued that reason why disadvantaged people suffer more illness is because they are exposed to social determinants. They are ill because society is set up to make them ill and the decisions that make society inequitable are systematically biased.

Models from psychology

Psychology has given medicine some highly effective models. The biopsychosocial model and the cognitive behavioural model have been very successful. The insights have led to new treatments and approaches and significantly improved care outcomes. Educators can use the opportunity to discuss these models as they may not occur elsewhere in the curriculum.

- The biopsychosocial model: This model of health and illness takes into account the biological, psychological and social factors that influence health. It is a more holistic approach to illness than the traditional biomedical model, which focuses only on the biological factors.

The biopsychosocial model argues that illness is caused by a complex interaction of biological, psychological and social factors. This insight that disease is caused by complexity is extraordinary and challenging to doctors. The medical (biomedical) model is the dominant paradigm in medicine and states the opposite. The medical model states that illness is caused by a specific biological problem, such as a virus or bacteria, that is simplicity.

The inconsistency between these two models makes the biopsychosocial model challenging to teach. The educator needs to help the students recognise that complexity can be as amenable to treatment as simplicity. A major prediction is that patients will get better results by addressing all their needs rather than just the biological needs.

This model has become a central pillar of primary care and has transformed care by GPs. It has led to patient centred care and new approaches to health care such as psychosocial progress. Psychosocial progress is the concept of making small changes to the person's health is more effective than a single change.

This has been proven in many areas such as diabetes and blood pressure management. Multi-disciplinary teams are based around the idea that specialists need to treat more than just the body. GPs have taken this further and become experts in complexity using the model to manage multimorbidity.

- The cognitive-behavioural model: This model focuses on the role of thoughts, feelings and behaviours in health and illness. It can be used to help patients identify and change unhelpful thoughts and behaviours that may be contributing to their illness.

The CBT model has had exceptional success and now is the first line psychological treatment for many mental health problems. The concepts are used in many primary care consultations and formal CBT is provided to a large proportion of those who require psychological treatment.

The CBT model has some minor issues for instance when it is used in people with a personality disorder who cannot tolerate the emotional effects. A modified technique called DBT has been created to allow those patients to also benefit from the approach.

- The psychodynamic model: This model focuses on the unconscious mind and how it can influence our thoughts, feelings and behaviours. It can be used to understand the underlying psychological factors that may be contributing to a patient's illness.

The psychodynamic model has been successful but is operator dependent. There are some practitioners who can use it reliably but many who cannot. The training is complex and it has been difficult to codify the insights so that they can be more widely used.

- The resilience model: This model focuses on the factors that help people bounce back from adversity. It is often used to help people build resilience and cope with the challenges of illness.

The resilience model is correct that resilience is reduced by failure to attend to Maslow's needs such as food and sleep as this depletes resources. It is mistaken because that resilience cannot be increased indefinitely. The evidence shows that when a person reaches their limits the most resilient thing to do is to leave.

Models from Anthropology.

Anthropology has been a rich source of insight because of the anthropologist's long term study of societies. They spend their time listening to and watching the people they study and have a deep understanding of their culture. This leads to findings that can be missed with more superficial observations.

- The biocultural model: This model views health and illness as the result of a complex interaction between biological, environmental and cultural factors. This model has been used to understand the spread of diseases, the development of treatment strategies and the impact of culture on health outcomes.

The biocultural model is based on the idea that biology and culture are inseparable. This means that our biology is shaped by our culture and our culture is shaped by our biology. The idea that human evolution was changed by our culture, diseases and the environment is persuasive. Resistance to diseases are the likely cause of many genetic variations.

The influence of culture on illness behaviour and beliefs can be seen in HIV and cancer. Other models do not fully explain elements such as the sexual practices and use of needles that led to HIV spread. Beliefs about cancer has cultural roots that are not explained by psychosocial models.

- The illness narrative: This model views illness as a story that is told by the patient, their family and their healthcare providers. The illness narrative can help to understand the patient's experience of illness, their treatment preferences and their cultural beliefs about health and illness.

The illness narrative gives a different view of illness as it follows the patient's experiences rather than symptoms. It is often used in training in primary care as a way of getting the student to listen to the patient rather than ask questions. The narrative often raises issues that would have been missed by a medical consultation.

There are parallels between the biopsychosocial model and the illness narrative. The illness narrative however is patient centred and experiential rather than task centred. This means that the medical student may miss important clinical or social details that might assist them in their treatment. Patients may not wish to or may not have the skills to share their stories.

- The medical anthropology of the body: This subfield of anthropology explores the cultural meanings of the body, illness and health. This subfield has been used to understand the ways in which culture shapes our understanding of the body, our experiences of illness and our choices about treatment.

The cultural understanding of medical matters is of great importance to understanding responses to illness. This knowledge has not been applied widely, to the detriment of medical practice. Doctors often do not understand their patients understanding and rely instead upon standardised cultural beliefs.

The gap between patients views of their illness and the doctors' perceptions of those views can be wide. The educator can share experiences of patient's views of the illness as examples of the gap. The BMJ has a section called 'what your patient is thinking' which can provide further examples. It is important to keep up to date with the latest ideas that are circulating about health.

- The anthropology of healing: This subfield of anthropology explores the different ways in which people around the world have sought to heal themselves and others. This subfield has been used to understand the different types of healing practices, the role of culture in healing and the ethics of cross-cultural healing.

Traditional healing practices often involve the use of herbs, massage and other forms of physical manipulation. The anthropology of healing has shown that traditional healing practices can be just as effective as biomedical healing practices. The patients value the attention that they receive in traditional health practice.

The dominance of the biomedical model has led to traditional healers and their arts being sidelined. This has meant that many countries have lost much of their healthcare resources and outcomes are worsened. The difficulties in training sufficient number of primary care doctors to deliver gold standard care have left these gaps unfilled.

There is rise of complementary and alternative medicine (CAM) despite not being as effective as allopathic medicine. Traditional Chinese medicine is a system of medicine uses herbs, acupuncture and other forms of physical manipulation to treat a variety of illnesses. Ayurveda is a system of medicine from India that uses herbs, diet and lifestyle changes to treat a variety of illnesses.

Educators can use this model to question whether the current biomedical model requiring highly trained doctors is the best for global health. The need for a wide range of healthcare professionals who can work together appears to be obvious. How do poor developing countries benefit from expensively trained doctors who leave to work in richer countries?

Arguably anthropologists have the best tools to deal with intractable problems such as the health effects of poverty, pollution and mental health. Their understanding of the nature of society goes beyond the sociologist's understanding of social systems. It looks at the culture of human society and ways we choose to live.

Conclusions.

Models from sociology, psychology and anthropology have provided valuable insights into the field of medicine. While some models have faced criticisms and limitations, they have contributed to a broader understanding of healthcare and patient care. Educators can utilise these models to encourage critical thinking, challenge biases and foster interdisciplinary perspectives among students.

Sociological models, such as the "sick role," offer valuable insights into illness behaviours and social expectations. However, they need further development and should be used cautiously to avoid stigmatising certain behaviours. The social construction of illness model highlights the influence of culture and society on our understanding of health, but it requires a more nuanced consideration of biological factors. The inequality model, although overshadowed by the social determinants of health model, still holds relevance, particularly in exploring the impact of social and environmental factors on health outcomes.

Psychological models have had a significant impact particularly on primary care. The biopsychosocial model has revolutionised healthcare by emphasising the importance of biological, psychological and social factors in understanding and treating illness. It has led to patient-centered care and the integration of approaches like cognitive-behavioural therapy (CBT) and mindfulness. The cognitive-behavioural model, specifically, has become a widely used treatment approach for various mental health problems, although modifications may be needed for specific populations. The psychodynamic model has shown promise, but its application is highly dependent on the skills and training of practitioners. The resilience model highlights the importance of building resilience, but it must be recognised that resilience training has its limits.

Anthropological models have provided unique perspectives on health and illness. The biocultural model recognises the complex interaction between biology, environment and culture in shaping health outcomes. The illness narrative approach encourages a patient-centered understanding of illness experiences, but it may not capture all clinical and social details. The medical anthropology of the body reveals the cultural meanings of the body and illness, which are often overlooked in medical practice. The anthropology of healing emphasises the value of traditional healing practices and raises questions about the dominance of the biomedical model and its impact on healthcare resources.

Overall, the models from sociology, psychology and anthropology have expanded our understanding of medicine beyond the biomedical paradigm. They offer valuable insights into the social, psychological, cultural and environmental factors that influence health and illness. By incorporating these models into medical education, educators can encourage critical thinking, promote patient-centered care and explore alternative approaches to healthcare.

Top tips.

Explore boundaries: Highlight the interdisciplinary nature of healthcare by incorporating insights from sociology, psychology and anthropology into medical education. Encourage students to appreciate the role of diverse factors in shaping health outcomes.

Complexity in medicine: Use models that emphasise complexity, such as the biocultural model, to better understand diseases and health issues that have multiple causative factors.

Potential insights: Discuss where insights into intractable health problems could emerge. The effect of poverty on health is unlikely to ever be solved by a medical explanation.

Chapter 35: DISABLED DOCTORS AND REASONABLE ADJUSTMENTS.

Doctors, like the general population, can experience disabilities that range from physical to psychological impairments, including hidden functional restrictions. Unfortunately, disabled doctors working in the healthcare system often face variable support and may even encounter discrimination. A significant challenge lies in the lack of understanding of disability among other healthcare staff.

Educators have a crucial role in fostering a comprehensive understanding of disability among students. They can achieve this by providing information about different types of disabilities, the challenges faced by disabled individuals and the importance of reasonable adjustments. By helping students develop a better understanding of disability, educators contribute to creating a more inclusive and supportive environment for disabled doctors.

Reasonable adjustments refer to accommodations made to ensure that disabled individuals can participate in activities on an equal basis with non-disabled individuals. In the context of healthcare, reasonable adjustments can be implemented to enable disabled doctors to practice medicine. Examples of such adjustments include flexible working arrangements, modifications to the physical environment and the provision of assistive technology.

Disability

The terms impairment, functional restriction and disability are often used interchangeably, but they have distinct meanings. In disability the doctor's impairments are the medical conditions that cause a change to the normal functioning of their systems. Functional restrictions on the other hand are the effects that those impairments have upon the doctor's ability to do tasks. Disability arises from the combination of impairments and functional restrictions, resulting in substantial limitations in interacting with the environment.

- Impairment is a loss or abnormality of body structure or function, including mental function. It is a medical condition that can cause limitations in a person's activities. For example, a person with arthritis may have a stiff joint and pain, which would be considered an impairment.

- Functional restriction is a limitation in the ability to perform an activity in the manner or within the range considered normal for a human being. It is the impact of an impairment on a person's ability to do things. For example, a person with arthritis may have difficulty walking, which would be considered a functional restriction.
- Disability is a combination of impairments and functional restrictions that substantially limits a person's ability to interact with the environment that they are in. It is the social consequence of an impairment. For example, a hospital without lifts could make it difficult for a doctor with arthritis to get around, which would be considered a disability.
- Reasonable adjustments are changes that can be made to remove or reduce the disadvantage that a person with a disability experiences. In the case of the doctor with arthritis who works in a hospital without lifts, some reasonable adjustments could include lifts, ground floor offices, personal assistant or increased time.

Educators can engage students in classifying different problems faced by disabled doctors into these categories—impairments, functional restrictions and disabilities. They can also prompt students to consider challenges encountered by all doctors and question whether the system also disables typically functioning doctors.

For instance, the discussion can revolve around the impact of continuous 24-hour work on a doctor's performance and potential mistakes. This exercise helps students recognise the porous boundary between disability and non-disability. Furthermore, it can lead to exploring the concept of reasonableness, such as considering cost-effective alternatives to expensive adjustments like installing lifts.

Are Reasonable Adjustments reasonable?

Many of the reasonable adjustments would improve the life of all doctors and the quality of care that they could offer. Whether a disabled doctor's request for adjustments is reasonable depends on a number of factors, including:

- The nature of the doctor's disability.
- The impact of the disability on the doctor's ability to do their job.
- The cost of the adjustments.
- The size and resources of the employer.
- The impact of the adjustments on other employees.

In general, an adjustment is considered reasonable if it:

- Removes or reduces the disadvantage caused by the disability.
- Is practicable to make.
- Is affordable.
- Does not harm the health and safety of others.

What is rarely considered is whether the reasonable adjustments will have benefits for the productivity of all staff. Any request for reasonable adjustments will be seen on its own as a response to that individual's needs. In the lifts example above the doctor who cannot use the stairs is seen as the exception. In fact, all the staff suffer if having to carry equipment up and downstairs.

When it comes to mental health the concept of reasonable adjustments is even more vague. A workplace that is toxic and dysfunctional will reduce the performance of all staff who work there. The doctor with a mental health disability may be the canary in the coal mine but the problem is not limited to that individual.

Another aspect of reasonable adjustments that is not considered is the effect on productivity of a happy and inclusive workplace. Although having a pleasant work environment is considered to be a bonus it can have benefits. It is easier to attract and retain talented doctors, patients and staff are more satisfied with their care and teamwork is increased.

The educators should explain that many of the reasonable adjustments would actually save money, improve productivity and reduce sickness. Many healthcare systems cause stress and anxiety which can lead to burnout, absenteeism and even mistakes that could harm patients.

Attitudes to disability in healthcare.

Attitudes towards disability in healthcare often assume that doctors with disabilities are unfit for practice if they require reasonable adjustments. Consequently, doctors may feel compelled to continue working without requesting adjustments, fearing being seen as unfit. The burden of hidden disability in healthcare is significant due to this reluctance to speak up.

Many disabled doctors do work slower than their able-bodied colleagues. This difference is more obvious than the steps that disabled doctors take to compensate. The disabled doctor is often more effective because getting things right first time has a higher priority. They can also show greater dedication because they see working as a privilege.

Educators can share personal experiences of working with disabled doctors and highlight their extraordinary qualities. They can explain that all doctors strive to have something that makes them stand out and this drive is even stronger for doctors with disabilities. Exceptional abilities can emerge as disabled doctors compensate for their impairments, offering valuable lessons for all doctors to learn from.

Examples of disabled doctors portrayed in TV shows and podcasts include The Good Doctor, ER, House, Greys Anatomy, New Amsterdam, The Resident, Doctors. There are podcasts from doctors who have disabilities (DocsWithDisabilities Podcast). There will also be local resources for the educator as an estimated 20% of doctors have disabilities.

Educators can help their students challenge their own preconceptions of disability. They could ask the students to imagine if they developed an impairment and what they would hope their workplace would provide. How would they feel if a reasonable request for adjustments was refused?

Reasonable Adjustments

Reasonable adjustments cannot be exhaustively listed since many are specific to the workplace environment or the doctor's specific impairments. Arguably the most important is education for colleagues. Some examples of reasonable adjustments that can be made for disabled doctors include:

- Training: Training for staff on how to interact with disabled patients and colleagues.
- Training for staff on how to use assistive technology or how to communicate with disabled patients.
- Assistive technology: Providing assistive technology, such as a screen reader or voice-to-text software. Providing visual aids to help with understanding complex concepts.
- Paperwork: Making changes to the way that paperwork is completed, such as providing electronic forms, magnifier, Braille, or large print.
- Physical environment: Making changes to the physical environment, such as providing accessible ramps or widened doorways. Providing a comfortable and accessible workspace.
- Support: Providing a mentor or buddy system to help the doctor adjust to the workplace and to provide support. Providing a scribe to take notes during consultations. Job sharing or having a co-worker who can help with tasks that require a lot of concentration.

- Role changes: Allowing the doctor to take on a different role within the practice, such as a research or teaching role, if their disability prevents them from practicing medicine in a traditional setting.
- Remote work: The ability to work from home on occasion.
- Social environment: Adjustments to social environments to avoid overstimulation.
- Work schedule: Providing a flexible work schedule that allows the doctor to adjust their hours to accommodate their disability.
- Workplace culture: A supportive work environment with reduced conflict in the workplace.
- Appointments: Allowing more time for appointments to allow a slower workload.
- Breaks: The ability to take breaks during the day to relax and de-stress.
- Mental health: Access to mental health services.

The educator can ask students if they have seen reasonable adjustments and how they felt about them. Students may have felt annoyed and that the adjustments were unfair or unnecessary. They may have felt proud that their institution was going above and beyond. They may not have seen any reasonable adjustments at all and watched colleagues struggling.

Disability rights.

Disability rights are protected under the Equality Act 2010, which requires employers to make reasonable adjustments for disabled employees. This applies to employers of all sizes and sectors, including self-employed individuals and those in the public sector. If a doctor believes they require reasonable adjustments to practice medicine, they should discuss their individual needs and circumstances with their employer.

If the employer refuses to make the adjustment, the doctor may have the option to appeal the decision through an employment tribunal. Other doctors can support their disabled colleagues by providing testimonies highlighting the financial benefits of reasonable adjustments.

An example might be that an office becomes unbearably hot in the summer for 3-4 weeks per year. A doctor could support their suffering colleagues by explaining that there are 4 members of staff and their productivity falls by one third during this time. They are on £10 per hour, working 30 hours a week which is a loss of £1200 in lost productivity. An air-conditioning system that costs £2000 would pay for itself in 2 years.

This example has an important feature, the staff in the example did not have impaired heat tolerance. They were disabled by the heat and the failure to provide adequate cooling. Without the doctor's input they would have had to wait until a disabled colleague with heat intolerance started work to make the necessary change.

Conclusion.

Disabled doctors face challenges within the healthcare system, including a lack of understanding and support from their colleagues. Educators play a vital role in fostering a comprehensive understanding of disability among medical students, by providing information about different types of disabilities, the challenges faced by disabled individuals and the importance of reasonable adjustments. Reasonable adjustments refer to accommodations made to ensure that disabled doctors can practice medicine on an equal basis with their non-disabled peers.

By promoting discussions and exercises that encourage students to classify problems faced by disabled doctors into impairments, functional restrictions and disabilities, educators can help break down barriers and create a more inclusive and supportive environment. It is important to recognise that many reasonable adjustments can benefit all doctors and improve the quality of care provided.

Attitudes towards disability in healthcare need to change, as disabled doctors are often seen as unfit for practice if they require reasonable adjustments. Educators can challenge preconceptions by sharing personal experiences of working with disabled doctors and highlighting their extraordinary qualities. By emphasising the drive and dedication of disabled doctors, educators can help students recognise that exceptional abilities can emerge through compensatory strategies, offering valuable lessons for all doctors to learn from.

Reasonable adjustments can depend on the specific workplace environment and the doctor's impairments. Examples of reasonable adjustments include providing training on disability awareness, wheelchair-accessible facilities, assistive technology, changes to paperwork processes, sign language interpreters, adjustments to the physical environment and providing a supportive work environment.

Disability rights are protected under the Equality Act 2010, which requires employers to make reasonable adjustments for disabled employees. Doctors who require reasonable adjustments should discuss their needs with their employer and, if necessary, appeal decisions through employment tribunals. Support from other doctors through testimonies highlighting the financial benefits of reasonable adjustments can strengthen the case for implementation.

In conclusion, by promoting understanding, advocating for reasonable adjustments and challenging preconceptions, educators and medical professionals can create a more inclusive and supportive healthcare environment for disabled doctors. Recognising the value and unique contributions of disabled doctors benefits not only the individuals themselves but also the overall healthcare system, leading to improved care and outcomes for patients.

Top Tips.

Study disability. The social model of disability sees disability as a problem with society. The social model argues that society is not designed to accommodate people with disabilities and that this can lead to discrimination and exclusion.

Reasonable adjustments: There is a porous boundary between disability and non-disability and anyone can have problems if the environment is hostile. Reasonable adjustments should be win-win and the changes should lead to a more inclusive environment.

Advocate. The educator is in a powerful position to recognise, share insights into disability and argue for change. Where reasonable adjustments would lead to financial benefits or improved patient care a strong argument can be made for their implementation.

Chapter 36: CHALLENGES AND FUTURE DIRECTIONS IN MEDICAL EDUCATION

The future of medical education is uncertain, but it is clear that the field is undergoing a period of significant change. In order to address these challenges, medical schools will need to find new ways to deliver education that is both affordable and effective. The future of medical education is likely to be shaped by a number of factors, such as the increasing use of technology, the growing emphasis on competency-based learning and the need to personalise education to meet the needs of individual students.

As the healthcare landscape continues to evolve, medical schools will need to adapt to meet the needs of patients and the demands of the profession. Medical schools will need to be adaptable and innovative in order to meet the challenges of the future. By embracing the trends, medical schools can help to ensure that the next generation of doctors is prepared to meet the challenges of the 21st century.

Challenges to medical education

Medical education is facing a number of challenges in the 21st century. These challenges include:

- The increasing complexity of medical knowledge and practice. The amount of medical knowledge that doctors need to know is constantly growing and the practice of medicine is becoming increasingly complex. This makes it difficult for medical schools to keep up with the latest advances and it can be challenging for students to learn everything they need to know in order to be competent physicians.

- The changing demographics of the patient population. The patient population is becoming more diverse, both in terms of age and ethnicity. This means that doctors need to be prepared to care for patients from a variety of backgrounds, with a variety of needs.

- The rising cost of medical education. The cost of medical education is rising, making it more difficult for people to afford to become doctors. This can lead to a shortage of doctors, which could have a negative impact on the healthcare system.

- The need to address the mental health of medical students and doctors. The stress of medical school and the practice of medicine can take a toll on the mental health of medical students and doctors. There is a need to provide more support for the mental health of these professionals.

- The need to prepare doctors for the future of medicine. The future of medicine is uncertain, but it is clear that there will be a need for doctors who are able to think critically and solve problems. Medical schools need to prepare doctors for the future by teaching them how to think critically and solve problems.

The educator can consider whether there is a common thread in these challenges. These challenges appear soluble but there appears to be a lack of willingness to make the necessary changes. The reasons appear to be lack of awareness or data, resistance to change and failure to provide seed funding for necessary changes.

As students represent the future of the profession the educator can flip the session. Ask the students to teach the educator what they want to see in the future. Asking them about their vision of what educational priorities should be and what steps they would like to take to reach that future. The educator can help them develop teamwork skills using a problem-based learning structure.

Setting a task such as 'Which is the most pressing problem facing medical education and how would you address it?' The group should then allocate roles based upon their skills and break down the issue into smaller pieces. They can present their findings to the educator and a plan to solve it.

Ranking Of Priorities

A common ranking of priorities for improvement in medical education is the cost of education, lack of diversity and then modernisation of the curriculum and mental health of students. After this comes improved training on public health, social determinants and primary care. Few students consider improved management and political training is a priority.

1. Cost of education. The cost of medical school is a major barrier for many students and it is only getting worse. The cost of medical school now includes tuition fees, living expenses and these are increasing. There is a lack of financial aid available for medical school and the aid that is available is often not enough to cover the full cost of tuition and living expenses.

2. Lack of diversity. The medical profession is still not as diverse as it should be. Medical schools are recruiting more students from underrepresented groups but the retention of these students is

higher. There are a number of factors that may contribute to the lack of diversity in the medical profession, including implicit bias and lack of a supportive environment for all students.

3. Modernisation of the curriculum. The medical curriculum is in need of an update. It needs to be more focused on the needs of patients in the 21st century and it needs to better prepare students for the challenges of practicing medicine in a changing healthcare environment. The curriculum is too full which prevents educators from developing training in these areas.

4. Mental health of students. The mental health of medical students is a serious concern. Many students experience stress, anxiety and depression during their training. Medical schools need to do more to provide support for students' mental health and reduce stigma. The demands of medical school can be overwhelming and students often feel isolated and unsupported.

5. Improved training on public health, social determinants and primary care. Medical students need to be better prepared to address the social determinants of health. They also need to be more familiar with the principles of public health and primary care. Public health is the science of protecting and improving the health of populations. Primary care is the first point of contact for patients with health problems. Students need the skills in these areas to be able to tackle the problems they will face in practice.

6. Improved management and political training. Medical students need to be better prepared to manage their careers and to advocate for change in the healthcare system. They need to be taught how to navigate the complex healthcare bureaucracy and how to influence policy decisions. Without the relevant training most students will avoid getting involved in important decisions.

The educator can summarise these priorities as a need for further training and increased skills. Understanding diversity can remove many of the barriers to retaining underrepresented groups, modernisation of the curriculum means tackling poorly addressed subjects. Learning about mental health and public health, management and politics and primary care can address the other priorities.

The responsibility for educational needs rests firmly with the educators themselves. They should be developing teaching materials so that students who are interested can self-study. They should be advocating for these areas to have their place in the curriculum. Identify where these ideas can be included within the curriculum by working with colleagues.

Future directions

Medical education will need to be adapted to align better with healthcare needs and incorporate new technologies. The way that education is delivered will need to adjust to the needs of an increasingly diverse workforce. Education has been struggling to properly equip new doctors with the required skills and many young doctors complain that they are unprepared for their roles.

Old ideas about doctors needing to be able to cope with extraordinary stress are being challenged. It is being recognised that diversity in medicine gives better results for patients from marginalised groups. By having a greater range of skills available in the healthcare workforce solutions can be found to apparently intractable problems.

The educator should discuss the students' ideas of what the future will or should hold for healthcare. These ideas will help the educator recognise further examples and understand the importance of these developments to the students.

- Incorporating new technologies into medical education. Technology is rapidly changing the way that healthcare is delivered and medical education needs to keep pace. Virtual reality, simulation and other technologies such as LLMs can be used to provide students with immersive learning experiences that prepare them for the realities of clinical practice.

- Competency-based approach to education. Traditional medical education is based on a content-based curriculum, which means that students are required to learn a certain amount of information in order to pass exams. However, this approach does not necessarily ensure that students are able to apply their knowledge in real-world settings. A competency-based approach, on the other hand, focuses on developing the skills and knowledge that students need to be competent practitioners.

- Interprofessional education is essential for preparing doctors to work effectively in today's healthcare environment. Patients are often seen by a team of different healthcare professionals and it is important for doctors to be able to communicate and collaborate effectively with these other professionals. Interprofessional education can help students to develop the skills and knowledge they need to work effectively in this type of environment.

- Lifelong learning is also essential for medical professionals, as the pace of change in healthcare is so rapid. New treatments and technologies are constantly being developed and doctors need to be able to keep up with these changes to provide the best possible care for their patients. Lifelong learning can help doctors to stay up-to-date on the latest medical knowledge and skills.

- Addressing social determinants of health. The social determinants of health are the factors that influence a person's health, such as their socioeconomic status, access to healthcare and living conditions. Medical education needs to do a better job of addressing these factors in order to produce doctors who are equipped to address the needs of their patients.

- Diversity and inclusion. Medical education is still aligned to the needs of white and male learners but new doctors are increasingly diverse. The dropout rate is increasing and medical education needs to do more to promote diversity and inclusion. This includes creating a more inclusive learning environment adapted for all students.

- Adapting to the changing healthcare landscape. The healthcare landscape is changing rapidly, with the rise of telemedicine, value-based care and other new models of care. Medical education needs to teach skills to prepare doctors for these changes so that they can be successful in the future.

- Mental health support. The mental health of medical students and doctors is a growing concern. Medical education can play a role in addressing this issue by providing students with mental health support and teaching them how to manage stress.

- Affordable education. The cost of medical education is a barrier for many students. Medical education can become more affordable by using innovative approaches and decreasing the spending in secondary care. Increased use of distance learning could disrupt the high cost model of medical education.

These areas have potential to change the way that medical education is delivered. The effects of LLMs are likely to dramatic and may give the possibility of making a real difference to the curriculum. Educators need to be actively developing educational materials in each of these areas to support future changes.

Conclusions.

The challenges faced by medical education in the 21st century are significant and multifaceted. These challenges include the increasing complexity of medical knowledge and practice, the changing demographics of the patient population, the rising cost of education, the need to address the mental health of students and doctors and the imperative to prepare doctors for the future of medicine.

To address these challenges, medical schools need to be adaptable, innovative and proactive. Incorporating new technologies into medical education, adopting a competency-based approach, promoting interprofessional education and fostering lifelong learning are key strategies for preparing future doctors. Furthermore, addressing social determinants of health, promoting diversity and inclusion, adapting to the changing healthcare landscape and providing mental health support are crucial considerations for medical education.

Educators play a vital role in shaping the future of medical education. They should engage with students to understand their visions and priorities for the future and foster a problem-based learning environment where students can actively contribute to educational improvements. Prioritising affordable education, advocating for necessary changes and developing teaching materials in collaboration with colleagues are important steps toward enhancing medical education.

The future of medical education holds great potential for positive transformation. By embracing the challenges and opportunities presented by new technologies, diverse workforce needs and evolving healthcare systems, medical education can produce competent, compassionate and well-prepared doctors who can effectively meet the healthcare needs of the 21st century.

Top tips.

Manage change: The world of education is currently being disrupted and educators need to be leading this change by removing resistance. These changes are likely to as great than in the next decade than the previous 1000 years.

Understand LLMs: Large language models LLMs are a complex and powerful new educational tool. They disrupt the current models of education by providing an AI solution for many assessments. Equally they can create a 2-sigma improvement in performance.

Improve medical education: There have been many pressures on medical education to improve in areas such as diversity, social aspects and medical competence. The current disruption is an opportunity to make some overdue changes to the curriculum.

Chapter 37: MEDICAL LAW

Medical law is the branch of law that deals with the legal aspects of the medical profession and the rights of patients. Medical law is highly complex and difficult to follow even for experts so the educator should focus on low hanging fruit. Filling forms is commonly performed badly but is necessary part of almost all doctors' professional lives.

Students can be encouraged to read the large amount of information that is available from the GMC. They can asked how confident they feel about the following areas and how relevant they feel the areas are to their practice. Typically consent and confidentiality are low on confidence and high on importance.

- Consent: The patient's right to consent to or refuse medical treatment. This is a fundamental right that is protected by law. Patients have the right to be informed about their treatment options and to make their own decisions about their care.

- Confidentiality: The doctor's duty to keep patient information confidential. This is another important right that is protected by law. Doctors have a duty to keep patient information confidential, except in certain limited circumstances.

- Negligence: The liability of doctors for their mistakes. Doctors are responsible for their actions and they can be held liable for negligence if they make a mistake that causes harm to a patient.

- End-of-life care: The legal issues surrounding death and dying. This is a complex and sensitive area of law and there are many different legal issues that can arise at the end of life.

- Genetics: The legal implications of genetic testing and research. Genetic testing and research can raise a number of legal issues, such as privacy, discrimination and informed consent.

- Healthcare regulation: The laws that govern the healthcare industry. The healthcare industry is heavily regulated and there are many different laws that govern the way that healthcare is delivered and the behaviour of doctors.

- Reproductive rights: The legal rights of patients to make decisions about their own reproductive health. This includes the right to abortion, contraception and assisted reproduction.

- Biomedical research: Biomedical research raises a number of legal issues, such as the use of human subjects, the protection of intellectual property and the regulation of new drugs and devices.

It is unlikely that students will be able to absorb more than a small fraction of this information. It is therefore important to get the students to look up the information so that they know how to access it quickly. The educator can then focus on those areas that are of more direct interest to the students.

Sources of law:

Use online legal material. There are many online legal databases that provide access to case law, legislation and other legal materials. Some of the most popular online legal resources include BAILLI and Legislation.gov.uk.

Read legal blogs and articles. There are many legal blogs and articles that discuss current legal issues. These can be a great way to stay up-to-date on the law and learn about new developments. Additionally, many legal blogs and articles provide links to relevant legal materials.

Practice legal research. The best way to learn how to locate relevant laws is to practice. Try searching for laws on a specific topic such as IVF. As you practice, you will become more familiar with the different types of legal materials and how to find them.

GMC guidance. Good Medical Practice is a summary of the key guidance for medical practice. There are also specific guidance on topics such as consent and confidentiality which expands on GMP.

Government guidance. Departments may also issue guidance to doctors such as the DWP on sickness certification and the Office for National statistic/passport office on death certificates.

Filling in legal forms.

An area of medical law which a doctor needs to have detailed knowledge is filling in legal forms. They need to understand the forms and their responsibilities to make reasonable check as well as any legal duties. Prescriptions and x-ray forms are two other legal forms that are commonly completed incorrectly.

- Death certification: Doctors are responsible for certifying the deaths of their patients. This involves completing a death certificate, which is a legal document that states the cause of death. Doctors need to be familiar with the legal requirements for death certification, as well as the different types of death certificates that are available.

- Assessment of capacity: Doctors may be called upon to assess the capacity of their patients to make decisions about their own care. This involves assessing the patient's ability to understand and retain information, to weigh up options and to make a decision that is in their best interests. Doctors need to be familiar with the legal test for capacity, as well as the different factors that can affect a patient's capacity.

- Fitness to work: Doctors may be asked to assess the fitness to work of their patients. This involves assessing the patient's physical and mental health, as well as their ability to perform their job duties. Doctors need to be familiar with the legal requirements for fitness to work assessments, as well as the different factors that can affect a patient's fitness to work.

- Consent: Doctors must obtain formal consent from patients before providing invasive treatment. This can be a complex process, as there are different types of consent and the requirements for consent can vary depending on the circumstances.

- Sectioning under the Mental Health Act: In some cases, doctors may need to section patients under the Mental Health Act. This is a legal process that allows doctors to detain patients who are a danger to themselves or others. Doctors need to be familiar with the requirements for sectioning under the Mental Health Act, as well as the different types of sections that are available.

There are other forms such as Abortion Act for termination of pregnancy, the GMC appraisal documentation and revalidation, consent forms for research and DNAR forms that a doctor may complete depending upon their roles. Other documents that they will need to understand are Lasting Power of Attorney and Advanced Medical Directive.

- DNAR Forms: These forms are used to document a patient's decision to refuse cardiopulmonary resuscitation (CPR) in the event of a cardiac arrest.

- Lasting Power of Attorney: This document allows a person to appoint someone else to make decisions on their behalf if they lose capacity in the future.

- Advanced Medical Directive: This document allows a person to specify their wishes for future medical treatment in the event that they lose capacity.

Completing the forms incorrectly can open the doctor to disciplinary action. There is increasing movement to improve doctors' performance in these areas such as the medical referee for death certification. The educator may wish to take the opportunity to test the students' knowledge on the more common of these forms. Students often have gaps in their knowledge of sick notes and prescriptions.

Coronial courts.

Coronial courts are responsible for investigating deaths that are sudden, unexpected, or violent. They can make a number of findings, including neglect, unlawful killing, death by misadventure, suicide and open verdict. These decisions can impact the doctor in specific circumstances as in the examples below.

- Neglect: This finding is made when a doctor fails to provide adequate care to a patient, resulting in their death. The failure must be gross and even basic level of care must be omitted.

- Unlawful killing: This finding is made when a doctor's actions are considered to be criminal, resulting in the death of a patient. Examples include gross negligence or reckless manslaughter.

- Death by misadventure: This finding is made when a patient's death is accidental but could have been prevented by the doctor's actions.

- Suicide: This finding is made when a patient's death is self-inflicted but the coroner can add comments about the doctor's actions.

- Open verdict: This finding is made when the coroner is unable to determine the cause of death but there may be adverse comments made about the doctor.

- Industrial disease. A doctor who is responsible for occupational health may be implicated in this death.

- RTC. The doctor may have failed to inform the DVLA that the patient was unfit to drive a car.

- Stillbirth. The doctor may have given a drug that caused premature labour or that was toxic to the foetus.

- Alcohol or drugs. The doctor may not have provided all the available treatments for instance due to long waiting lists.

- Natural causes. Although any negligence could make a natural cause such as infection an unnatural death a delay insufficient to change the course of the disease could be criticised.

- Narrative verdicts. This is a conclusion setting out the facts surrounding the death in more detail and explaining the reasons for the decision. These can discuss the actions of several people including doctors.

Whilst the coroner is not permitted to blame an individual practitioner for the death, they can make damning findings. A finding of neglect is more serious than clinical negligence and should be avoided. The coronial law is archaic, the decisions can appear random and they are not published.

These difficulties make it difficult to teach the subject and the educator may prefer instead to consider the process. 'Who died, when and where did they die and how did they come by their death and then come to a conclusion about their death'. The question 'how did they come by their death' is phrased awkwardly for a reason.

Coroners cannot determine guilt or innocence so can only investigate the medical cause. They will rely upon the postmortem so if it finds a death by natural causes then many inquests will be ended. There are section 2 inquests which take a broader view but coroners are usually limited to understanding the mechanism of death.

Where a series of errors contributed to the death the coroner will only consider those errors that had causative potential. If the deceased would have died anyway or if the error did not cause the death they will not further investigate these errors. This is frustrating to families who may believe that there has been a cover up.

Educators can use the question 'how did they come by their death' to discuss how to complete a death certificate. The death certificate must be completed in a way that explains how the person came to die. This means that the logical steps must be included for instance as in this fictious death certificate in a murder.

1a. Exsanguination.

1b. Knife wound to the heart.

2. Multiple stab wounds with blood loss.

The death certificate would not include the delay of 40 minutes of the ambulance, the difficulties siting a venous line and his previous anaemia. The death certificate would not mention that the exsanguination caused no output or that the cardiac massage caused several ribs to fracture.

These events did not cause the patient's death or contribute significantly to it and should not be included. If the patient recovered circulation and had a further collapse due to incompatible blood the cause of death might change or this event might need to be included in section 2 as it is likely to have contributed to the death.

Educators can help the students understand how coroners come to their conclusions and develop their own death certificate skills. The tasks must be engaging and the students must have plenty of time to discuss their ideas. Medical law is complex and often counter intuitive making retaining information more challenging.

Fit note law.

The following are quotes from the DWP and statute.

Getting the most out of the fit note guidance DWP.

> *Your assessment about whether your patient is fit for work is about their fitness for work in general and is not job-specific. Your liability for the advice you provide goes no further than your responsibility to carry out a suitable clinical assessment of your patient's health condition.*

> *Your patient's employer is responsible for undertaking a suitable risk assessment to accommodate your clinical judgment. Your assessment should still be based on your clinical judgement about the functional effects of your patient's health condition and you should issue a fit note only if your patient has a health condition which impacts on their general fitness for work.*

> *My patient has a personal or social problem and is asking for a fit note (for example caring for relatives). What should I do? You can issue fit notes only to cover your patient's own health condition.*

The Social Security (Medical Evidence) and Statutory Sick Pay (Medical Evidence) (Amendment) Regulations 2010

> *4. A doctor's statement must be based on an assessment made by that doctor.*

> *6. Subject to rule 8, the condition in respect of which the doctor is advising the patient is not fit for work or, as the case may be, which has caused the patient's absence from work shall be specified as precisely as the doctor's knowledge of the patient's condition at the time of the assessment permits.*

> *7. Where a doctor considers that a patient may be fit for work the doctor shall state the reasons for that advice and where this is considered appropriate, the arrangements which the patient might make, with their employer's agreement, to return to work.*

> *8. The condition may be specified less precisely where, in the doctor's opinion, disclosure of the precise condition would be*

*prejudicial to the patient's well-being, or to the patient's position
with their employer.*

The words used in both the DWP advice and the statute law are vague and
may cause confusion. The educator should discuss what the students
consider are the meanings and then discuss whether they agree with those
below. The importance of complying with the law can also be discussed.

- Suitable clinical assessment: A medical assessment that is
  appropriate for the patient's condition. This assessment should
  consider the patient's physical and mental health, as well as their
  ability to work. Would a telephone call be sufficient?

- All work test: A test that assesses the patient's ability to perform any
  work-related duties. This means that a person who is fit for light or
  amended duties should be told that they are fit for work and asked
  to speak to their employer.

- Risk assessment: The risk assessment is the responsibility of the
  employer not the doctor. The doctor can specify amended duties but
  the employer is responsible for determining if that can be
  accommodated in the workplace. In effect this means that doctor
  can say someone is fit and the employer can sign them off.

- Functional effects: The doctor must record the physical and mental
  effects of the patient's condition on their ability to work. This
  includes the impact of the condition on the patient's ability to
  perform their work duties, as well as their ability to cope with the
  demands of the job. It is not sufficient to just state a diagnosis the
  doctor must consider whether that diagnosis impacts on any work-
  related activities such as mobility, lifting etc.

- Specified as precisely: This reinforces that the doctor is obliged to
  provide all details they have as to the person's inability to work.
  This could include inconsistencies that the doctor has seen.

- Arrangements to return to work: The sick note should include
  phased return to work, altered hours, amended duties or it may
  include recommendations for adaptations to the workplace.

Students need to consider what effect failure to follow the legal guidelines
might have on their patients. Delayed return to work has health as well as
financial implications. The failure to request appropriate adaptations may
lead to further sickness and loss of employment.

Failing to make a suitable clinical assessment may lead to the doctor missing
a treatable problem. A patient off work for another reason may develop
mental health problems which deteriorates and prevents return to work.

Failing to specifically address functional restrictions may result in the employer breaching their duties under the Equality Act.

Conclusions.

Medical law encompasses a wide range of legal aspects that are crucial for healthcare professionals to understand. The complexity of medical law can pose challenges for educators and students alike. Therefore, it is important to prioritise the essential areas and encourage students to familiarise themselves with the available information from reputable sources such as the General Medical Council (GMC).

Some key areas of medical law that should be emphasised include consent, confidentiality, negligence, end-of-life care, genetics, healthcare regulation, reproductive rights and biomedical research. These topics address rights of patients, legal responsibilities of doctors and the regulations that govern the healthcare industry.

Filling in legal forms correctly is a vital skill for doctors, as errors in documentation can have serious consequences and may lead to disciplinary action. Forms such as death certification, assessment of capacity, fitness to work assessments, consent forms, sectioning under the Mental Health Act and various other documents require careful attention and understanding.

Coronial courts play a significant role in investigating sudden, unexpected, or violent deaths. While they cannot assign guilt or innocence, they can make findings such as neglect, unlawful killing, death by misadventure, suicide, open verdicts and narrative verdicts. Understanding the process and purpose of coronial courts can help doctors navigate these situations and improve their skills in completing death certificates accurately.

Fit note law, as outlined by the Department for Work and Pensions (DWP) and statutory regulations, guides doctors in assessing their patients' fitness for work. It is important for doctors to conduct suitable clinical assessments, specify the patient's condition precisely, consider functional effects on work ability and provide recommendations for a safe return to work. Compliance with the law in issuing fit notes can have a significant impact on patients' well-being, their employment status and the overall effectiveness of healthcare.

Overall, medical law is a complex and nuanced field that requires continuous learning and adaptation. Educators should aim to engage students in discussions and practical exercises to enhance their understanding of medical law concepts and their application in real-world scenarios. By focusing on essential areas, promoting access to relevant information and fostering critical thinking, educators can help prepare healthcare professionals to navigate the legal landscape effectively and provide high-quality care while minimising legal risks.

Top tips.

Prioritise Essential Areas: Emphasise key aspects of medical law, such as consent, confidentiality, negligence, end-of-life care and reproductive to provide a foundational understanding.

Legal forms: Completing legal forms provides examples of the law for students to consider and develop practical skills in following legal guidelines.

Sources of law: Train students to access legal materials online to develop the skills in locating relevant laws. Many are accessible through Google but can be difficult to understand.

Chapter 38: POLITICAL ISSUES IN MEDICAL EDUCATION

Teaching about politics is challenging and teaching about political issues in medical education is arguably impossible. Students can only engage if they have - an interest in educational issues, an interest in political processes and an understanding of what can be done. For even the most talented educators helping students gain these interests is not possible.

Some educators would argue that the issues are important to students because they should help future students. They have a responsibility to pass on all that has been done for them to future students. Sitting on committees or becoming leaders is a way of achieving this. An alternative approach is to ask the students to classify the important to them, the health service, the public and the government of the following areas.

Political issues in medical education can be broadly categorised into four areas:

- Standards. The standards of medical education are influenced by political factors that change the structure, content and delivery of medical education. This includes factors such as whether government funding is sufficient, who is responsible for accreditation standards and the influence of professional medical associations.

- Ideology. The ideology of medical education refers to the ways in which political ideology and debate shape the way that medicine is taught and practiced. This includes issues such as public health and the effects of reforms in healthcare systems.

- Funding. Politics can determine the funding for medical education and thus the number of medical school and training places and even the length of the course. Political issues in this area include the amount of government funding for medical education, the role of medical bodies and public pressure.

- Curriculum. Issues related to the content and delivery of medical education. Political issues are what to include in the curriculum, the use of technology such as generative AI and what to leave out of medical training.

I asked BARD who suggested that there were all of high importance to all parties apart from Ideology. This approach allows the students to engage with the materials without having to be interested in the subject. The next topic is equally dull as medical leaders often have a poor reputation.

Area	Importance to medical students in training	Importance to the NHS	Importance to the public	Importance to the government
Standards	8	7	6	7
Ideology	6	5	4	5
Funding	10	9	8	9
Curriculum	9	8	7	8

The question to engage the students is what should medical education leaders do?

Medical Education Leaders.

Medical education leaders are a diverse group of doctors, nurses, administrators and other healthcare professionals who play a key role in shaping the future of medicine. They are found in positions of authority in a wide variety of bodies. They can be leading unions, hospitals, royal colleges, educational institutions, regulatory bodies and government agencies.

Medical education leaders are essential to ensuring that medical education meets the needs of patients and the public. They are also responsible for shaping the future of medicine by identifying and addressing emerging education challenges. They set out education strategies, develop training, advocate for education, promote education innovation and equity for students.

Political change is slow, so the impact of leaders' work may not be immediately apparent. People often only notice the problems, not the successes. Expectations of what doctors should learn have exceeded any reasonable expectations. The students should be able to identify the following areas.

- Expert advice for the medical curriculum. Medical education leaders can help policymakers understand the current and future needs in the healthcare system, such as the need for more primary care providers or specialists in certain areas. They can also provide information on the cost of medical education and the impact of different policies on the supply of doctors.

- Help to build consensus among stakeholders. Medical education leaders can help to bring together different stakeholders in the healthcare system, such as medical schools, hospitals and government agencies, to discuss and agree on the best way to improve medical education. This can be particularly important in countries with a decentralised healthcare system, where there are many different stakeholders with different interests.

- Advocate for improvements to medical education. Medical leaders can advocate for policies that support high-quality medical education, such as policies that increase funding for medical schools, make medical education more affordable, or improve the quality of clinical training. They can also work to raise awareness of the importance of medical education and the need for political support.

Medical education leaders in the UK have been effective at providing expert advice to developing the curriculum, building consensus on improving medical education and advocating for improving education. They have a strong track record of working with policymakers, medical schools and other stakeholders to ensure that medical education is meeting the needs of the healthcare system.

The educator can ask what areas of medical education are problematic and need action. Here the students should be able to engage with the task without difficulty. Using a brainstorm approach can increase the energy and finish the session leaving the students with interesting thoughts about what a better education system would look like.

Political Medical Education Issues.

There are many areas where there are questions as to whether medical education is meeting the needs of the students. These examples may not be universally accepted and it is worth ensuring that each student is listened to. The debates in each area are interesting but should be considered by the students when reading these notes after the session rather than in group.

- The cost of medical education. The cost of medical education has been rising steadily in recent years, making it increasingly difficult for students to afford to attend medical school. This has led to calls for increased government funding for medical education, as well as for changes to the way that medical schools are financed.

- The role of government regulation in medical education. Some argue that government regulation is necessary to ensure that medical education is effective, while others argue that it is heavy handed and does not address real problems that exist such as gaps in knowledge.

- The content of the medical school curriculum. There is a debate whether the curriculum should include more basic knowledge or more clinical experience. Some doctors feel that both are insufficient for the role of the modern doctor.

- The use of technology in medical education. There is a debate about the use of technology in medical education. Some argue that technology such as generative AI can be used to transform the quality of medical education, while others argue that it can have adverse effects such as increasing plagiarism.

- Climate change. Medical students understand that climate change will alter the patterns of disease and increase the risk of heat stress diseases. They also have personal concerns about the way that healthcare contributes to pollution and carbon emissions. Some will be concerned that they have not been prepared for the economic instability that may come from increasing migration.

- The role of diversity and inclusion in medical education. It is agreed that medical schools should be more diverse. There are concerns that many aspects of medical education can make it difficult for those with disabilities or different cultures to fit in and obstruct the progress of many talented students.

- The role of social factors in medical education. There is a growing recognition that social factors such as poverty, housing and education all play a significant role in health. The solutions to many of these factors are political rather than medical. This in turn has led to medical school under pressure to provide more education on both social and political aspects of social change.

These are just some of the political issues that have been debated in medical education. As the healthcare landscape continues to evolve, it is likely that new political issues will emerge. The decisions in these areas are made by the people in power but they need expertise to make the right decisions.

Problems with politics

Some students may find these discussions to be too negative or depressing. It is important to balance the discussion of problems with a focus on solutions. Some students may find this topic to be too abstract or theoretical. It is important to make sure that the discussion is relevant to the students' own experiences.

This discussion can be controversial. It is important to be respectful of all viewpoints. These sessions can be chaotic and unproductive. It is important to have a clear structure and to facilitate the discussion effectively. These sessions can be frustrating if there are no easy solutions. It is important to emphasise the importance of incremental progress. Can be controversial, depending on the topics that are discussed.

- Can lead to heated debates, which may not be productive.
- Can be overwhelming for students, as they may feel that they are not able to make a difference.
- Can be seen as too idealistic, as students may not believe that they can make a difference in the system.
- Can be seen as too political, as students may not want to get involved in the debate about medical education reform.
- Can be unrealistic, as students may not have the power to implement the solutions that they propose.
- Can be overwhelming for students, as they may feel that they are not able to make a difference.

Discussion of problematic areas can also be controversial and it is important to be sensitive to the different perspectives of students. It is also important to make sure that the discussion is constructive and that it does not devolve into a debate. Discussing the role of medical education leaders can be somewhat abstract and it may not be as engaging for students as discussing more concrete topics.

It is also important to make sure that the discussion does not become too focused on the personalities of individual leaders. Brainstorming sessions can be time-consuming and it is important to make sure that the discussion is productive. It is also important to be realistic about the challenges of implementing change and to avoid setting unrealistic expectations.

Small steps to political solutions.

Politics is not an esoteric concept, it is part of any discussion between doctors about the systems. A few doctors will want to take things further and get involved with activism. Others will want to write about their insights and attempt to influence others.

It is not possible to perform professional duties without trying to understand the issues and discussing them with others. The educator needs to explain to the student that they are only expected to have a view on the issues. They do not need to spend hours discussing them with everyone.

There will be times when it is right for them to share their views. They have a professional duty to engage when asked to do so. Students should understand that their contribution is vital to the proper development of medical education. As a profession we are collectively responsible for the outcomes.

There is a fallacy that medical education leaders should be solely responsible for finding solutions and making decisions. The truth is that 100 doctors have ideas that are far cleverer than any individual leader. The fallacy is that a leader can be effective without listening to others.

- Understand the issues. This involves gathering information about the problem, its causes and its potential solutions. It is important to be as objective as possible in this step and to avoid letting personal biases cloud your judgment.
- Discuss. Once you have a good understanding of the issues, you need to communicate your findings to others. This can be done through writing, speaking, or other forms of communication. The goal is to raise awareness of the problem and to build support for potential solutions.
- List potential solutions. Once you have communicated the understanding, you need to start brainstorming potential solutions. This is where your creativity can come in handy. There is no one-size-fits-all solution to political problems, so it is important to come up with a variety of options.
- Question medical leaders. Doctors often have a chance to meet and question medical leaders. This is important because leaders have the expertise to assess the feasibility and effectiveness of your solutions. Their feedback can help you to refine your solutions and to make them more likely to succeed.
- Mediate: Many political issues can become polarised. Listening to both sides can help identify areas of common interest and potential solutions that meet both side's demands.
- Writing: The written word can be powerful as it reaches a wider audience, the wording is careful and the ideas are easier to understand. However it does put the writer into the public notice and can lead to attacks and criticism.

- Political relationships: Many doctors who are concerned about issues will not want to take direct action. They can however help advise and support leaders. They can listen to others and feedback the concerns raised to the leader.
- Activism: Direct action through campaigning, protests, public debate and political involvement such as getting elected is only appropriate for a small number of doctors. Although joining a union and taking strike action is a form of political activism many doctors are reluctant even to take these steps.

The educator can ask where on this list the student feels comfortable. The student can defend their position by saying 'I am happy to discuss the problem but I do not have solutions to offer'. They can say 'I am happy to listen to both sides but do not want to have political relationships'.

Understanding the hierarchy of political action can help create boundaries. A doctor may want to find solutions but leave it to others to implement them. They can decline positions of power and instead provide advice to others who have power. They may prefer to provide their insights in writing rather than orally.

Conclusions.

Political issues in medical education are complex and multifaceted. They encompass a wide range of areas, including standards, ideology, funding and curriculum. These issues significantly influence the structure, content and delivery of medical education, ultimately shaping the future of medicine. While teaching about political issues in medical education can be challenging, it is crucial for educators to engage students in understanding these topics and their importance.

Medical education leaders play a vital role in addressing political issues and shaping medical education to meet the needs of patients and the public. They provide expert advice, help build consensus among stakeholders and advocate for improvements in medical education. Their work may not always be immediately apparent, but their efforts contribute to the development of high-quality medical education and the overall healthcare system.

There are several problematic areas in medical education that require attention. These include the rising cost of medical education, the role of government regulation, the content of the curriculum, the use of technology, the impact of climate change, the importance of diversity and inclusion and the recognition of social factors in healthcare. The aim of the teaching is give the message political issues are important medical education keeps pace with the evolving healthcare landscape.

In conclusion, political issues in medical education are vital to consider and address. It is crucial for medical educators, leaders and policymakers to collaborate and make informed decisions that enhance the quality and relevance of medical education. By doing so, we can strive towards a better education system that equips future healthcare professionals with the necessary knowledge, skills and understanding to meet the healthcare challenges of the future.

Top tips.

Problematic Areas: Discussion of problematic areas in medical education, including rising costs, government regulation, curriculum content and technology use can increase engagement. Other students will prefer to discuss climate change, diversity and inclusion and recognition of social factors in healthcare.

Personal Boundaries: Politics can be polarising and disempowering. Helping students identify their comfort boundaries with political issues can prevent them from being overwhelmed. Paradoxically it can also increase engagement as they feel safer when discussing the issues.

Solutions: Engage students in brainstorming sessions and discussions about potential solutions to the identified issues in medical education. Encourage students to think critically about what small steps they would like to take. Highlight the importance of collaboration with leaders to achieve improvements.

Chapter 39: CONTINUING MEDICAL EDUCATION (CME)

Teaching how to organise Continuing Medical Education is based on identifying key skills. These skills include how to identify learning needs, areas of interest and emerging issues. All doctors have gaps in their knowledge and skills but may develop a blind spot. Finding areas of interest gives the learner a greater feeling of control.

Emerging areas of interest are a more difficult sell to learners. The area may not develop and the learner may feel that their learning was wasted. They may prefer to wait until their patients raise the issue and then look into the area. Explaining that being aware of the areas does not take much time and makes them appear up to date may reduce their objections.

Educators can find teaching about learning styles meets resistance to engagement. Medics have their own ways of learning and object to being taught new methods. Some will be, perhaps reasonably, angry that they were not given teaching about how to learn previously in the course. Resistance can be reduced by acknowledging the learner's feelings.

Analysing which activities will give the maximum benefit can be very personal to students. They will often base their opinions on their own preferences, fears and learning styles. Asking a group to provide pros and cons of each activity for that learning area can help overcome this resistance.

How to plan CME.

Educators can start with a simple task, to use the following steps to plan learning for one goal. The students can be instructed to choose a goal in a particular area or to create an imaginary goal. The task to follow each of the steps and produce a plan of action.

1. Start by identifying your learning goals. What do you want to learn from your CME activities? Do you want to stay up-to-date on the latest medical knowledge? Do you want to develop new skills? Do you want to learn about a new area of medicine? Once you know what you want to learn, you can start to look for CME activities that will help you achieve your goals.
2. Consider your learning style. Some people learn best by reading, while others learn best by watching videos or attending live events. There are many different types of CME activities

available and choosing an activity that feels comfortable improves learning.

3. Choose a variety of activities. There are many different types of CME activities available, so don't limit yourself to one type. Consider attending conferences, taking online courses, or reading medical journals if they will give better results.

4. Get feedback. After you complete a CME activity, take some time to reflect on what you learned. Did the activity meet your goals? Did you find it helpful? This feedback will help you make better decisions about your future CME.

It should be possible for every student to produce 4 phrases to represent their thinking for each step. For example, based upon the above steps, 1. learn a language, 2. Speaking to people. 3. Online conversation. 4. Can you get it for free? Asking the students to work in pairs can help with the final task. The step that the students find hardest should be the learning goal.

It can be helpful to ask different students to share their plans and their solutions to the problem. The educator should focus on students who appear to be struggling at this stage. Using an imaginary goal can help students who have learned helplessness. They are afraid that engaging with the exercise will lead to more work.

Educators should be aware of their own feelings as they may recognise that a student has learning needs that they were not aware of. This can cause a feeling of dissonance and guilt that they have not recognised this earlier. The correct response is to read about learning styles and reflect about their previous experiences with students.

Learning styles.

Learning is most enjoyable when it matches the brain structure of the individual. This type of diversity overlaps with learning problems such as ASD, ADHD, dyslexia and OCD. These problems are also based upon the brain structure and are largely genetically determined. This can be compared with asking a left-handed person to use their right hand to write.

- Visual learners: Visual learners learn best by seeing information. They may prefer to read textbooks, watch videos, or use mind maps to help them learn. They often are able to learn large amounts of information and remember the information precisely. They may struggle see connections in the information that they have learned.

- Auditory learners: Auditory learners learn best by hearing information. They may prefer to listen to lectures, take notes, or discuss concepts with others. They are often eloquent and able to phrase their answers in sophisticated ways.

- Kinaesthetic learners: Kinaesthetic learners learn best by doing. They may prefer to participate in hands-on activities, lab experiments, or role-playing exercises. They may find written examinations more difficult but are often skilled in clinical skills.

- Logical learners: Logical (or systems) learners learn best by thinking through information. They may prefer to solve problems, analyse data, or create models. They may struggle with writing what they have learned in a coherent text. They often perform badly until they have fully understood the material leading to a step wise improvement.

There are strengths and weaknesses with each learning style and the educator can recommend resources in overcoming difficulties. There is generic advice on these areas however it is important to have a full diagnostic assessment if the student is disabled by their learning styles. This can help the student obtain specialist support and identify what reasonable adjustments can be provided by the university or workplace.

It is important to stress that whilst learning is easiest using the student's learning style this does mean that they cannot learn in other ways. Research has confirmed that a good fit between the learning approach and the material is more important than fitting the student's style.

Collaboration styles

Collaboration can be a very effective way for learners to learn and grow and can have additional benefits. Learners can develop social skills, deepen their learning and develop critical thinking as they listen to other people's points of view. Learners have different preferred collaboration styles and these can make it difficult to create a single learning experience.

The educator can improve the learning for all students by explaining the style that they have chosen and its advantages. Often the learning topic indicates the right collaboration style to use so the students can see the reasoning. Where the educator is unsure about the correct style it can be worth asking the students for the preferences.

- Narrative learners. Narrative learners collect stories that explain what they are learning. These stories engage the learner's emotions and imagination and connect the different elements into a coherent whole. Story learning is also a natural way of sharing the person's understanding with others. Story learning can be beneficial for students who are visual learners, as they can see the story unfold in their minds.

- Social learners: This type of learning involves interacting with others, such as working in groups, collaborating on projects, or discussing concepts with others. They use social rewards to maintain engagement for longer periods of learning and to improve retention of memories. This type of learning can help them to solidify their understanding of new material, as well as to develop their communication and teamwork skills. Social learning appears more effective for students who are auditory learners who are good at clarifying things they do not understand.

- Competitive learners learn by competing with others. They prefer games, challenges, or other activities where they can interact socially and test their skills against others. This type of learning can help them to develop a sense of achievement, as well as to learn from their mistakes and improve their skills over time. Competitive learning can be beneficial for all learners, but it may be particularly helpful for kinaesthetic learners who enjoy physical activity and challenges.

- Analytical learners. Analytical learners learn quickly when they have access to debate and discussion. This is not always possible as many learners avoid this type of challenging interaction. LLMs provide a stimulating and challenging environment for exploring different ideas, perspectives and feedback and provide a substitute for analytic learners. Logical learners often prefer to debate with an individual than work in a group and can use the LLM to explore different ideas and perspectives.

There is overlap between the types of learning styles and collaboration styles. That does not mean that a collaboration style with not work for a student with a different learning style. They may find the different style allows them to work outside of their usual skill base and draw upon other skills. Or they may simply enjoy the challenge in the knowledge that they are not expected to do well.

The collaboration styles are of particular use when teaching hard to teach topics. They alter the way that the students engage and learn turning a disadvantage into an advantage. For instance a subject where all the answers appear similar can become a series of choices of actions when presented as a competition.

How to identify learning needs (PDP).

PDPs have a problem. Most students passively assess their learning needs, they only react when they find a gap in their knowledge. In passive assessment is that the student will identify the need on Monday, read up about it by Wednesday and implement by Friday. This promotes lifelong learning as long as they remain aware of what they do not know.

This means that although what they are learning is important and changes practice it is not recorded in the PDP. The educator should explain that short term learning is far more effective so is not less important than long term learning. Reflective sentences can increase the chance that a student will record passive learning.

The following are examples of active assessment and can be used to create personal development plans PDP to show at appraisal.

- Self-assessment: Doctors can reflect on their own practice and identify areas where they feel they need more knowledge or skills. This can be done through a variety of methods, such as self-assessment questionnaires, performance reviews, or feedback from colleagues.

- Practice audits: Doctors can review their own patient records or conduct practice audits to identify areas where they are providing suboptimal care. This can help to identify gaps in knowledge or skills that need to be addressed through CME.

- Complaints. Many complaints have a learning need buried in the text. It is important to reflect on the whole of the complaint rather than just the key areas. Responding to a complaint with additional learning improves professionalism.

- Peer review: Doctors can participate in peer review activities to receive feedback from their colleagues on their clinical practice. This can help to identify areas where they need to improve their knowledge or skills.

- Literature reviews: Doctors can review the medical literature to identify new developments in their field. This can help them to stay up-to-date on the latest evidence-based practices and identify areas where they need to improve their knowledge or skills.

- CME providers: CME providers can offer a variety of tools and resources to help doctors identify their learning needs. These tools can include self-assessment questionnaires, practice audits and literature reviews.

- Changes in the healthcare landscape: Doctors can stay up-to-date on changes in the healthcare landscape to identify areas where they need to learn new skills or knowledge. This includes things like new medical advances, changes in reimbursement and new regulations.

The importance of identifying long term learning aims is that learning is both organic and revolutionary. Learning the next me-to drug in a class may be no more complex than reading the name a few times. Learning about a new class of drugs may take much longer and need a variety of activities.

Educators can share experiences of revolution such as when statins were effective in primary prevention or H Pylori treatment prevented ulcers. They can share how colleagues resisted using the new technology for years. The adoption curve can be used to show how there are few early adopters years before most doctors change practice.

How to find new areas to study?

Some students enjoy learning and look for new opportunities, there are techniques to help them find new areas. These techniques are also important later in a doctor's career when they want to study something new.

The key advantages are that the areas increase motivation and interest in the area. They give opportunities to do things that are outside of the doctor's usual experiences. The involve meeting new people and learning about humility. They can open new doors and new career prospects.

- Think about the boundaries between medical specialties. There are many areas of medicine that intersect with each other and you may be surprised at how much you can learn by exploring these boundaries. For example, if you are a general practitioner, you might be interested in learning more about the overlap between primary care and public health.

- Look at the syllabus for an examination. If you are preparing for a CME examination, the syllabus will often provide you with a list of topics that you need to know. This can be a great way to identify new areas of study that you might not have considered otherwise.

- Read about non-medical areas that could give useful skills. There are many non-medical areas that can be helpful for doctors, such as business, law and public health. By reading about these areas, you can gain new skills that can be applied to your medical practice.

- Come up with research questions and look for the answer. Even if you are not interested in conducting research, you can come up with research questions that will help you learn more about a particular area of medicine. This is a great way to stay up-to-date on the latest developments in your field.

- Write an article on a subject you want to learn more about. This is a great way to consolidate your knowledge and share your learning with others. You can write an article for a medical journal, a blog, or even just for yourself. This will force you to learn more about the subject and to think critically about it.

- Talk to colleagues about new areas they have heard about. Your colleagues are a great source of information about new areas of study. They may have heard about new developments in their own field or in other fields that could be relevant to you. By talking to them, you can learn about these new areas and decide if they are of interest to you.

- Read medical and other journals looking for developments. Medical journals are a great way to stay up-to-date on the latest developments in medicine. You can also read journals from other fields that may be relevant to your practice. By reading these journals, you can learn about new areas of study that you may not have been aware of before.

- Network at conferences and listen to the questions raised. Conferences are a great way to meet other healthcare professionals and learn about new areas of study. You can also listen to the questions that are being raised at conferences to get a sense of what other people are interested in learning about.

- Look for a competency that you are weak on and make a plan. If there is an area of your practice that you are not confident in, you can make a plan to improve your skills in that area. This could involve reading books or articles, taking courses, or observing other healthcare professionals.

- Read about basic science discoveries that could be applied to medicine. Basic science discoveries can often lead to new treatments and diagnostic tools. By staying up-to-date on basic science research, you can learn about new areas of study that may be relevant to your practice.

The educator can ask the students to rate these approaches on the likelihood that they will ever use them. This makes the ideas more personal and allows them to engage with them whilst feeling that they have a choice. The objective is to help students see the range of choices available and identify their preferences.

Conclusions.

Teaching how to organise Continuing Medical Education (CME) requires identifying key skills such as recognising learning needs, areas of interest and emerging issues. It is important to address doctors' gaps in knowledge and skills while also considering their preferences and learning styles. Educators should acknowledge and reduce resistance to engagement by empathising with learners' feelings and involving them in the decision-making process.

When planning CME, doctors should identify their learning goals, consider their learning style, choose a variety of activities and seek feedback to improve future learning experiences. Collaborative learning can be effective in promoting social skills, deepening learning and developing critical thinking. Understanding different collaboration styles and aligning them with the learning topic can enhance the overall learning experience.

To identify learning needs, doctors can engage in self-assessment, practice audits, peer reviews, literature reviews and staying updated with changes in the healthcare landscape. It is essential to recognise that learning is both organic and revolutionary and identifying long-term learning aims can lead to transformative changes in medical practice.

Finding new areas of study can be achieved by exploring the boundaries between medical specialties, examining examination syllabi, reading about non-medical areas for acquiring additional skills, asking research questions, writing articles, networking with colleagues, staying updated through journals and conferences and focusing on improving weak competencies. These techniques not only expand knowledge but also promote motivation, interest and career prospects.

In conclusion, Continuing Medical Education should be tailored to individual learning styles, preferences and needs. By embracing diverse learning and collaboration styles, actively assessing learning needs and exploring new areas of study, doctors can foster continuous growth and provide better care to their patients.

Top tips.

Embrace collaborative learning: Highlight the benefits of collaborative learning and the use of social, analytical, narrative and competitive techniques. Although students have a preference for one technique the correct choice depends upon the material.

Address resistance to learning: Although most doctors have extensive learning experience they will still have areas of resistance. They may resist adopting new learning methods or considering new areas of study or feel that they have learned enough. Encourage doctors to diversify their CME activities so that it does not feel like learning.

Reflection: It is important for doctors to reflect on how much learning that they are actually doing. Short-term learning is an example of undercounted learning because the learning need is addressed within a few days. Other underappreciated learning activities are discussion with peers and general reading.

Chapter 40: THE DISSERTATION, THESIS OR ESSAY.

Students at every level are asked to write a long form essay that shows that a medic has understood a particular area of medicine. The skills required vary from low level ability to write in a clear and concise manner, analyse data or even to conduct independent research. The length will vary from 10-20 pages for an essay to 100-200 pages for a dissertation.

Writing a dissertation is a collaborative effort between the learner and supervisor. The supervisor is responsible for providing guidance and support to the student throughout the writing process. This means that the supervisor must read the students work and ask relevant questions. The student is responsible for conducting the research, collecting the data and writing the dissertation.

The student will need to develop research skills and the supervisor needs to monitor the student's needs. These skills may be taught formally, as the student requires or the student may be referred to sources for self-learning. The thesis should be broken into steps so that the student can focus on each stage separately.

Supervisors are key to the process but must balance the needs of multiple students, managing their own time as well as providing constructive feedback. They need to build rapport with students, manage conflict and provide timely feedback. This can make whether a student progresses depend upon the time management skills of their supervisor.

Writing a thesis.

The supervisor may need to follow the university's programme when asking for feedback on how you are getting on. You should provide a document for each stage, both showing how far you have got but also as a basis of the final document. The question for study can be used to generate a number of possible titles for your project.

- Choose a question for study. Your research question should be something that you are genuinely interested in and that you can answer with the resources available to you. You should review the literature summarising existing research on your topic. Once you have chosen a research question, you need to think about the feasibility of any proposals you may have. This includes considering the resources available to you, such as time, money and access to data.

You can discuss with your supervisor this list which will help you develop an overview of your research question and why it is important. The supervisor can help you identify methods of approaching the question by asking about previous literature. The key is for the supervisor to ask you questions which make you think harder about your topic.

- Develop a Research proposal. A research proposal is a document that outlines your research question, your methods and your expected outcomes. A research proposal will help you to stay focused and on track. Your research proposal should include the following sections: Methods: This section should describe how you plan to collect and analyse your data. Expected outcomes: This section should state what you hope to achieve with your research. Alternatives: This section should discuss any alternative approaches to your research.

The research proposal should be written as potential methodologies for the final paper. You can then run thought experiments for each of the different methodologies and the likely outcomes. The supervisor can then discuss with you as to the methodology you think will work best and ask you questions about possible barriers.

- Research methods. Researching involves finding and evaluating sources, conducting interviews and collecting data. When finding sources, it is important to use a variety, including academic journals, books and websites. You should also evaluate your sources critically to ensure that they are reliable and credible. When conducting interviews, it is important to prepare a list of questions in advance and to take notes during the interview. When collecting data, it is important to use a variety of methods, such as surveys, experiments and observations.

You will need to learn any research methods that are necessary for your topic. This may mean attending a course, working with a trainer or self-study. You need to identify any gaps in your skill base and your supervisor will check where you are with the necessary skills. They may ask you whether you want to try a different approach if you are trying to learn too many new skills at once.

You will be directly applying any new research skill to your project for instance gathering data. You should allocate enough time to practicing any new skill so you feel confident. The supervisor will ask if you are having any problems and can trouble-shoot if you are getting stuck. Keep in touch with your supervisor so that they can understand what you are achieving.

- Analysing data. Use statistical techniques to interpret your results and to draw conclusions. You should synthesise the data with your knowledge. When analysing your data, it is important to be objective and to avoid making any assumptions. You should also be aware of the limitations of your data and of the potential for bias and include these in the conclusions.

You will need further skills when analysing data although there are good statistical packages you need to check that your data is suitable. You may find problems in the data and you may need to repeat parts of the data collection or write the paper discussing the problems. You may simply not have enough time to get more data and will need use criticism when discussing your poor-quality data.

- Writing up. Organise your thoughts, writing in a clear and concise style and get feedback on your drafts. When writing up your thesis, it is important to follow the guidelines provided by your university or academic department. You should also make sure to cite your sources properly.

You will already have the title, most of the introduction, the methodology, reference list and most of the results written and can simply copy and paste them in. You will need to write the discussion, refine the previously written sections and write an abstract. If you are struggling with any of these it is worth going back to the previous stage and considering where you have gone wrong.

The supervisor cannot really help you with writing up but should be asked to review each section as they are finished and ask questions. These questions can help you polish the section, improving the clarity and removing irrelevancies. When you put the sections together you will have a complete research paper that delivers what you intended.

Asking students questions.

The supervisor needs to develop strong questioning skills. Learning how to ask good questions is as challenging as learning any skill. A supervisor may not have learned how to ask good questions and must undergo training. There are no formal courses or training so the supervisor should use practice and self reflection.

- Insightful questioning. Supervisors need ask their students questions that stimulate and make them look deeper at their work.

This is a skill that requires creativity, emotional insight and common sense. Asking questions is less about what logically is missing and more about what feels like it is missing from the work.

- Emotional insight. The supervisor should be mindful of their own emotions when asking questions. If they are feeling angry, bored, or uninterested, it is important to reflect on why they are feeling that way. These emotions can be a valuable source of insight into what is missing from the student's work.
- Positive questions. When deciding on the right question the supervisor should consider whether their question shows insight, is positive and encouraging and leave it open to the student how to respond. Questions that are too abstract or critical or can be answered simply are unhelpful.
- Missing details. Students can fail to understand the size of the task, whether they are using an accepted technique, whether their report is too vague and ambiguous and whether they can get any reasonable results. It can be difficult to work out what is missing and the supervisor should take time to reflect so that they can identify the gaps.

The supervisor should check that the questions they have asked have been effective. This can be comparing a follow draft of the writing task or by talking to the student or asking for feedback. It is essential for a new supervisor to develop this skill quickly so that they can be useful to their student.

The signs of good questioning is that the student has addressed an area of weakness in a follow up draft. The process of improvement is slow and the student is not likely to have addressed multiple issues. Ineffective questioning can include multiple vague questions, questions which have not led to improvement and signs of confusion in the student.

Roles of a supervisor.

Supervisors play a vital role in the success of their students. Supervision involves a wide set of roles that can be difficult to manage. The supervisor needs to ensure that the student has the tools to complete the tasks, support when having problems, boundaries to acceptable behaviour and feedback on progress.

The supervisor needs to consider whether any action they take falls within one of these groups. If it does not it is likely that the supervisor is stepping outside of their roles and risks the student's work being excluded. The educator can help doctors who are learning to be supervisors consider examples of behaviours. The doctors can then give their opinion on whether they are within or without their role and why.

Feedback on progress.

- Provide feedback on research area and research questions: Supervisors can provide valuable feedback on students' research area and research questions. They can help students to refine their research questions, to ask important questions that can be answered with the available data.

- Help manage research timelines: Supervisors can help students to develop realistic research timelines and to track their progress. They can also help students to identify potential problems and to develop solutions.

- Monitor progress: Supervisors can monitor students' progress and to provide feedback on their work. They can also help students to identify areas where they need improvement and to develop a plan for improvement.

- Agree a feedback process and timeframes: Supervisors should agree a feedback process and timeframes with students. This ensures that students receive timely and constructive feedback on their work.

- Write requested references: Supervisors can write requested references. This can help students to demonstrate their research experience and to obtain employment or further study opportunities.

Tools to complete the tasks.

- Provide guidance on the student's professional development: Supervisors can provide guidance on students' professional development. They can help students to identify relevant conferences and workshops to attend and to develop their CV and cover letters.

- Suggesting research methods and theoretical models: Supervisors can suggest research methods and theoretical models that are appropriate for students' research questions. They can also help students to understand the strengths and weaknesses of different research methods and theoretical models.

- Arrange training for presentation skills e.g., oral examinations and conference presentations: Supervisors can arrange training for presentation skills such as public speaking. This can help students to develop their confidence and to deliver effective presentations.

- Advise on resubmission, public engagement and publishing research: Supervisors can advise students on resubmission, public engagement and publishing research. They can help students to identify appropriate journals, to prepare their manuscripts for submission and to promote their research.

Support when having problems.

- Help students identify research questions and design research projects: Supervisors have the knowledge and experience to help students identify interesting and feasible research questions. They can also help students to design research projects that are well-structured and methodologically sound.

- Problem solve research barriers: Supervisors can help students to problem solve research barriers. This can include helping them to find research participants, to access data, or to troubleshoot technical problems.

- Interpreting examiners' comments: Supervisors can help students to interpret examiners' comments. This can help students to understand the strengths and weaknesses of their work and to develop a plan for improvement.

- Provide guidance on academic English: Supervisors can provide guidance on academic English. They can help students to improve their writing skills, to use appropriate grammar and punctuation. Academic English allows the student to use the correct way of describing their results.

Boundaries to acceptable behaviour.

- Advise on research integrity and ethical research practices: Supervisors advise students on research integrity and ethical research practices. They can help students to understand the ethical guidelines for research and to conduct their research in an ethical manner.

- Ensure that core data analysis is performed by the student: Supervisors must ensure that core data analysis is performed by the student. This is so students are not using other people's data analysis and plagiarising.

- Ensure that students understand any methods used by those assisting them: Supervisors have a responsibility to ensure that students understand any methods used by those assisting them. This ensures that students are able to critically evaluate the methods used in their research and explain the results.

- Assist with presentation and editorial matters but not content: Supervisors can assist with presentation and editorial matters. The supervisor can help them to present their work in a clear and concise manner. Supervisors should not assist with content to ensure that students are able to take ownership of their ideas.

- Assist compliance with academic regulations and guidelines: Supervisors have a responsibility to assist students with complying with academic regulations and guidelines. This ensures that students are aware of the rules and regulations that apply to their research and that they are able to complete their research in a compliant manner.

Educators can test the doctor's knowledge to ensure that they are able to identify the supervisor's roles. As the doctor may have some time between the training and their first researcher it is probably more important to focus on their own needs from their supervisors. This helps improving engagement and they can use reflection of their own experiences.

The complexity of the supervisor's role means that some supervisors are overcautious in the help that they offer. This can lead to poorer results from students who lack the tools or have more problems. Students can become stuck and unable to progress without assistance.

Conclusions.

The process of writing a dissertation or thesis is a collaborative effort between the student and the supervisor. The supervisor plays a crucial role in providing guidance, support and feedback to ensure the successful completion of the research project. The supervisor should assist the student in developing research skills, monitoring progress and managing timelines. They should also provide constructive feedback on drafts and help the student in areas such as research design, data analysis and writing skills.

Effective questioning by the supervisor is essential to stimulate critical thinking and deeper exploration of the research topic. Supervisors should ask insightful, positive and open-ended questions to help students identify areas of improvement and address any missing details in their work.

Supervisors have multiple roles, including providing feedback on progress, offering guidance on professional development, suggesting research methods and assisting with resubmission, public engagement and publishing research. They should also support students when they face problems or barriers during the research process, helping them to troubleshoot and find solutions.

Establishing boundaries is important, ensuring that core data analysis is performed by the student and that the supervisor's assistance is limited to presentation and editorial matters rather than content. Additionally, supervisors should ensure compliance with academic regulations and ethical research practices.

The complexity of the supervisor's role requires a balance between providing adequate support and empowering students to take ownership of their work. Supervisors should continuously reflect on their own questioning skills and seek feedback to improve their effectiveness.

Overall, the supervisor's role is vital in guiding and supporting students throughout the dissertation or thesis writing process, ultimately contributing to the students' academic and professional development.

Top tips.

Research steps: Break down the research into a series of steps that logically build the document through tasks. Each completed step will create a draft of part of the document as well as progress the project.

Acquire Research Skills: When necessary, learn new research methods and techniques relevant to the topic. Allocate sufficient time to practice and gain confidence in applying these skills to the project.

Questions: As a supervisor, develop strong questioning skills to stimulate deeper exploration of the student's work. Ask questions that are positive, insightful and leave room for the student to respond thoughtfully.

Chapter 41: FINAL COMMENTS

The value of a book on the PGCME is that it provides a resource to doctors who wish to become an educator. It might introduce some doctors to medical education who would not otherwise have considered it. There are many insights in this book many of which are drawn from experience rather than LLMs. If they assist the reader they should be used and if they do not they should be discarded.

There are many lists which is deliberate as well as reflecting the style of LLMs. For each list I have tried to provide a rational for that list as well as a way of using it. Some are steps in a recipe, others are check lists and still others are to hand to the students.

I hope that the experiment was successful, that I and the LLMs were able to collaborate and produce something of value. Feedback would be gratefully received whether critical or complementary. Feedback is the only true way of appraising the experiment and I will be writing an article with the final results in a year or so time.

I have criticisms of the book, there is no index, this is because the book is highly structured and is not designed to be a reference book. There are no references, this is to keep the book to a reasonable size, it is already too long. There are typos, this is because I do not have access to an LLM that can read a whole book and provide me with a list.

The book is personal at times, this is my writing style and I have not yet learned to avoid it. There are some errors, this is because my memory is not always perfect or I missed them when proof reading. Only a few topics have lesson plans, this is because they are specialist.

There is no example of a standard medical topic, this is because I could not think how to do it. Each topic needs to be crafted and developed over time using the methods that I described. Any model example would defeat the purpose of the book by suggesting that there was a one-size-fits-all approach.

Readers will have many more criticisms but I hope that the additional details such as top tips, chapter description, hook, objectives and alternative title will add something special. Perhaps the clarity of the language will make up for the lack of visuals. Students of the PGCME will no doubt recognise the books strengths and weaknesses and I hope will share their insights.

Dr Mark Innes Burgin 2023

www.ingramcontent.com/pod-product-compliance
Lightning Source LLC
Chambersburg PA
CBHW071231050326
40690CB00011B/2070